ORBAN'S
Oral histology and
embryology

# ORBAN'S
# Oral histology and embryology

*Edited by*

## S. N. BHASKAR, B.D.S., D.D.S., M.S., Ph.D.

Major General, U.S. Army; Assistant Surgeon General and Chief,
Dental Corps, U.S. Army; Diplomate, American Board
of Oral Pathology; Diplomate, American Board
of Oral Medicine, Washington, D.C.

*with 607 illustrations, including 4 color plates*

EIGHTH EDITION

# The C. V. Mosby Company

SAINT LOUIS  1976

EIGHTH EDITION

Library of Congress Cataloging in Publication Data

Orban, Balint Joseph, 1899-1960, ed.
  Orban's Oral histology and embryology.

  Includes bibliographies and index.
  1. Mouth.  2. Teeth.  3. Jaws.  4. Salivary
glands.  I. Bhaskar, S. N.  II. Title.  III. Title:  Oral histology and embryology.  [DNLM:
1.  Mouth—Anatomy and histology.  2.  Mouth—
Embryology.  3.  Tooth—Anatomy and histology.
4.  Tooth—Embryology.  WU101 064]
RK280.072  1976      611'.0189'31       75-31628
ISBN 0-8016-4608-1


CB/CB/B  9  8  7  6  5  4

# Contributors

**Gary C. Armitage, D.D.S., M.S.**

Assistant Professor, Division of Periodontology, School of Dentistry, University of California, San Francisco, California

**James K. Avery, D.D.S., Ph.D.**

Professor, Oral Biology, University of Michigan School of Dentistry; Professor, Anatomy, University of Michigan School of Medicine, Ann Arbor, Michigan

**S. N. Bhaskar, B.D.S., D.D.S., M.S., Ph.D.**

Major General, U.S. Army; Assistant Surgeon General and Chief, Dental Corps, U.S. Army; Diplomate, American Board of Oral Pathology; Diplomate, American Board of Oral Medicine, Washington, D.C.

**Baldev Raj Bhussry, B.D.S., M.S., Ph.D.**

Department of Anatomy, Schools of Medicine and Dentistry, Georgetown University, Washington, D.C.

**Arthur R. Hand, D.D.S.**

Laboratory of Biological Structure, National Institute of Dental Research, National Institutes of Health, Bethesda, Maryland

**Malcolm C. Johnston, D.D.S., M.Sc.D., Ph.D.**

Laboratory of Developmental Biology and Anomalies, National Institute of Dental Research, Bethesda, Maryland

**Shakti P. Kapur, M.Sc., Ph.D.**

Department of Anatomy, Schools of Medicine and Dentistry, Georgetown University, Washington, D.C.

**A. H. Melcher, M.D.S., H.D.D., Ph.D.**

Professor and Director, Medical Research Council Group in Periodontal Physiology, Faculty of Dentistry, University of Toronto, Toronto, Ontario, Canada

**Irving B. Stern, D.D.S.**

Professor and Chairman, Department of Periodontology; Director of Graduate Periodontology, School of Dental Medicine, Tufts University, Boston, Massachusetts

**A. Richard Ten Cate, B.Sc., B.D.S., Ph.D.**

Professor and Chairman, Division of Biological Sciences, Faculty of Dentistry, University of Toronto, Toronto, Ontario, Canada

**Branislav Vidić, S.D.**

Professor of Anatomy, Schools of Medicine and Dentistry, Georgetown University, Washington, D.C.

**James A. Yaeger, D.D.S., Ph.D.**

Department of Oral Biology, School of Dental Medicine, University of Connecticut Health Center, Farmington, Connecticut

*To*

**Balint  J.  Orban**

superb  teacher,
amiable  colleague,  and
dear  friend

# Preface

This eighth edition of *Orban's Oral Histology and Embryology* has undergone a major revision. The contributors to this edition were carefully chosen and represent the very best in their area of interest. The subject matter as presented is the current status of our knowledge in the field.

Oral histology is a basic science. It brings the student into intimate contact with the tissues that are to be the subject of his manipulation for the rest of his professional life. Knowledge of oral histology, therefore, is essential for good dental practice. The general practitioner as well as the specialist must draw upon it to understand disease, to prevent disease, and above all to plan for its correct therapy. Lack of a sound knowledge of normal and abnormal histology is an impediment in the training of a dentist and reduces him to a mere technician.

The eighth edition of *Orban's Oral Histology and Embryology* is presented to the undergraduate and graduate student with the hope that it will give him a better understanding of the tissues he is called upon to heal.

**S. N. Bhaskar**

# Contents

# Color plates

ORBAN'S
Oral histology and
embryology

# 1 Development of face and oral cavity

This chapter deals primarily with the development of the human face and oral cavity. Consideration is also given to information about underlying mechanisms that is derived from experimental studies conducted on developing subhuman embryos. Much of the experimental work has been conducted on amphibian and avian embryos. Evidence derived from these and more limited studies on other vertebrates including mammals indicates that the early facial development of all vertebrate embryos is similar. Many events occur, including cell migrations, interactions, differential growth, and differentiation, all of which lead to progressively maturing structures (Fig. 1-1). Progress has also been made with respect to abnormal developmental alterations that give rise to some of the most common human malformations (Fig. 1-15). Further information on the topics discussed can be obtained by consulting the references at the end of the chapter.

## ORIGIN OF FACIAL TISSUES

After fertilization of the ovum, a series of cell divisions gives rise to an egg cell mass known as the *morula* in mammals. In most vertebrates, including man, the major portion of the egg cell mass forms the extraembryonic membranes and other supportive structures such as the placenta. As little as one fourth of the cells of the egg cell mass assemble into a single layer, which will form the embryo. Cell movements then convert this *embryonic disc* into two layers with an intervening space. An additional, well-integrated movement of actively migrating cells from the upper of the two layers leads to the formation of a third layer of cells, which occupies the intervening space. The uppermost of these three "germ" layers is called the *ectoderm;* the middle layer, the *mesoderm;* and the lowest layer, the *endoderm* (Fig. 1-2, A). Thus, at this stage, three distinct populations of embryonic cells have arisen largely through division and migration. They follow distinctly separate courses during later development.

Migrations, such as those described above, create new associations between

1

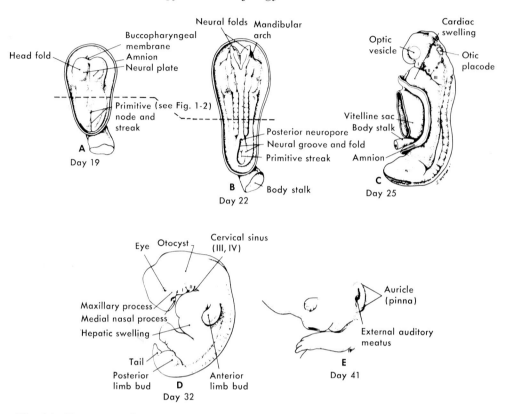

**Fig. 1-1.** Emergence of facial structures during development of human embryo. **A** and **B**, Dorsal views of earlier stages. **C** and **D**, Visceral arches are designated by roman numerals. Broken lines in **A** and **B** represent the section planes of Fig. 1-2. **E**, Lateral view of face at 41 days. (From Allen, F.: Essentials of human embryology, Oxford, 1969, Oxford University Press.)

cells, which, in turn, allow unique possibilities for subsequent development through interactions between the cell populations. Such interactions have been studied experimentally by isolating the different cell populations or tissues and recombining them in different ways in culture or in transplants. From such studies it is known, for example, that a median strip of mesoderm cells extending throughout the length of the embryo induces *neural plate* formation within the overlying ectoderm (Fig. 1-2). The nature of such inductive stimuli is presently unknown. Sometimes, cell-to-cell contact appears to be necessary, whereas in other cases (as in neural plate induction) the inductive influences appear to be able to act between cells separated by considerable distances and to consist of diffusible substances. It is known that inductive influences need only be present for a short time, after which the responding tissue is capable of independent development. For example, an induced neural plate isolated in culture will roll up into a tube, which then differentiates into the brain, spinal cord, and other structures.

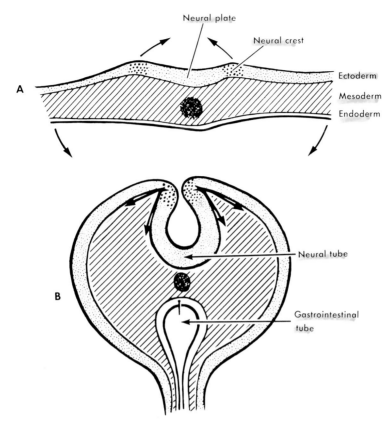

**Fig. 1-2.** Scheme of neural and gastrointestinal tube formation in higher vertebrate embryos. (Section planes are illustrated in Fig. 1-1.) **A,** Cross section through three-germ-layer embryo. Similar structures are seen in both head and trunk regions. Neural crest cells are initially located at the junction between the neural and surface ectoderm. *Arrows,* Directions of folding processes. **B,** Neural tube, which later forms the major components of the brain and spinal cord, and gastrointestinal tube will separate from the embryo surface after fusions are completed. *Arrows,* Directions of crest cell migrations, which are initiated at about end of third week in human embryo. (From Johnston, M. C., et al.: Clinics in Plastic Surg. **2:** 50-75, 1975.)

A unique population of cells develops from the ectoderm along the lateral margins of the neural plate. These are the neural crest cells. They undergo extensive migrations, usually beginning at about the time of tube closure (Fig. 1-2), and give rise to a variety of different cells that form components of many tissues. The crest cells that migrate in the trunk region form mostly neural, endocrine, and pigment cells, whereas those that migrate in the head and neck also contribute extensively to skeletal and connective tissues (i.e., cartilage, bone, dentin, dermis, etc.). In the trunk, all skeletal and connective tissues are formed by mesoderm. Of the skeletal or connective tissue of the facial region, it appears that tooth enamel (an acellular skeletal tissue) is the only one not formed by

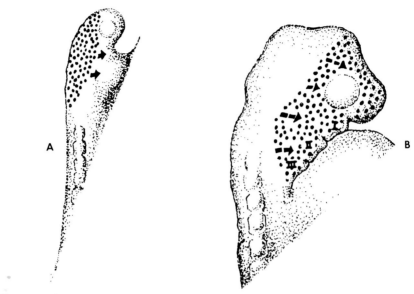

**Fig. 1-3.** Scheme of subectodermal distribution of neural crest cells *(large stipples)* during, **A**, and toward the completion, **B**, of migration. *Arrows*, Direction of migration. First three visceral arches are indicated by roman numerals.

crest cells. The enamel-forming cells are derived from ectoderm lining the oral cavity.

The migration routes that cephalic (head) neural crest cells follow are illustrated in Fig. 1-3. They move around the sides of the head beneath the surface ectoderm, en masse, as a sheet of cells. They form all the mesenchyme* in the upper facial region, whereas in the lower facial region they surround mesodermal cores already present in the visceral arches. The pharyngeal region is then characterized by grooves (clefts) in the lateral pharyngeal wall endoderm and ectoderm that approach each other and appear to have effectively segmented the mesoderm into a number of bars that become surrounded by crest mesenchyme (Fig. 1-6, A).

Toward the completion of migration, the trailing edge of the crest cell mass appears to attach itself to the neural tube at locations where sensory ganglia of the fifth, seventh, ninth, and tenth cranial nerves will form. In the trunk sensory ganglia, supporting (e.g., Schwann) cells and all neurons are derived from neural crest cells. On the other hand, many of the sensory neurons of the cranial sensory ganglia originate from surface ectoderm.

Eventually, capillary endothelial cells derived from mesoderm cells invade the crest cell mesenchyme, and it is from this mesenchyme that the supporting

---

*Mesenchyme is defined here as the loosely organized embryonic tissue in contrast to epithelium, which is compactly arranged.

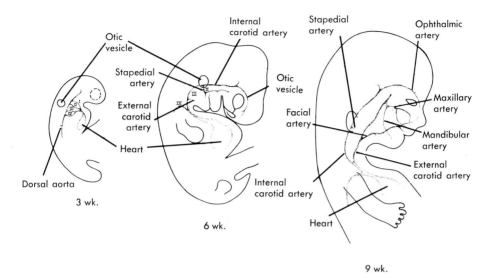

**Fig. 1-4.** Development of arterial vascular system proceeds through three successive stages. *I-IV,* Aortic arch vessels. During intermediate stage the stapedial artery and its branches supply most of the facial region. The external carotid artery (6-week specimen) grows forward to fuse with the stapedial artery and, after separation from the more proximal portion of the stapedial artery, takes over the arterial supply to most of the facial region (9-week specimen). (From Ross, R. B., and Johnston, M. C.: Cleft lip and palate, Baltimore, 1972, The Williams & Wilkins Co.)

cells of the developing blood vessels are derived. Initially, these supporting cells include only pericytes, which are closely apposed to the outer surfaces of endothelial cells. Later additional crest cells differentiate into the fibroblasts and smooth muscle cells that will form the vessel wall. The developing blood vessels become interconnected to form vascular networks. These networks undergo a series of modifications, examples of which are illustrated in Fig. 1-4, before they eventually form the mature vascular system. The underlying mechanisms are not clearly understood.

Almost all the myoblasts that subsequently fuse with each other to form the multinucleated striated muscle fibers are derived from mesoderm. The myoblasts that form the hypoglossal (tongue) muscles are derived from somites located beside the developing hindbrain. Somites are condensed masses of cells derived from mesoderm located adjacent to the neural tube. The extrinsic ocular muscles originate from similar, more anterior mesoderm (Fig. 1-5), which fails to condense in higher vertebrates. These prospective myoblasts (still not recognizable as premuscle cells) must undergo extensive migrations (Fig. 1-5). The supporting connective tissue found in facial muscles is derived from neural crest cells. Much of the development of the masticatory and other facial musculature is closely related to the final stages of visceral arch development and will be described later.

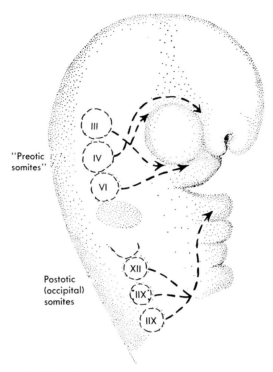

**Fig. 1-5.** Migration paths followed by prospective skeletal muscle cells. Somites or comparable structures from which the muscle cells are derived are indicated by the number of the cranial nerve that provides the motor innervation. (From Ross, R. B., and Johnston, M. C.: Cleft lip and palate, Baltimore, 1972, The Williams & Wilkins Co.)

A number of other structures in the facial region, such as glands and the enamel organ of the tooth bud, are derived from epithelium that grows (invaginates) into underlying mesenchyme. Again, the connective tissue components in these structures (e.g., fibroblasts, odontoblasts, and the cells of tooth-supporting tissues) are derived from neural crest cells.

## DEVELOPMENT OF FACIAL PROCESSES

Upon the completion of the initial crest cell migration and the vascularization of the derived mesenchyme, a series of outgrowths or swellings termed "facial processes" initiate the next stages of facial development (Fig. 1-6). The growth and fusion of upper facial processes produces the primary and secondary palates. As will be described below, other processes developing from the first two visceral arches considerably alter the nature of these arches.

*Development of nasal placodes, frontonasal processes, primary palate, and nose.* Before crest cell migration, the surface ectoderm lies in apposition to portions of the developing forebrain. Inductive influences originating from the forebrain initiate the formation of the nasal placodes in the apposed ectoderm. Pla-

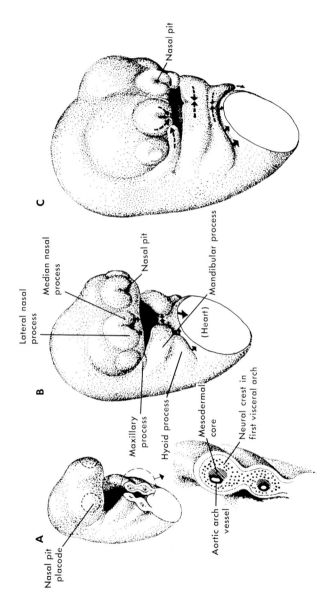

**Fig. 1-6.** Scheme of development of facial processes. After completion of crest cell migration, **A**, facial process development begins, **B**, and is completed after the fusion of the processes with each other or with other structures, **C**. Details are given in text. Heart and adjacent portions of visceral arches have been removed in **A**, and most of the heart has been removed in **B** and **C**. *Arrows*, Directions of growth.

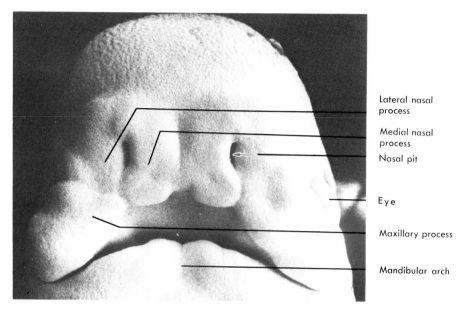

Lateral nasal
process

Medial nasal
process

Nasal pit

Eye

Maxillary process

Mandibular arch

**Fig. 1-7.** Scanning electron micrograph of primary palate in a ferret embryo just after time of fusion between medial nasal and lateral nasal processes. Mesenchyme of maxillary process coalesces with that of lateral and medial nasal processes. Note nasal pit, eye, and mandibular arch. (Courtesy A. J. Steffek, Chicago, and D. Mujwid, Chicago.)

codes are recognizable as ectodermal thickenings, and they give rise to a variety of structures such as the lens of the eye and the inner ear epithelium. The nasal placodes will later form the sensory epithelium for olfaction. After induction, mesenchymal cells separate the nasal placodal ectoderm from the underlying forebrain. The thickening nasal placodes appear to interact with mesenchymal cells that aggregate along their undersurfaces. It is not clear whether this interaction is related to placodal invagination.

After the nasal placode invaginates to form a pit, the medial and lateral nasal processes (also termed the frontonasal processes) appear on each side (Figs. 1-6 and 1-7). They contact each other below the developing nasal pit (Figs. 1-6 to 1-8) during the fourth week of pregnancy in man and a portion of the adhering epithelium breaks down so that the mesenchyme of the two processes becomes continuous (Fig. 1-8). Fluid accumulates between the cells of the persisting epithelium behind the point of epithelial breakdown (Fig. 1-8, *F*). Eventually, these fluid-filled spaces coalesce to form the initial nasal passageway connecting the olfactory pit with the roof of the primitive oral cavity (Fig. 1-8, *I*). The tissue below the passageway that separate it from the most anterior portion of the primitive oral cavity is the *primary palate*. In later development, the primary palate will form portions of the upper lip, anterior maxilla, and upper incisor teeth.

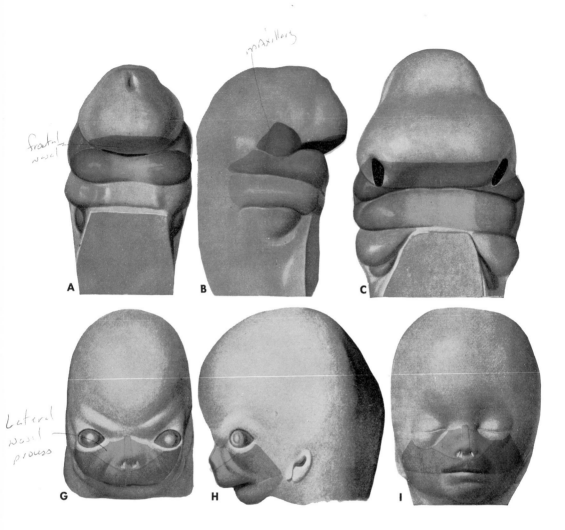

Handwritten annotations on figure: *maxillary* (top), *frontal nasal* (left, near A), *Lateral Nasal process* (left, near G)

**Plate 1.** Schematic development of human face. **A** and **B**, Embryo 3 mm. in length, third week. The frontonasal process *(dull green)* is undivided. It is anterior to mandibular arch *(yellow)*, hyoid arch, and third branchial arch. **C**, Embryo 6.5 mm. in length, fourth week. Nasal pits divide the frontonasal process into the medial nasal process *(dull green)* and lateral nasal processes *(reddish)*. **D**, Embryo 9 mm. in length, fifth week. Fusion of *medial nasal* with the *lateral nasal* and *maxillary processes* has narrowed entrance into nasal pit. **E**, Embryo 9.2 mm. in length, sixth week. Fusion of medial and lateral nasal processes has further narrowed the nostrils. Medial nasal process is reduced in relative width. Eyes are at lateral edges of face.

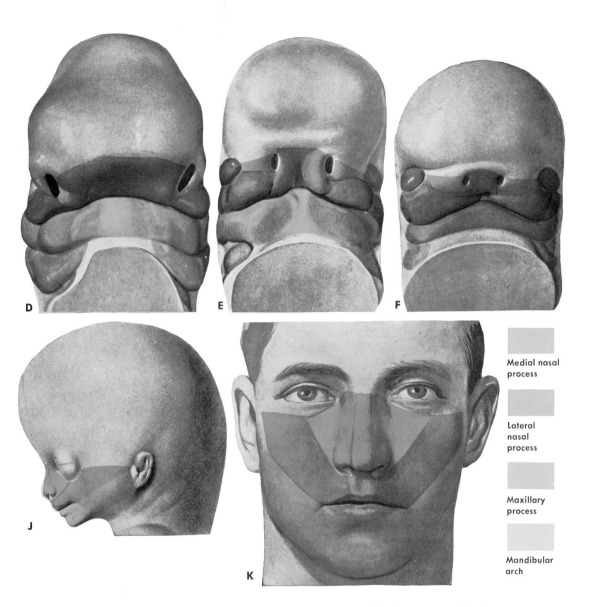

Labels on right side of figure:

Medial nasal process

Lateral nasal process

Maxillary process

Mandibular arch

**F**, Embryo 14.5 mm. in length, seventh week. Nasal area is slightly prominent. Nasal septum is further reduced in relative width. Eyes are on anterior surface of face. **G** and **H**, Embryo 18 mm. in length, eighth week. Lidless eyes are on anterior surface of face. Their distance is relatively reduced, and the mandible is short. **I** and **J**, Embryo 60 mm. in length, twelfth week. Lids are closed. Nostrils are closed by epithelial proliferation. Relation of the mandible to the maxilla is normal. **K**, Adult face: approximate derivatives of medial nasal process (*dull green*), lateral nasal processes (*reddish*), maxillary processes (*bright green*), and mandibular arch (*yellow*). (Modified from Sicher, H., and Tandler, J.: Anatomie für Zahnärtze [Anatomy for dentists], Berlin, 1928, Julius Springer Verlag.)

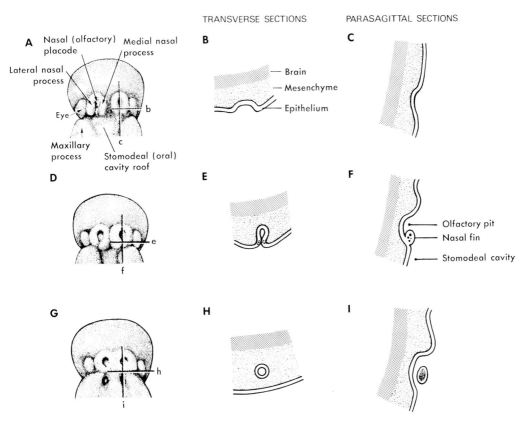

TRANSVERSE SECTIONS    PARASAGITTAL SECTIONS

**A** Nasal (olfactory) placode    Medial nasal process
Lateral nasal process
Eye
Maxillary process    Stomodeal (oral) cavity roof

**B**    — Brain
— Mesenchyme
— Epithelium

**C**

**D**    **E**    **F**    — Olfactory pit
— Nasal fin
— Stomodeal cavity

**G**    **H**    **I**

**Fig. 1-8.** Different stages of primary palate development in human embryo where it occurs at about end of fourth week. **A, D,** and **G,** Primary palate from in front and below, with mandibular arch removed. Planes for transverse sections, **B, E,** and **H,** and parasagittal sections, **C, F,** and **I,** are also illustrated. Lower portions of medial and lateral nasal processes come into contact, **D** and **E,** producing an epithelial nasal fin or seam, **F.** Portion of the epithelial seam breaks down (cell death, *dots* in **E** and **F**), and this portion of the seam becomes replaced by mesenchyme. Opening of a passageway through the epithelium separating olfactory pit and stomodeal cavity completes formation of initial nasal passage, **F** and **I.** (From Johnston, M. C., et al.: Clinics in Plastic Surg. 2:50, 1975.)

The outlines of the developing external nose can be seen in Fig. 1-7. Although disproportionately large, the basic form of the nose is easily recognizable. Subsequent alterations in form lead to a progressively more mature structure (Fig. 1-1, *E*). Plate 1 is a schematic illustration of the contribution of various facial processes to the development of the external face.

*Development of pituitary gland, maxillary processes, and secondary palate.* The pituitary gland develops as a result of inductive interactions between the ventral forebrain and oral ectoderm and is derived, in part, from both tissues (Fig. 1-9). Crest cells that migrate to the pituitary gland and later form its connective tissue components are continuous with the crest cells that later form the

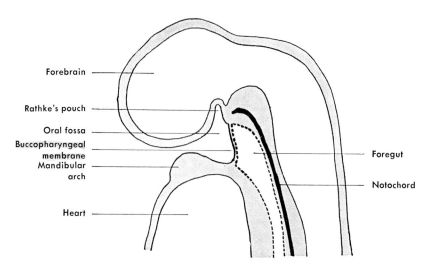

**Fig. 1-9.** Diagram of median section through head of 3½-week human embryo. Oral fossa is separated from foregut by a double layer of epithelium, the buccopharyngeal membrane. Oral ectoderm lining Rathke's pouch forms anterior portion of pituitary gland.

mesenchyme of the maxillary process (Fig. 1-13). As the primary palate is forming, the maxillary processes grow forward under the eye, and the mesenchymal cells it contains eventually coalesce with those of the median and lateral nasal processes (Figs. 1-6 and 1-7).

New outgrowths from the medial edges of the maxillary processes form the shelves of the secondary palate. These palatal shelves grow downward beside the tongue (Figs. 1-10 and 1-11) at which time the tongue partially fills the nasal cavities. At about the end of the eighth gestational week, the shelves elevate, make contact, and fuse with each other about the tongue (Fig. 1-11). In the anterior region, the shelves are brought to the horizontal position by a rotational (hingelike) movement. In the more posterior regions, the shelves appear to alter their position by changing shape (remodeling) as well as by rotation. Available evidence indicates that the shelves are incapable of elevation until the tongue is first withdrawn from between them. Although the motive force for shelf elevation is not clearly defined, contractile elements may be involved.

Fusion of palatal shelves requires alterations in the epithelium of the medial edges that begins prior to elevation. These alterations consist of cessation of cell division, which appears to be mediated through distinct underlying biochemical pathways, including a rise in cyclic AMP levels. There is also loss of some surface epithelial cells (Fig. 1-12) and production of extracellular surface substances, particularly glycoproteins, that appear to enhance adhesion between the shelf edges as well as between the shelves and interior margin of the nasal septum (Fig. 1-11). Finally, the adhering epithelia, together with their basement membranes, break down and are replaced by mesenchyme. Epithelial cell debris is

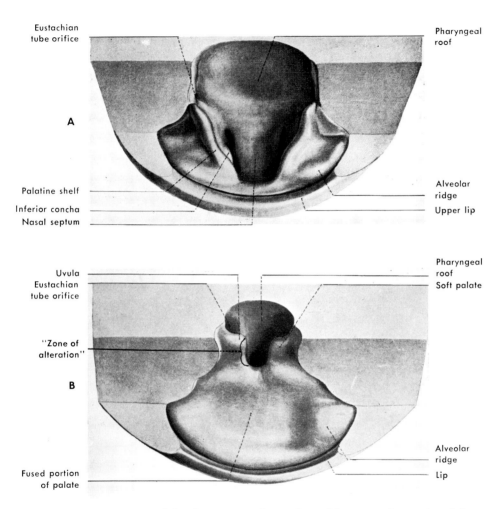

Eustachian
tube orifice

Pharyngeal
roof

**A**

Palatine shelf

Inferior concha

Nasal septum

Alveolar
ridge

Upper lip

Uvula

Eustachian
tube orifice

Pharyngeal
roof

Soft palate

"Zone of
alteration"

**B**

Alveolar
ridge

Fused portion
of palate

Lip

**Fig. 1-10.** Reconstructions of developing secondary palate of human embryos viewed from below. **A,** Reconstruction of roof of primitive oral and pharyngeal cavities of 8-week human embryo. Primary palate and internal surface of the maxillary process form a horseshoe-shaped incomplete roof of oral cavity. In the center, oral cavity communicates with nasal cavities. At edges of maxillary processes, palatal shelves develop. **B,** Reconstruction of palate of slightly older human embryo. Palatal shelves are fused in area of hard palate. Fusion has not reached soft palate and uvula. The nature of the "zone of alteration" is described in Fig. 1-12. (From Sicher, H., and Tandler, J.: Anatomie für Zahnärzte [Anatomy for dentists]. Berlin, 1928, Julius Springer Verlag.)

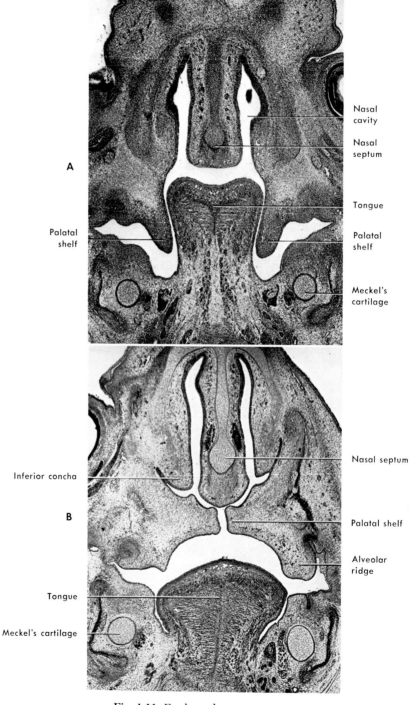

Fig. 1-11. For legend see opposite page.

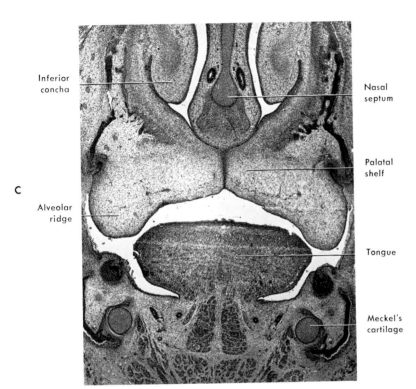

Inferior
concha

Nasal
septum

Palatal
shelf

C

Alveolar
ridge

Tongue

Meckel's
cartilage

**Fig. 1-11.** Coronal sections through secondary palates of human embryos showing progressive stages of development. **A,** Frontal section through head of 8-week embryo. Tongue is high and narrow between vertical palatal shelves. Meckel's cartilage is the first visceral arch cartilage. **B,** Frontal section through head of slightly more advanced embryo. Tongue has left the space between the palatal shelves and lies flat and wide within the mandibular arch. Palatal shelves have assumed a horizontal position. **C,** Frontal section through head of embryo slightly older than that in **B.** Horizontal palatal shelves are fusing with each other and with nasal septum. Secondary palate separates nasal cavities from oral cavity. (**A** and **B,** Courtesy P. Gruenwald, Richmond, Va.)

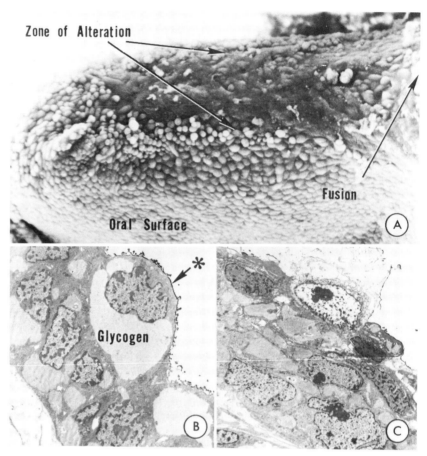

**Fig. 1-12.** Scanning and transmission electron micrographs of palatal shelf of human embryo at the same stage of development as reconstruction in Fig. 1-10, *B*. **A,** Posterior region of palatal shelf viewed from below and from opposite side. Fusion will occur in the "zone of alteration," the location of which is indicated in Fig. 1-10, *B*. **B** and **C,** Transmission electron micrographs of specimen in **A.** Surface cells of oral epithelium in **B** contain large amounts of glycogen, whereas those of zone of alteration in **C** are undergoing degenerative changes and many of them are presumably desquamated into the oral cavity fluids. *Asterisk* in **B** indicates heavy metal deposited on embryo surfaces for scanning electron microscopy. (**A** to **C,** From Waterman, R. E., and Meller, S. M.: Anat. Rec. **180:**11, 1974.)

phagocytosed by mesenchymal cells. Not all the epithelial cells are lost in this process; some remain indefinitely in clusters ("cell rests") along the fusion line. Eventually, most of the hard palate and all of the soft palate forms from the secondary palate (see Chapter 8).

*Development of visceral arches.* The first (mandibular) and second (hyoid) visceral arches undergo further developmental changes. As the heart recedes caudally, both arches send out bilateral processes that fuse with their opposite members in ventral midline (Figs. 1-6 and 1-13). Contained within each arch is

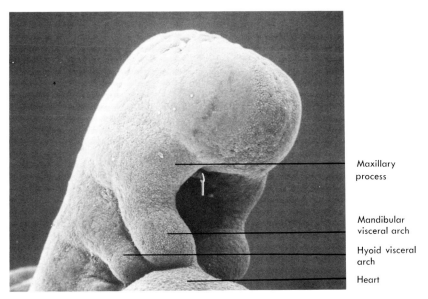

Maxillary
process

Mandibular
visceral arch

Hyoid visceral
arch

Heart

**Fig. 1-13.** Scanning electron micrograph of a ferret embryo showing an intermediate stage of visceral arch development. Eventually both mandibular and hyoid visceral arches will fuse in the ventral midline as the heart recedes caudally. *Arrow,* Opening to Rathke's pouch is located at medial edge of maxillary process, which is just beginning to form a recognizable structure. (Courtesy A. J. Steffek, Chicago, and D. Mujwid, Chicago.)

a mesodermal core with a surrounding layer of neural crest cells. Growth of the caudal (lower) edge of the hyoid arch forms a skirtlike extension (Fig. 1-6, *B* and *C*) that covers the remnants of the remaining visceral arches. In higher vertebrate embryos, the hyoid arch eventually fuses with the lower neck. The mesoderm in this portion of the hyoid arch forms the platysma muscle.

Nerve fibers from the fifth, seventh, ninth, and tenth cranial nerves extend into the mesoderm of the first four visceral arches. The mesoderm of the definitive mandibular and hyoid arches gives rise to the fifth and seventh nerve musculature, while mesoderm associated with the less well developed third and fourth arches forms the ninth and tenth nerve musculature. There is some evidence that myoblast cells that differentiate in the visceral arches actually originate from mesoderm more closely associated with the neural tube (as do the cells that form the hypoglossal and extrinsic eye musculature, Fig. 1-5). They would then migrate into the visceral arches and replace the mesodermal cells that initiated blood vessel formation earlier (see p. 5). If this origin for "visceral arch" myoblasts is confirmed, all myoblasts forming striated muscle fibers of the facial region would then originate from mesoderm adjacent to the neural tube.

Groups of visceral arch myoblasts that are destined to form individual muscles each take a branch of the appropriate visceral arch nerve. Myoblasts from the second visceral arch, for example, take branches of the seventh cranial nerve

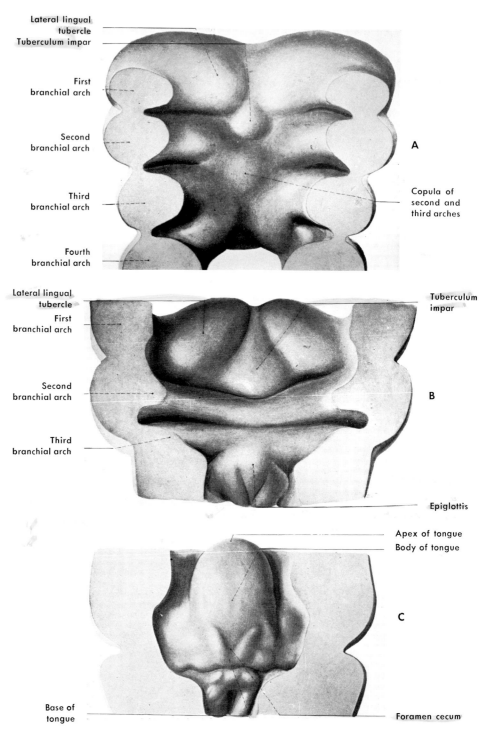

Fig. 1-14. Development of tongue in human embryo. Anterior (ventral) wall of the pharynx and floor of the oral cavity are seen from within. Embryo ages: **A,** Third week. **B,** Fourth week. **C,** Sixth week. For further explanation, see text. (From Sicher, H., and Tandler, J.: Anatomie für Zahnärzte [Anatomy for dentists], Berlin, 1928, Julius Springer Verlag.)

and migrate very extensively throughout the head and neck to form the contractile components of the "muscles of facial expression." Myoblasts from the first arch contribute mostly to the muscles of mastication, while those from the third and fourth arches contribute to the pharyngeal and soft palate musculature. As noted earlier, connective tissue components of each muscle in the facial region are provided by mesenchymal cells of crest origin.

The crest mesenchymal cells of the visceral arches gives rise to skeletal components such as the temporary visceral arch cartilages (e.g., Meckel's cartilage, Fig. 1-11), middle ear cartilages, and mandibular bones. Also visceral arch crest cells form connective tissues such as dermis and the connective tissue components of the tongue.

The tongue forms in the ventral floor of the pharynx after arrival of the hypoglossal muscle cells. The significance of the lateral lingual tubercles (Fig. 1-14) and other swellings in the forming tongue has not been carefully documented. It is known that the anterior two thirds of the tongue is covered by ectoderm whereas endoderm covers the posterior one third. The thyroid gland forms by invagination of the most anterior endoderm (thyroglossal duct). A residual pit (the foramen cecum, Fig. 1-14, *C*) left in the epithelium at the site of invagination marks the junction between the anterior two thirds and posterior one third of the tongue, which are, respectively, covered by epithelia of ectodermal and endodermal origin. It is also known that the connective tissue components of the anterior two thirds of the tongue are derived from first-arch mesenchyme whereas those of the posterior one third are derived from the second-arch mesenchyme.

The epithelial components of a number of glands are derived from the endodermal lining of the pharynx. In addition to the thyroid, these include the parathyroid and thymus. The epithelial components of the salivary and anterior pituitary glands are derived from oral ectoderm.

Finally, a lateral extension from the inner groove between the first and second arch gives rise to the eustachian tube, which connects the pharynx with the ear. The external ear or pinna is formed at least partially from tissues of the first and second arches (Fig. 1-1, *E*).

## FINAL DIFFERENTIATION OF FACIAL TISSUES

The extensive cell migrations referred to above bring cell populations into new relationships and lead to further inductive interactions, which, in turn, lead to progressively more differentiated cell types. For example, some of the crest cells coming into contact with pharyngeal endoderm are induced by the endoderm to form visceral arch cartilages (see Chapter 8). Other crest cells that have migrated in the vicinity of the pharyngeal endoderm on their way to the oral cavity are preconditioned by the endoderm and will react with oral ectoderm and differentiate into tooth papilla mesenchyme.

In many instances, such as those cited above, only crest mesenchymal cells

incomplete. Most of this variation results from variable degrees of fusion and may be explained by variable degrees of mesenchyme in the facial processes. Some of the variation may represent different initiating events.

Clefts involving only the secondary palate ("cleft palate," Fig. 1-15) constitute, after clefts involving primary palate, the second most frequent facial malformation in man. Cleft palate can also be produced in experimental animals with a wide variety of chemical agents or other manipulations affecting the embryo. Usually, such agents retard or prevent shelf elevation. In other cases, however, it is shelf growth that is retarded so that although elevation occurs the shelves are too small to make contact. There is also some evidence that indicates that failure of the epithelial seam occurs after the application of some environmental agents. Cleft formation could then result from rupture of the persisting seam, which would not have sufficient strength to prevent such rupture indefinitely.

Less frequently, other types of facial clefting are observed. In most instances they can be explained by failure of fusion between facial processes of reduced size, and similar clefts can be produced experimentally. Examples include failure of fusion between the maxillary process and frontonasal processes (Fig. 1-6) leading to oblique facial clefting and failure of fusion between the bilateral mandibular processes leading to clefts of the mandible.

*Hemifacial microsomia.* Hemifacial microsomia is the third most common facial malformation. Affected individuals have underdevelopment and other abnormalities of the temporomandibular joint, middle and external ear, and other structures in this region such as the parotid gland and muscles of mastication. The defect is almost invariably unilateral.

Recent studies strongly suggest that hemifacial microsomia results from hemorrhage at the point of fusion between the external carotid and stapedial arteries. The stapedial artery supplies much of the facial region during an early embryonic stage. The newly developing external carotid takes over most of this function by fusing with the stapedial, after which the proximal portion of the latter artery regresses (Fig. 1-4). Thalidomide and other chemical agents cause hemorrhage at the point of fusion and later result in malformations similar to hemifacial microsomia. Malformations similar to hemifacial microsomia also occur as part of the thalidomide syndrome in man.

*Treacher Collins' syndrome.* Treacher Collins' syndrome (mandibulofacial dysostosis) is an inherited disorder that results from the action of dominant gene and may be almost as common as hemifacial microsomia. The syndrome consists of underdevelopment of the tissues derived from the maxillary, mandibular, and hyoid processes. The external and middle ear is often defective and clefts of the secondary palate sometimes are found. Defects of a similar nature result from the action of an abnormal gene in mice and can also be produced experimentally with excessive doses of vitamin A.

*Labial pits.* Small pits may persist on either side of the midline of the lower lip. They are caused by the failure of the embryonic labial pits to disappear.

*Lingual anomalies.* Median rhomboid glossitis, an innocuous, red, rhomboidal smooth zone of the tongue in the midline in front of the foramen cecum, is considered the result of persistence of the tuberculum impar. Lack of fusion between the two lateral lingual prominences may produce a bifid tongue. Thyroid tissue may be present in the base of the tongue. Part of the thyroglossal duct may persist and form cysts at the base of the tongue.

*Developmental cysts.* Epithelial rests in lines of union of facial or oral processes or from epithelial organs, that is, vestigial nasopalatine ducts, may give rise to cysts lined with epithelium.

Branchial cleft (cervical) cysts or fistulas may arise from the rests of epithelium in the visceral arch area. They usually are laterally disposed on the neck. Thyroglossal duct cysts may occur at any place along the course of the duct, usually at or near the midline.

Cysts may arise from epithelial rests after the fusion of medial and lateral nasal processes. They are called globulomaxillary cysts and are lined with pseudostratified columnar epithelium and squamous epithelium. They may, however, develop as primordial cysts from a supernumerary tooth germ.

Anterior palatine cysts are situated in the midline of the maxillary alveolar process. Once believed to be from remnants of the fusion of two processes, they may be primordial cysts of odontogenic origin and their true nature is a subject of discussion.

Nasolabial cysts, originating in the base of the wing of the nose and bulging into the nasal and oral vestibule and the root of the upper lip, sometimes causing a flat depression on the anterior surface of the alveolar process, are also explained as originating from epithelial remnants in the cleft-lip line. It is, however, more probable that they derive from excessive epithelial proliferations that normally, for some time in embryonic life, plug the nostrils. It is also possible that they are retention cysts of vestibular nasal glands or that they develop from the epithelium of the nasolacrimal duct.

## REFERENCES

Balinsky, B. I.: An introduction to embryology, ed. 3, Philadelphia, 1970, W. B. Saunders Co.

Bartelmez, G. W.: Neural crest in the forebrain of mammals, Anat. Rec. **138:**269, 1960.

Gasser, R. F.: The development of the facial muscles in man, Am. J. Anat. **120:**357, 1967.

Hamilton, W. J., and Mossman, H.: Human embryology, ed. 4, Cambridge, 1972, W. Heffer & Sons, Ltd.

Hazelton, R. B.: A radioautographic analysis of the migration and fate of cells derived from the occipital somites of the chick embryo with specific reference to the hypoglossal musculature, J. Embryol. Exp. Morphol. **24:**455, 1970.

Johnston, M. C.: Abnormal organogenesis of facial structures. In Wilson, J. G., and Fraser, F. C., editors: Handbook of teratology, Philadelphia, 1975, W. B. Saunders Co.

Johnston, M. C., and Listgarten, M. A.: The migration interaction and early differentiation of oro-facial tissues. In Slavkin, H. S., and Bavetta, L. A., editors: Developmental aspects of oral biology, New York, 1972, Academic Press Inc.

Kraus, B. S., Kitamura, H., and Latham, R. A.: Atlas of the developmental anatomy of the face, New York, 1966, Harper & Row, Inc.

Langman, J.: Medical embryology, ed. 2, Baltimore, 1969, The Williams & Wilkins Co.

Nishimura, H.: Incidence of malformations in abortions. In Fraser, F. C., and McKusick, V. A., editors: Congenital malformations, Amsterdam, 1969, Exerpta Medica Press.

Poswillo, D.: The pathogenesis of the first and second branchial arch syndrome, Oral Surg. **35**:302, 1973.

Pourtois, M.: Morphogenesis of the primary and secondary palate. In Slavkin, H. S., and Bevetta, L. A., editors: Developmental aspects of oral biology, New York, 1972, Academic Press Inc.

Pratt, R. M., and Martin, G. R.: Epithelial cell death and elevated cyclic AMP during palatal development, Proc. Nat. Acad. Sci. U. S. A. **72**:814, 1975.

Ross, R. B., and Johnston, M. C.: Cleft lip and palate, Baltimore, 1972, The Williams & Wilkins Co.

Sicher, H., and Tandler, J.: Anatomie für Zahnärzte [Anatomy for dentists], Berlin, 1928, Julius Springer Verlag.

Sperber, G. H.: Craniofacial embryology, Bristol, 1973, John Wright & Sons, Ltd.

Streeter, G. L.: Developmental horizons in human embryos, Contrib. Embryol. **32**:133, 1948.

Trasler, D. G.: Pathogenesis of cleft lip and its relation to embryonic face shape in A/Jax and C57BL mice, Teratology **1**:33, 1968.

Waterman, R. E., and Meller, S. M.: A scanning electron microscope study of secondary palate formation in the human, Anat. Rec. **175**:464, 1973.

Weston, J. A.: The migration and differentiation of neural crest cells, Adv. Morphog. **8**:41, 1970.

# 2 Development and growth of teeth

The primitive oral cavity, or stomodeum, is lined with ectoderm. At its deeper aspect it contacts the blind upper end of the endoderm-lined foregut. The union of the ectodermal and endodermal layers is called the *buccopharyngeal membrane* (Fig. 1-9). At about 27 days this membrane ruptures and the stomodeum establishes a connection with the foregut.

The primitive oral cavity is therefore lined by ectoderm that consists of a basal layer of columnar cells and a surface layer of flattened cells. Each tooth develops from a tooth bud that forms from the lining of the oral cavity. A tooth bud consists of three parts: (1) an *enamel organ,* which is derived from the oral ectoderm; (2) a *dental papilla,* which is derived from the mesenchyme; and (3) a *dental sac,* which is also derived from the mesenchyme (Fig. 2-8). The enamel organ produces the tooth enamel, the dental papilla produces the tooth pulp and the dentin, and the dental sac produces the cementum and the periodontal ligament.

Two or 3 weeks after the rupture of the buccopharyngeal membrane, when the embryo is about 6 weeks old, the first sign of tooth development is seen. In the oral ectoderm, which will, of course, give rise to the oral epithelium, certain areas of basal cells begin to proliferate at a more rapid rate than do the cells of the adjacent areas (Fig. 2-3). This leads to the formation of a band of epithelium that runs along the outline of the future dental arches and is called the *dental lamina.*

**23**

At certain points on the dental lamina, each representing the location of one of the ten mandibular and ten maxillary deciduous teeth, the ectodermal cells multiply still more rapidly and form a little knob that presses slightly into the underlying mesenchyme (Figs. 2-2 and 2-4). Each of these little downgrowths from the dental lamina represents the beginning of the enamel organ of the tooth bud of a deciduous tooth. Not all of these enamel organs start to develop at the same time, and the first to appear are those of the anterior mandibular region.

As cell proliferation continues, each enamel organ increases in size and changes in shape. As it develops, it takes on a shape that somewhat resembles a cap, with the outside of the cap directed toward the oral surface (Figs. 2-5 and 2-7).

Inside of the cap (i.e., inside the depression of the enamel organ), the mesenchymal cells increase in number. The tissue appears more dense than the surrounding mesenchyme and represents the beginning of the dental papilla. Surrounding the combined enamel organ and dental papilla, the third part of the tooth bud forms. It is called the *dental sac,* and it consists of mesenchymal cells and fibers that surround the dental papilla and the enamel organ (Fig. 2-8).

During and after these developments the shape of the enamel organ continues to change. The depression occupied by the dental papilla deepens until the enamel organ assumes a shape resembling a bell. As these developments take place, the dental lamina, which had thus far connected the enamel organ to the oral epithelium, breaks up, and the tooth bud loses its connection with the epithelium of the primitive oral cavity.

## DEVELOPMENTAL STAGES

Despite the obvious fact that tooth development (as the development of any other organ) is a continual process, it is not only traditional but also didactically necessary to divide the developmental history of a tooth into several "stages." They are named after the shape of the epithelial part of the tooth germ and are the bud, cap, and bell stages (Fig. 2-1, A to C).

### Dental lamina and bud stage

*Dental lamina.* The first sign of human tooth development is seen during the sixth week of embryonic life (11 mm. embryo). At this stage the oral epithelium consists of a basal layer of high cells and a surface layer of flattened cells. The glycogen droplets in their cytoplasm are lost in routine preparations, giving them an empty appearance. The epithelium is separated from the connective tissue by a basement membrane. Certain cells in the basal layer of the oral epithelium begin to proliferate at a more rapid rate than do the adjacent cells. An epithelial thickening arises in the region of the future dental arch and extends along the entire free margin of the jaws (Figs. 2-2 and 2-3). It is the primordium of the ectodermal portion of the teeth and is known as the dental lamina. Mitotic figures are seen not only in the epithelium but also in the subjacent mesoderm (Fig. 2-3).

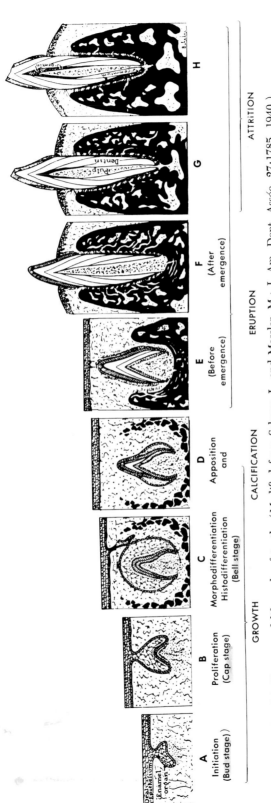

Fig. 2-1. Diagram of life cycle of tooth. (Modified from Schour, I., and Massler, M.: J. Am. Dent. Assoc. 27:1785, 1940.)

A
Initiation
(Bud stage)

B
Proliferation
(Cap stage)

C
Morphodifferentiation
Histodifferentiation
(Bell stage)

D
Apposition
and

E
(Before emergence)

F
(After emergence)

G

H

GROWTH

CALCIFICATION

ERUPTION

ATTRITION

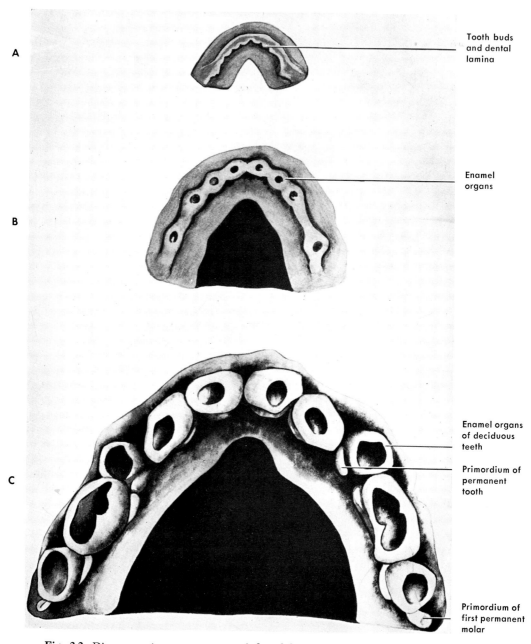

Tooth buds
and dental
lamina

Enamel
organs

Enamel organs
of deciduous
teeth

Primordium of
permanent
tooth

Primordium of
first permanent
molar

**Fig. 2-2.** Diagrammatic reconstruction of dental lamina and enamel organs of mandible. **A,** 22 mm. embryo, bud stage (eighth week). **B,** 43 mm. embryo, cap stage (tenth week). **C,** 163 mm. embryo, bell stage (about 4 months). The primordia of permanent teeth are seen as thickenings of dental lamina on lingual side of each tooth germ. Distal extension of dental lamina with primordium of first molar.

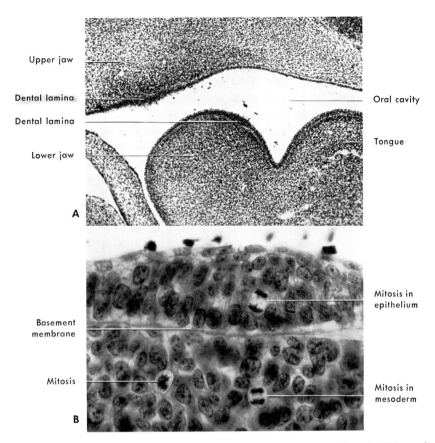

Fig. 2-3. Initiation of tooth development. Human embryo 13.5 mm. in length, fifth week. **A,** Sagittal section through upper and lower jaws. **B,** High magnification of thickened oral epithelium. (From Orban, B.: Dental histology and embryology, Philadelphia, 1929, P. Blakiston's Son & Co.)

*Tooth buds (primordia of teeth).* Simultaneous with the differentiation of the dental lamina, there arise from it in each jaw, round or ovoid swellings at ten different points, corresponding to the future position of the deciduous teeth; they are the primordia of the enamel organs, the tooth buds (Fig. 2-4). Thus the development of the tooth germs is initiated, and the cells continue to proliferate faster than the adjacent cells do. The dental lamina is shallow, and microscopic sections often show the tooth buds close to the oral epithelium.

## Cap stage

As the tooth bud continues to proliferate, it does not expand uniformly into a larger sphere. Unequal growth in the different parts of the bud leads to formation of the cap stage, which is characterized by a shallow invagination on the deep surface of the bud (Figs. 2-2, *B,* and 2-5).

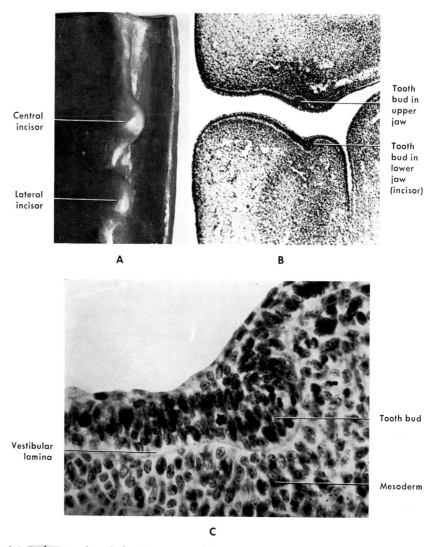

Fig. 2-4. Bud stage of tooth development, proliferation stage. Human embryo 16 mm. in length, sixth week. **A,** Wax reconstruction of germs of lower central and lateral incisors. **B,** Sagittal section through upper and lower jaws. **C,** High magnification of tooth germ of lower incisor in bud stage. (From Orban, B.: Dental histology and embryology, Philadelphia, 1929, P. Blakiston's Son & Co.)

*Outer and inner enamel epithelium.* The peripheral cells of the cap stage are cuboidal, line the convexity of the "cap," and are called the outer enamel (dental) epithelium. The cells on the concavity of the "cap" are tall and represent the inner enamel (dental) epithelium (Figs. 2-6 and 2-7).

*Stellate reticulum (enamel pulp).* The cells in the center of the epithelial enamel organ, situated between the outer and inner epithelia, begin to separate

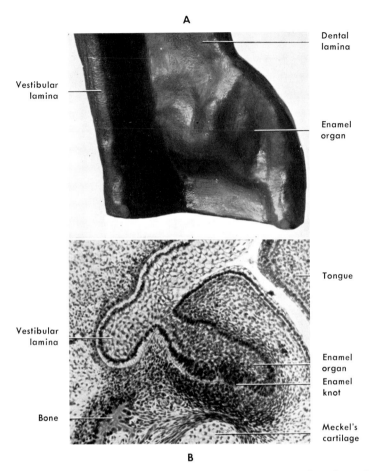

**Fig. 2-5.** Cap stage of tooth development. Human embryo 31.5 mm. in length, ninth week. **A,** Wax reconstruction of enamel organ of lower lateral incisor. **B,** Labiolingual section through the same tooth. (From Orban, B.: Dental histology and embryology, Philadelphia, 1929, P. Blakiston's Son & Co.)

by an increase of the intercellular fluid and arrange themselves in a network called the stellate reticulum (Figs. 2-8 and 2-9). The cells assume a branched reticular form. The spaces in this reticular network are filled with a mucoid fluid rich in albumin, giving the stellate reticulum a cushionlike consistency that later supports and protects the delicate enamel-forming cells.

The cells in the center of the enamel organ are densely packed and form the *enamel knot* (Fig. 2-5). This knot projects in part toward the underlying dental papilla, so that the center of the epithelial invagination shows a slightly knoblike enlargement that is bordered by the labial and lingual enamel grooves (Fig. 2-5). At the same time there arises in the increasingly high enamel organ a vertical extension of the enamel knot, called the *enamel cord* (Fig. 2-8). Both are temporary structures that disappear before enamel formation begins.

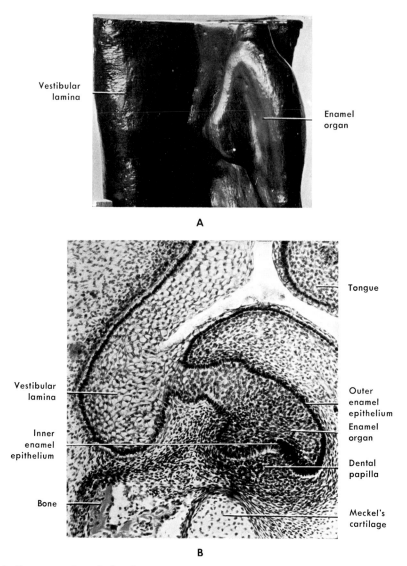

Fig. 2-6. Cap stage of tooth development. Human embryo 41.5 mm. in length, tenth week. **A,** Wax reconstruction of enamel organ of lower central incisor. **B,** Labiolingual section through the same tooth. (From Orban, B.: Dental histology and embryology, Philadelphia, 1929, P. Blakiston's Son & Co.)

*Dental papilla.* Under the organizing influence of the proliferating epithelium of the enamel organ, the mesenchyme, partially enclosed by the invaginated portion of the inner enamel epithelium, proliferates. It condenses to form the dental papilla, which is the formative organ of the dentin and the primordium of the pulp (Figs. 2-5 and 2-6). The changes in the dental papilla occur concomitantly with the development of the epithelial enamel organ. Although the

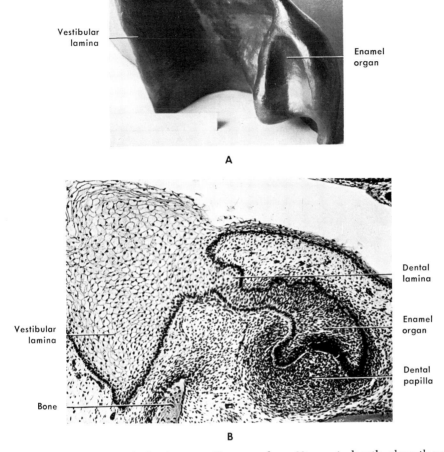

Fig. 2-7. Cap stage of tooth development. Human embryo 60 mm. in length, eleventh week. **A,** Wax reconstruction of enamel organ of lower lateral incisor. **B,** Labiolingual section through the same tooth. (From Orban, B.: Dental histology and embryology, Philadelphia, 1929, P. Blakiston's Son & Co.)

epithelium exerts a dominating influence over the adjacent connective tissue, the condensation of the latter should not be considered to be a passive crowding by the proliferating epithelium. The dental papilla shows active budding of capillaries and mitotic figures, and its peripheral cells adjacent to the inner enamel epithelium enlarge and later differentiate into the odontoblasts.

*Dental sac.* Concomitant with the development of the enamel organ and the dental papilla, there is a marginal condensation in the mesenchyme surrounding the enamel organ and dental papilla. In this zone, gradually a denser and more fibrous layer develops, which is the primitive dental sac.

The epithelial enamel organ, the dental papilla, and the dental sac are the formative tissues for an entire tooth and its supporting structures.

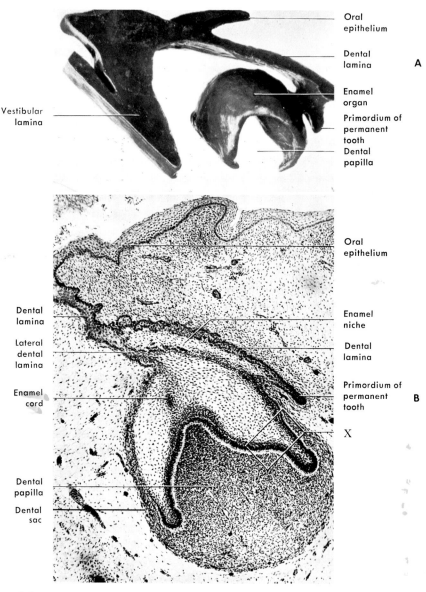

Oral
epithelium

Dental
lamina    **A**

Enamel
organ

Primordium of
permanent
tooth
Dental
papilla

Vestibular
lamina

Oral
epithelium

Dental
lamina

Enamel
niche

Lateral
dental
lamina

Dental
lamina

Enamel
cord

Primordium of
permanent    **B**
tooth

X

Dental
papilla

Dental
sac

**Fig. 2-8.** Bell stage of tooth development. Human embryo 105 mm. in length, fourteenth week. **A,** Wax reconstruction of lower central incisor. **B,** Labiolingual section of the same tooth. x, See Fig. 2-9. (From Orban, B.: Dental histology and embryology, Philadelphia, 1929, P. Blakiston's Son & Co.)

## Bell stage

As the invagination of the epithelium deepens and its margins continue to grow, the enamel organ assumes a bell shape (Figs. 2-2, *C,* and 2-8).

***Inner enamel epithelium.*** The inner enamel epithelium consists of a single layer of cells that differentiate prior to amelogenesis into tall columnar cells, the ameloblasts (Figs. 2-8 and 2-9). They are 4 to 5 microns in diameter and about 40 microns high. In cross section they assume a hexagonal shape similar to that seen later in transverse sections of the enamel rods.

The cells of the inner enamel epithelium exert an organizing influence on the underlying mesenchymal cells, which differentiate into odontoblasts.

***Stratum intermedium.*** Several layers of squamous cells, called stratum intermedium, appear between the inner enamel epithelium and the stellate reticulum (Fig. 2-9). This layer seems to be essential to enamel formation. It is absent in the part of the tooth germ that outlines the root portions of the tooth but does not form enamel.

***Stellate reticulum.*** The stellate reticulum expands further, mainly by increase of the intercellular fluid. The cells are star shaped, with long processes that anastomose with those of adjacent cells (Fig. 2-9). Before enamel formation begins, the stellate reticulum shrinks by loss of the intercellular fluid. Its cells then are hardly distinguishable from those of the stratum intermedium. This change begins at the height of the cusp or the incisal edge and progresses cervically (Figs. 3-37 and 4-29).

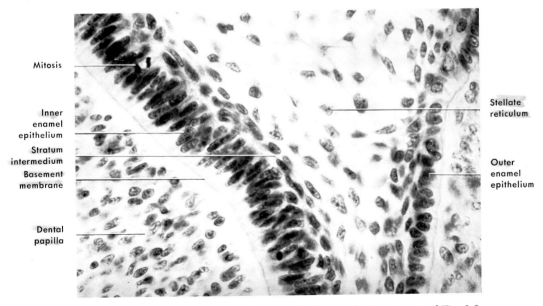

Fig. 2-9. Layers of epithelial enamel organ at high magnification. Area X of Fig. 2-8.

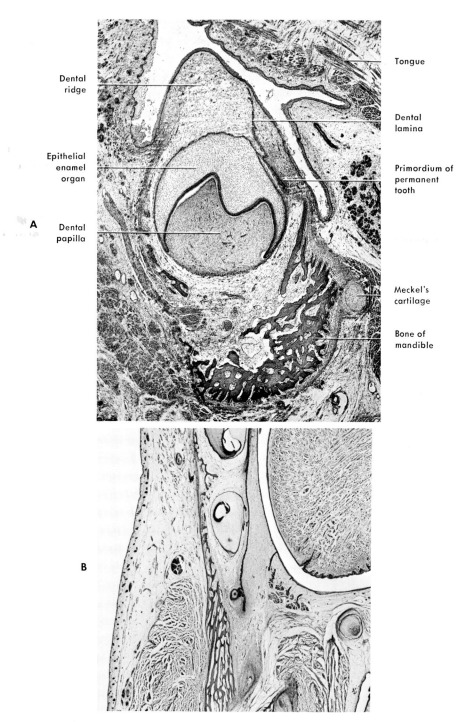

Dental ridge

Tongue

Epithelial enamel organ

Dental lamina

**A**

Primordium of permanent tooth

Dental papilla

Meckel's cartilage

Bone of mandible

**B**

**Fig. 2-10. A,** Advanced bell stage of tooth development. Human embryo 200 mm. in length, about 18 weeks. Labiolingual section through deciduous lower first molar. **B,** Horizontal section through human embryo about 20 mm. in length showing extension of dental lamina distal to second deciduous molar and formation of permanent first molar tooth germ. (**B** from Bhaskar, S. N.: Synopsis of oral histology, St. Louis, 1962, The C. V. Mosby Co.)

*Outer enamel epithelium.* The cells of the outer enamel epithelium flatten to a low cuboid form. At the end of the bell stage, preparatory to and during the formation of enamel, the formerly smooth surface of the outer enamel epithelium is laid in folds. Between the folds the adjacent mesenchyme of the dental sac forms papillae that contain capillary loops and thus provide a rich nutritional supply for the intense metabolic activity of the avascular enamel organ.

*Dental lamina.* In all teeth except the permanent molars the dental lamina proliferates at its deep end to give rise to the enamel organs of the permanent teeth (Figs. 2-10 and 2-11).

*Dental papilla.* The dental papilla is enclosed in the invaginated portion of the enamel organ. Before the inner enamel epithelium begins to produce enamel, the peripheral cells of the mesenchymal dental papilla differentiate into odonto-

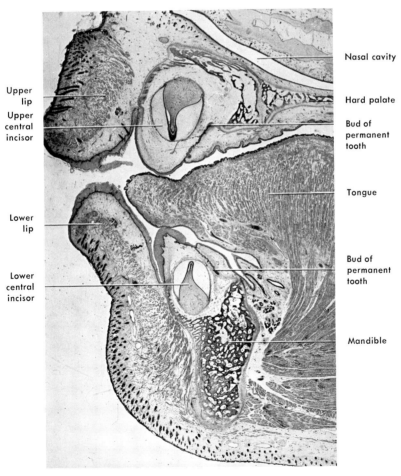

Fig. 2-11. Sagittal section through head of human fetus 200 mm. in length, about 18 weeks, in region of central incisors.

blasts under the organizing influence of the epithelium. They assume a cuboid and later a columnar form and acquire the specific potentiality to produce dentin.

The basement membrane separating the enamel organ and the dental papilla just preceding dentin formation is called *membrana preformativa*.

*Dental sac.* Before formation of dental tissues begins, the dental sac shows a circular arrangement of its fibers and resembles a capsular structure. With the development of the root, the fibers of the dental sac differentiate into the periodontal fibers that become embedded in the cementum and the alveolar bone.

*Advanced bell stage.* During the advanced bell stage the boundary between inner enamel epithelium and odontoblasts outlines the future dentinoenamel junction (Figs. 2-8 and 2-10). In addition, the basal margin of the enamel organ gives rise to the epithelial root sheath of Hertwig.

*Function of dental lamina.* The functional activity of the dental lamina and its chronology may be considered in three phases. The first phase is concerned with the initiation of the entire deciduous dentition that occurs during the second month in utero (Fig. 2-2, *A* and *B*). The second phase deals with the initiation of the successors of the deciduous teeth. It is preceded by the growth of the free end of the dental lamina (successional lamina), lingual to the enamel organ of each deciduous tooth, and occurs from about the fifth month in utero for the permanent central incisors to 10 months of age for the second premolar (Fig. 2-2, *C*). The third phase is preceded by the extension of the dental lamina distal to the enamel organ of the second deciduous molar and the formation of permanent molar tooth germs (Figs. 2-2 and 2-10, *B*). The permanent molars arise directly from the distal extension of the dental lamina. The time of initiation is at about 4 months of fetal life for the first permanent molar, the first year for the second permanent molar, and the fourth to fifth year for the third permanent molar.

It is thus evident that the total activity of the dental lamina extends over a period of about 5 years. Any particular portion of it functions for a much briefer period, since only a relatively short time elapses after initiation before the dental lamina begins to disintegrate at that particular location. However, the dental lamina may still be active in the third molar region after it has disappeared elsewhere except for occasional epithelial remnants. The distal proliferation of the dental lamina is responsible for the location of the germs of the permanent molars in the ramus of the mandible and in the tuberosity of the maxilla.

*Fate of dental lamina.* During the cap stage the dental lamina maintains a broad connection with the enamel organ, but in the bell stage it begins to break up by mesenchymal invasion, which first penetrates its central portion and divides it into the lateral lamina and the dental lamina proper. The mesenchymal invasion is at first incomplete and does not perforate the dental lamina (Fig. 2-8). The dental lamina proper proliferates only at its deeper margin, which becomes a free end situated lingually to the enamel organ and forms the primordium of the permanent tooth (Figs. 2-8 and 2-11). The epithelial connection of the enamel organ with the oral epithelium is severed by the proliferating mesoderm. Remnants of the dental lamina persist as epithelial pearls or islands within the jaw as well as in the gingiva.

*Vestibular lamina.* Labial and buccal to the dental lamina, another epithelial thickening develops independently and somewhat later. It is the vestibular lamina, also termed the *lip furrow band* (Figs. 2-6 and 2-7). It subsequently hollows and forms the oral vestibule between the alveolar portion of the jaws and the lips and cheeks (Figs. 2-10 and 2-11).

### Hertwig's epithelial root sheath and root formation

The development of the roots begins after enamel and dentin formation has reached the future cementoenamel junction. The enamel organ plays an important part in root development by forming Hertwig's epithelial root sheath, which molds the shape of the roots and initiates dentin formation. Hertwig's root sheath consists only of the outer and inner enamel epithelia, without a stratum intermedium and stellate reticulum. The cells of the inner layer remain short and normally do not produce enamel. When these cells have induced the differentiation of connective tissue cells into odontoblasts and the first layer of dentin has been laid down, the epithelial root sheath loses its continuity and its close relation to the surface of the tooth. It remnants persists as epithelial rests of Malassez in the periodontal ligament.

There is a pronounced difference in the development of Hertwig's epithelial root sheath in teeth with one root and in those with two or more roots. Prior to the beginning of root formation, the root sheath forms the epithelial diaphragm (Fig. 2-12). The outer and inner enamel epithelia bend at the future cementoenamel junction into a horizontal plane, narrowing the wide cervical opening of the tooth germ. The plane of the diaphragm remains relatively fixed during the development and growth of the root (Chapter 11). The proliferation of the cells of the epithelial diaphragm is accompanied by proliferation of the cells of the connective tissue of the pulp, which occurs in the area adjacent to the diaphragm. The free end of the diaphragm does not grow into the connective tissue, but the epithelium proliferates coronally to the epithelial diaphragm (Fig. 2-12, *B*). The differentiation of odontoblasts and the formation of dentin follow the lengthening of the root sheath. At the same time the connective tissue of the dental sac surrounding the sheath proliferates and divides the continuous double epithelial layer (Fig. 2-12, *C*) into a network of epithelial strands (Fig. 2-12, *D*). The epithelium is moved away from the surface of the dentin so that connective tissue cells come into contact with the outer surface of the dentin and differentiate into cementoblasts, which deposit a layer of cementum onto the surface of the dentin. The rapid sequence of proliferation and destruction of Hertwig's root sheath explains the fact that it cannot be seen as a continuous layer on the surface of the developing root (Fig. 2-12, *D*). In the last stages of root development

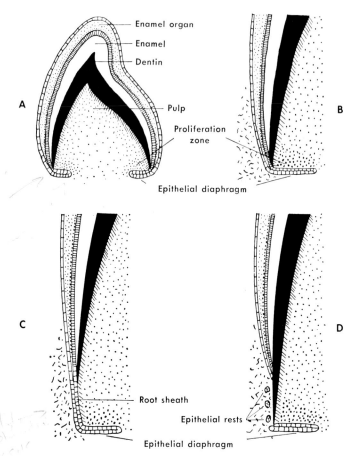

**Fig. 2-12.** Diagrams showing three stages in root development. **A,** Section through a tooth germ. Note epithelial diaphragm and proliferation zone of pulp. **B,** Higher magnification of cervical region of **A. C,** "Imaginary" stage showing elongation of Hertwig's epithelial sheath coronal to diaphragm. Differentiation of odontoblasts in elongated pulp. **D,** In area of proliferation, dentin has been formed. Root sheath is broken up into epithelial rest and is separated from dentinal surface by connective tissue. Differentiation of cementoblasts.

the proliferation of the epithelium in the diaphragm lags behind that of the pulpal connective tissue. The wide apical foramen is reduced first to the width of the diaphragmatic opening itself and later is further narrowed by apposition of dentin and cementum at the apex of the root.

Differential growth of the epithelial diaphragm in multirooted teeth causes the division of the root trunk into two or three roots. During the general growth of the enamel organ the expansion of its cervical opening occurs in such a way that long tonguelike extensions of the horizontal diaphragm develop (Fig. 2-13). Two such extensions are found in the germs of lower molars and three in the germs of upper molars. Before division of the root trunk occurs, the free ends of

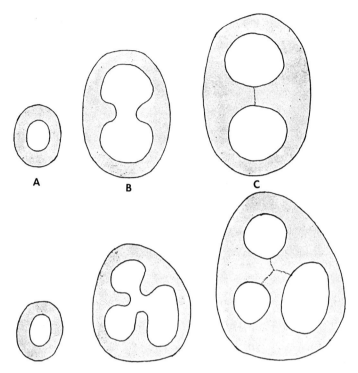

**Fig. 2-13.** Three stages in development of tooth with two roots and one with three roots. Surface view of epithelial diaphragm. During growth of tooth germ the simple diaphragm, **A,** expands eccentrically so that horizontal epithelial flaps are formed. **B.** Later these flaps proliferate and unite (*dotted lines* in **C**) and divide the single cervical opening into two or three openings.

these horizontal epithelial flaps grow toward each other and fuse. The single cervical opening of the coronal enamel organ is then divided into two or three openings. On the pulpal surface of the dividing epithelial bridges, dentin formation starts (Fig. 2-14, *A*), and on the periphery of each opening, root development follows in the same way as described for single-rooted teeth (Fig. 2-14, *B*).

If cells of the epithelial root sheath remain adherent to the dentin surface, they may differentiate into fully functioning ameloblasts and produce enamel. Such droplets of enamel, called *enamel pearls,* are sometimes found in the area of furcation of the roots of permanent molars. If the continuity of Hertwig's root sheath is broken or is not established prior to dentin formation, a defect in the dentinal wall of the pulp ensues. Such defects are found in the pulpal floor corresponding to the furcation or on any point of the root itself if the fusion of the horizontal extensions of the diaphragm remains incomplete. This accounts for the development of accessory root canals opening on the periodontal surface of the root (Chapter 5).

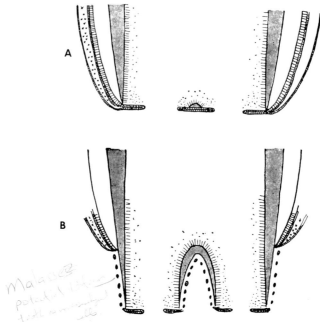

**Fig. 2-14.** Two stages in development of two-rooted tooth. Diagrammatic mesiodistal sections of lower molar. **A,** Beginning of dentin formation at bifurcation. **B,** Formation of two roots in progress. (Details as shown in Fig. 2-12.)

## HISTOPHYSIOLOGY AND CLINICAL CONSIDERATIONS

A number of physiologic growth processes participate in the progressive development of the teeth (Table 1). Except for their initiation, which is a momentary event, these processes overlap considerably, and many are continuous over several histologic stages. Nevertheless, each tends to predominate in one stage more than in another.

For example, the process of histodifferentiation characterizes the bell stage, in which the cells of the inner enamel epithelium differentiate into functional ameloblasts. However, proliferation still progresses at the deeper portion of the enamel organ.

*Initiation.* The dental lamina and tooth buds represent that part of the oral epithelium that has potencies for tooth formation. Specific cells contain the entire growth potential of certain teeth and respond to those factors that initiate tooth development. Different teeth are initiated at definite times. Initiation is set off by unknown factors, just as the growth potential of the ovum is set off by the fertilizing spermatozoon.

Teeth may develop in abnormal locations, e.g., in the ovary (dermoid tumors or cysts) or in the hypophysis. In such instances the tooth undergoes stages of development similar to those in the jaws.

**Table 1.** Stages in tooth growth

| *Morphologic stages* | *Physiologic processes* |
|---|---|
| Dental lamina ⟵⟶ | Initiation |
| Bud stage | |
| Cap stage | Proliferation |
| Bell stage (early) | Histodifferentiation |
| Bell stage (advanced) | Morphodifferentiation |
| Formation of enamel and dentin matrix | Apposition |

A lack of initiation results in the absence of teeth, which may involve single teeth, most frequently the permanent upper lateral incisors, third molars, and lower second premolars, or there may be a complete lack of teeth (anodontia). On the other hand, abnormal initiation may result in the development of single or multiple supernumerary teeth.

**Proliferation.** Enhanced proliferative activity ensues at the points of initiation and results successively in the bud, cap, and bell stages of the odontogenic organ. Proliferative growth causes regular changes in the size and proportions of the growing tooth germ (Figs. 2-3 and 2-7).

During the stage of proliferation the tooth germ has the potentiality to progress to more advanced development. This is illustrated by the fact that explants of these early stages continue to develop in tissue culture through the subsequent stages of histodifferentiation and appositional growth. A disturbance or experimental interference has entirely different effects, according to the time of occurrence and the stage of development that it affects.

**Histodifferentiation.** Histodifferentiation succeeds the proliferative stage. The formative cells of the tooth germs developing during the proliferative stage undergo definite morphologic as well as functional changes and acquire their functional assignment (the appositional growth potential). The cells become restricted in their potencies. They give up their capacity to multiply as they assume their new function; this is a law that governs all differentiating cells. This phase reaches its highest development in the bell stage of the enamel organ, just preceding the beginning of formation and apposition of dentin and enamel (Fig. 2-8).

The organizing influence of the inner enamel epithelium on the mesenchyme is evident in the bell stage and causes the differentiation of the adjacent cells of the dental papilla into odontoblasts. With the formation of dentin, the cells of the inner enamel epithelium differentiate into ameloblasts, and enamel matrix is formed opposite the dentin. Enamel does not form in the absence of dentin, as demonstrated by the failure of transplanted ameloblasts to form enamel when no dentin is present. Dentin formation therefore precedes and is essential to enamel formation. The differentiation of the epithelial cells precedes and is essential to the differentiation of the odontoblasts and the initiation of dentin formation.

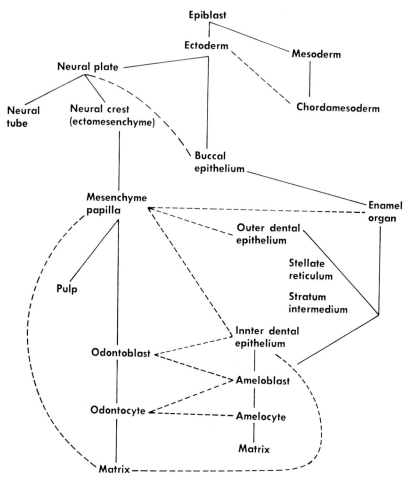

**Fig. 2-15.** Outline of development of a tooth. *Broken lines,* Known or suspected interactions that occur between tissues. The data suggesting placement of these lines derive from transplantations and in vitro studies. The words "amelocyte" and "odontocyte" are employed only to indicate that these cells may possess different capabilities for interaction with other tissues after their overt differentiation. (Courtesy Dr. William E. Koch.)

The in vitro studies on tooth development have provided vital information concerning the interaction of dermal-epidermal components of tooth tissues upon differentiation of odontoblasts and ameloblasts. The importance of the basement membrane at this interface has been recognized. However, the criteria for the development of this complex organ system will have to wait till the precise role of stellate reticulum, stratum intermedium, and outer dental epithelium is defined. The following model (Fig. 2-15) has been suggested for the interactions that may occur between tissues during the development of a tooth.

In vitamin A deficiency the ameloblasts fail to differentiate properly. Consequently, their organizing influence upon the adjacent mesenchymal cells is disturbed, and atypical dentin, known as osteodentin, is formed.

*Morphodifferentiation.* The morphologic pattern or basic form and relative size of the future tooth is established by morphodifferentiation, i.e., by differential growth. Morphodifferentation therefore is impossible without proliferation. The advanced bell stage marks not only active histodifferentiation but also an important stage of morphodifferentiation of the crown by outlining the future dentinoenamel junction (Figs. 2-8 and 2-10).

The dentinoenamel and dentinocemental junctions, which are different and characteristic for each type of tooth, act as a blueprint pattern. In conformity with this pattern the ameloblasts, odontoblasts, and cementoblasts deposit enamel, dentin, and cementum and thus give the completed tooth its characteristic form and size. For example, the size and form of the cuspal portion of the crown of the first permanent molar are established at birth and occur prior to the formation of hard tissues.

The frequent statement in the literature that endocrine disturbances affect the size or form of the crown of teeth is not tenable unless such effects occur during morphodifferentiation, i.e., in utero or in the first year of life. Size and shape of the root, however, may be altered by disturbances in later periods. Clinical examinations show that the retarded eruption that occurs in persons with hypopituitarism and hypothyroidism results in a small clinical crown that is often mistaken for a small anatomic crown.

Disturbances in morphodifferentiation may affect the form and size of the tooth without impairing the function of the ameloblasts or odontoblasts. New parts may be differentiated (supernumerary cusps or roots), twinning may result, a suppression of parts may occur (loss of cusps or roots), or the result may be a peg or malformed tooth (e.g., Hutchinson's incisor) with enamel and dentin that may be normal in structure.

*Apposition.* Apposition is the deposition of the matrix of the hard dental structures. It will be described in separate chapters on enamel, dentin, and cementum. This chapter deals with certain aspects of apposition in order to complete the discussion of the physiologic processes concerned in the growth of teeth.

Appositional growth of enamel and dentin is a layerlike deposition of an extracellular matrix. This type of growth is therefore additive. It is the fulfillment of the plans outlined at the stages of histodifferentiation and morphodifferentiation. Appositional growth is characterized by regular and rhythmic deposition of the extracellular material, which is of itself incapable of further growth. Periods of activity and rest alternate at definite intervals.

The matrix is deposited by the cells along the site outlined by the formative cells at the end of morphodifferentiation, determining the future dentinoenamel and dentinocemental junctions, and according to a definite pattern of cellular activity that is common to all types and forms of teeth.

## REFERENCES

Avery, J. K.: Embryology of the teeth, J. Dent. Res. 30:490, 1951.

Avery, J. K.: Primary inductions of tooth formation, J. Dent. Res. 33:702, 1954. (Abstract.)

Bhaskar, S. N.: Synopsis of oral pathology, ed. 3, St. Louis, 1969, The C. V. Mosby Co.

Diamond, M., and Applebaum, E.: The epithelial sheath, J. Dent. Res. 21:403, 1942.

Fisher, A. R.: The differentiation of the molar tooth germ of the mouse in vivo and in vitro with special reference to cusp development, Ph.D. thesis, University of Bristol, 1957.

Fleming, H. S.: Homologous and heterologous intraocular growth of transplanted tooth germs, J. Dent. Res. 31:166, 1952.

Gaunt, W. A.: The vascular supply to the dental lamina during early development, Acta Anat. 37:232, 1959.

Glasstone, S.: Regulative changes in tooth germs grown in tissue culture, J. Dent. Res. 42: 1364, 1963.

Hoffman, R., and Gillette, R.: Mitotic patterns in pulpal and periodontal tissue in developing teeth, Fortieth General Meeting of the International Association of Dental Research, St. Louis, 1962.

Johnson, P. L., and Bevelander, G.: The role of the stratum intermedium in tooth development, Oral Surg. 10:437, 1957.

Koch, W. E.: Tissue interaction during in vitro odontogenesis. In Slavkin, H. S., and Bavetta, L. A., editors: Developmental aspects of oral biology, New York, 1972, Academic Press Inc.

Kollar, E. J.: Histogenetics of dermal-epidermal interactions. In Slavkin, H. S., and Bavetta, L. A., editors: Developmental aspects of oral biology, New York, 1972, Academic Press Inc.

Kraus, B. S.: Calcification of the human deciduous teeth, J. Am. Dent. Assoc. 59:1128, 1959.

Lefkowitz, W., and Swayne, P.: Normal development of tooth buds cultured in vitro, J. Dent. Res. 37:1100, 1958.

Marsland, E. A.: Histological investigation of amelogenesis in rats, Br. Dent. J. 91:251, 1951; 92:109, 1952.

Orban, B.: Growth and movement of the tooth germs and teeth, J. Am. Dent. Assoc. 15:1004, 1928.

Orban, B.: Dental histology and embryology, Philadelphia, 1929, P. Blakiston's Son & Co.

Orban, B., and Mueller, E.: The development of the bifurcation of multirooted teeth, J. Am. Dent. Assoc. 16:297, 1929.

Schour, I., and Massler, M.: Studies in tooth development: the growth pattern of human teeth, J. Am. Dent. Assoc. 27:1785, 1918, 1940.

Sicher, H.: Tooth eruption: axial movement of teeth with limited growth, J. Dent. Res. 21:395, 1942.

# 3 Enamel

## HISTOLOGY

### Physical characteristics

Enamel forms a protective covering of variable thickness over the entire surface of the crown. On the cusps of human molars and premolars the enamel attains a maximum thickness of about 2 to 2.5 mm., thinning down to almost a knife edge at the neck of the tooth. The shape and contour of the cusps receive their final modeling in the enamel.

Because of its high content of mineral salts and their crystalline arrangement, enamel is the hardest calcified tissue in the human body. The function of the enamel is to form a resistant covering of the teeth, rendering them suitable for mastication. The structure and hardness of the enamel render it brittle, which is particularly apparent when the enamel loses its foundation of sound dentin. The specific gravity of enamel is 2.8.

Another physical property of enamel is its permeability. It has been found with radioactive tracers that the enamel can act in a sense like a semipermeable membrane, permitting complete or partial passage of certain molecules: $^{14}$C-labeled urea, I, etc. The same phenomenon has also been demonstrated by means of dyestuffs.

The color of the enamel-covered crown ranges from yellowish white to grayish white. It has been suggested that the color is determined by differences in the translucency of enamel, yellowish teeth having a thin, translucent enamel through which the yellow color of the dentin is visible and grayish teeth having a more opaque enamel. The translucency may be attributable to variations in the degree of calcification and homogeneity of the enamel. Grayish teeth frequently show a slightly yellowish color at the cervical areas, presumably because the thinness of the enamel permits the light to strike the underlying yellow dentin and be reflected. Incisal areas may have a bluish tinge where the thin edge consists only of a double layer of enamel.

### Chemical properties

The enamel consists mainly of inorganic material (96%) and only a small amount of organic substance and water (4%). The inorganic material of the enamel is similar to apatite. The bar graph in Fig. 3-1 indicates the composition by volume of mineralized tissues in which odontoblast processes have been replaced with peritubular dentin (sclerotic dentin) and the equivalent situation in bone in which osteocyte lacunae are filled with mineral.

The origins shown at the left of Fig. 3-1 reflect the facts that enamel matrix mineralization begins immediately after it is secreted and that the lag in min-

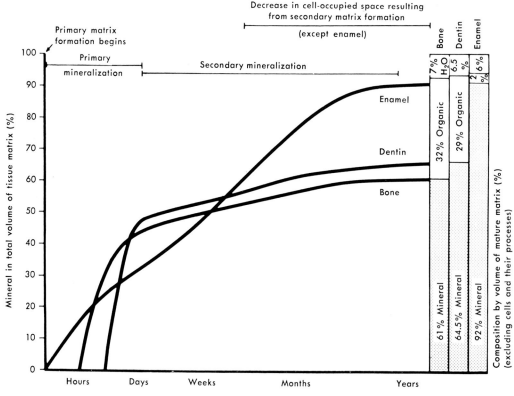

**Fig. 3-1.** Formation, mineralization, and maturation of some mineralized tissues. (Figures for bone from Robinson, R. A.: In Rodahl, K., Nicholson, J. T., and Brown, E. M., editors: Bone as a tissue, New York, 1960, The Blakiston Division, McGraw-Hill Book Co., Inc., pp. 186-250. Figures for dentin and enamel from Brudevold, F.: In Sognnaes, R. F., editor: Chemistry and prevention of dental caries, Springfield, Ill., 1962, Charles C Thomas, Publisher, pp. 32-88.)

eralization after matrix formation is greater in dentin than in bone. Enamel primary mineralization and secondary mineralization (maturation) increase mineral content in a relatively smooth curve. In both bone and dentin, well over one half of the mineral accumulates rapidly (primary mineralization). The curves then flatten as secondary mineralization occurs. The curves continue to rise slowly as cell-occupied space is filled with mineralized matrix (secondary matrix formation) in bone and dentin.

The relative *space occupied* by the organic framework and the entire enamel is almost equal. Fig. 3-2 illustrates this by comparing a stone and a sponge of approximately *equal size*. The stone represents the mineral content, and the sponge represents the organic framework of the enamel. Although their sizes are almost equal, their weights are vastly different. The stone is more than 100 times heavier than the sponge, or expressed in percentage, the weight of the sponge is less than 1% of that of the stone.

The nature of the organic elements of enamel is incompletely understood. In development and histologic staining reactions the enamel matrix resembles keratinizing epidermis. More specific methods have revealed sulfhydryl groups and other reactions suggestive of keratin. However, chemical analyses of the matrix of mature enamel indicate that the amino acid composition is not closely related to keratin and is distinctly different from collagen. Proteins can be isolated in several different fractions, and they generally contain high percentages of serine, glutamic acid, and glycine. Roentgen-ray diffraction studies reveal that the molecular structure is typical of the group of proteins called cross-$\beta$-proteins. In addition, histochemical reactions have suggested that the enamel-forming cells of developing teeth also contain a polysaccharide-protein complex and that an acid mucopolysaccharide enters the enamel itself at the time when calcification becomes a prominent feature. Tracer studies have indicated that the enamel of erupted teeth of rhesus monkeys can transmit and exchange radioactive isotopes originating from the saliva and the pulp. Considerable investigation is still required to determine the normal physiologic characteristics and the age changes that occur in the enamel.

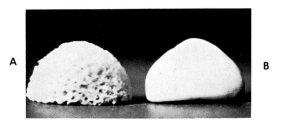

Fig. 3-2. A sponge, **A**, and a stone, **B**, are comparable to the organic and mineral elements of enamel. Their sizes are approximately equal, but their weights differ greatly. (From Bodecker, C. F.: Dent. Rev. **20**:317, 1906.)

### Structure

*Rods.* The enamel is composed of enamel rods or prisms, rod sheaths, and in some regions a cementing interprismatic substance. The number of enamel rods has been estimated as ranging from 5 million in the lower lateral incisors to 12 million in the upper first molars. From the dentinoenamel junction the rods run somewhat tortuous courses outward to the surface of the tooth. The length of most rods is greater than the thickness of the enamel because of the oblique direction and the wavy course of the rods. The rods located in the cusps, the thickest part of the enamel, are longer than those at the cervical areas of the teeth. It is stated generally that, as observed with the light microscope, the diameter of the rods averages 4 microns, but this measurement necessarily varies, since the outer surface of the enamel is greater than the dentinal surface where the rods originate. It is claimed that the diameter of the rods increases from the dentinoenamel junction toward the surface of the enamel at a ratio of about 1:2.

The enamel rods normally have a clear crystalline appearance, permitting

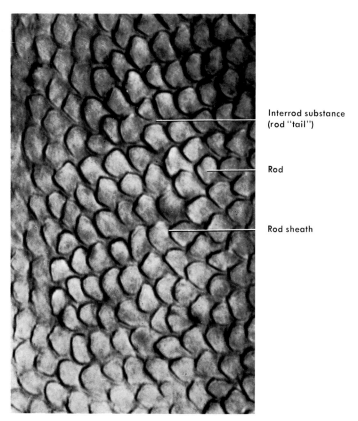

Interrod substance
(rod "tail")

Rod

Rod sheath

**Fig. 3-3.** Decalcified section of enamel of human tooth germ. Rods cut transversely have appearance of fish scales.

light to pass through them. In cross section under the light microscope they occasionally appear hexagonal. Sometimes they appear round or oval. In cross sections of human enamel, many rods resemble fish scales (Fig. 3-3).

*Submicroscopic structure.* Since many features of enamel rods are below the limit of resolution of the light microscope, many questions concerning their morphology can only be answered by electron microscopy. Although many areas of human enamel seem to contain rods surrounded by rod sheaths and separated by interrod substance (Fig. 3-4), a more common pattern is a keyhole- or paddle-shaped prism in human enamel (Fig. 3-5). When cut longitudinally (Fig. 3-6), sections pass through the "heads" or "bodies" of one row of rods and the "tails" of an adjacent row. This produces an appearance of rods separated by interrod substance. These rods measure about 5 microns in breadth and 9 microns in length. Rods of this shape can be packed tightly together (Fig. 3-7), and enamel with this structure explains many bizarre patterns seen with the electron micro-

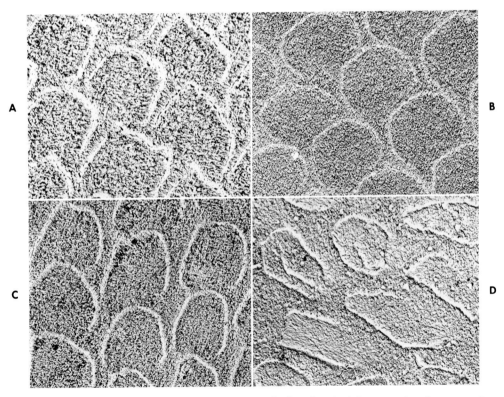

**Fig. 3-4.** Electron micrographs of replicas of polished and etched human subsurface enamel. Rods are cut in cross section. Various patterns are apparent. **A,** "Keyholes." **B,** "Staggered arches." **C,** "Stacked arches." **D,** Irregular rods near the dentinoenamel junction. (Approximately ×3000.) (From Swancar, V. R., Scott, D. B., and Njemirovskij, Z.: J. Dent. Res. **49:**1025, 1970. Copyright by the American Dental Association. Reprinted by permission.)

scope. The "bodies" of the rods are nearer occlusal and incisal surfaces, whereas the "tails" point cervically.

Studies with polarized light and roentgen-ray diffraction have indicated that the apatite crystals are arranged approximately parallel to the long axis of the prisms, although deviations of up to 40 degrees have been reported. Careful electron microscope studies have made it possible to describe more precisely the orientation of these crystals. They are approximately parallel to the long axes of the rods in their "bodies" or "heads" and deviate about 65 degrees from this axis as they fan out into the "tails" of the prisms (Fig. 3-8). Since it is extremely

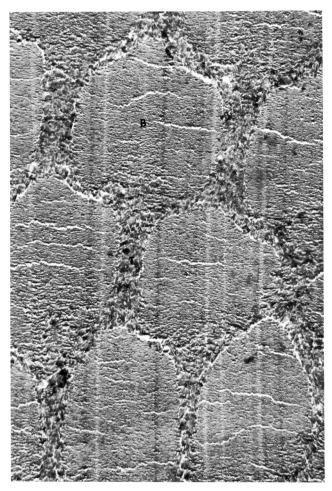

**Fig. 3-5.** Electron micrograph of cross sections of rods in mature human enamel. Rods are keyhole shaped, and crystal orientation is different in the "bodies," *B*, than in the "tails," *T*. (Approximately ×5000.) (From Meckel, A. H., Griebstein, W. J., and Neal, R. J.: Arch. Oral Biol. **10**:775, 1965.)

difficult to prepare a section that is exactly parallel to the long axes of the crystals, there is some question about their length, but they are estimated to vary between 0.05 and 1 micron. When cut in cross section, the crystals of human enamel are somewhat irregular in shape (Fig. 3-9) and have an average thickness of about 300 Å (angstrom units) and an average width of about 900 Å.

Early investigators using electron microscopy described a network of fine organic fibrils running throughout the rods and interrod substance. Recent improvements in preparative methods have disclosed that the organic matrix probably forms an envelope surrounding each apatite crystal (Fig. 3-10). In electron

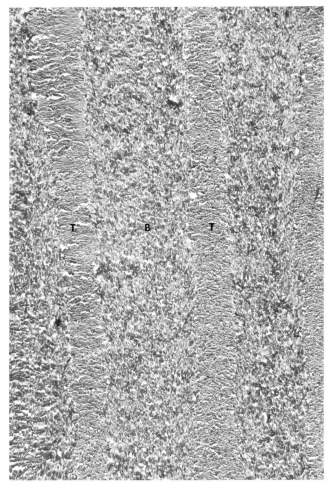

**Fig. 3-6.** Electron micrograph of longitudinal section through mature human enamel. Alternating "tails," *T*, and "bodies," *B*, of the rods are defined by abrupt changes in crystal direction where they meet. (Approximately ×5000.) (From Meckel, A. H., Griebstein, W. J., and Neal, R. J.: Arch. Oral Biol. **10**:775, 1965.)

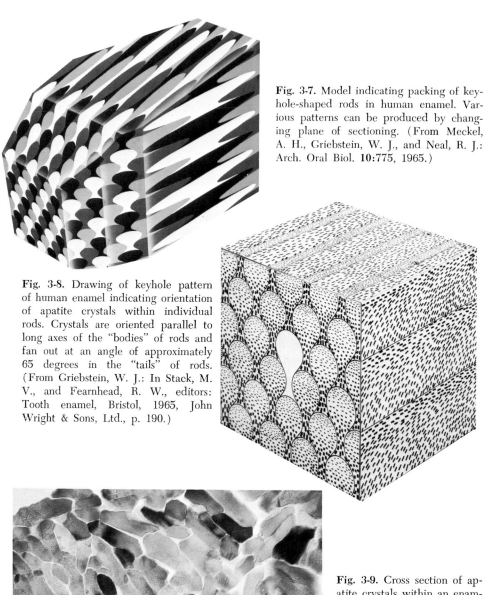

Fig. 3-7. Model indicating packing of key-hole-shaped rods in human enamel. Various patterns can be produced by changing plane of sectioning. (From Meckel, A. H., Griebstein, W. J., and Neal, R. J.: Arch. Oral Biol. **10**:775, 1965.)

Fig. 3-8. Drawing of keyhole pattern of human enamel indicating orientation of apatite crystals within individual rods. Crystals are oriented parallel to long axes of the "bodies" of rods and fan out at an angle of approximately 65 degrees in the "tails" of rods. (From Griebstein, W. J.: In Stack, M. V., and Fearnhead, R. W., editors: Tooth enamel, Bristol, 1965, John Wright & Sons, Ltd., p. 190.)

Fig. 3-9. Cross section of apatite crystals within an enamel rod in human enamel. Crystals are tightly packed and irregular in shape. (Approximately ×168,000.) (From Frazier, P. D.: J. Ultrastruct. Res. **22**:1, 1968.)

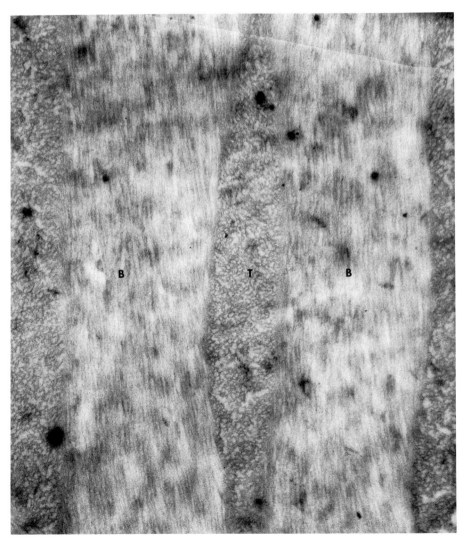

**Fig. 3-10.** Electron micrograph of decalcified section of immature bovine enamel. Although shape of rods in bovine enamel is not clearly established, this electron micrograph reproduces the pattern one would expect in longitudinal sections through human enamel. Organic sheaths around individual apatite crystals are oriented parallel to long axes of rods in their "bodies," *B*, and more nearly perpendicular to long axes in their "tails," *T*. (Approximately ×38,000.) (From Travis, D. F., and Glimcher, M. J.: J. Cell Biol. **23**:447, 1964.)

micrographs the surfaces of rods are visible because of abrupt changes in crystal orientation from one rod to another. For this reason the crystals are not as tightly packed and there may be more space for organic matrix at these surfaces. This accounts for the rod sheath visible in the light microscope (Fig. 3-3).

*Striations.* Each enamel rod is built up of segments separated by dark lines that give it a striated appearance (Fig. 3-11). These transverse striations demarcate rod segments and become more visible by the action of mild acids. The striations are more pronounced in enamel that is insufficiently calcified. The rods are segmented because the enamel matrix is formed in a rhythmic manner. In man these segments seem to be a uniform length of about 4 microns.

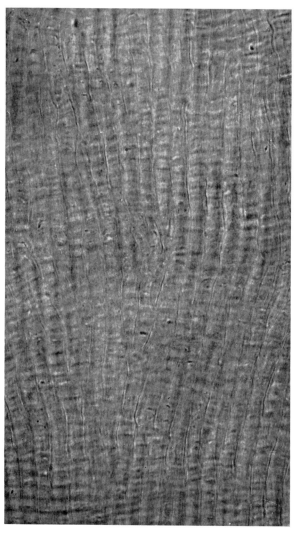

**Fig. 3-11.** Ground section through enamel. Rods cut longitudinally. Cross striation of rods.

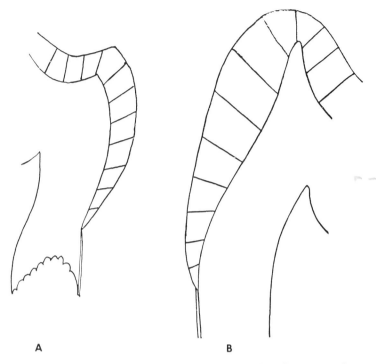

**Fig. 3-12.** Diagrams indicating general direction of enamel rods. **A,** Deciduous tooth. **B,** Permanent tooth.

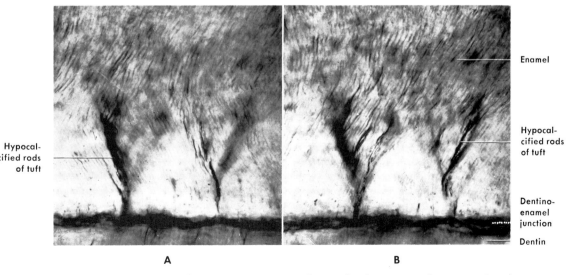

**Fig. 3-13.** Horizontal ground section through enamel near the dentinoenamel junction. **A** and **B** show change in direction of rods in two adjacent layers of enamel, which is made visible by a change in focus of microscope.

*Direction of rods.* Generally the rods are oriented at right angles to the dentin surface. In the cervical and central parts of the crown of a deciduous tooth they are approximately horizontal (Fig. 3-12, *A*). Near the incisal edge or tip of the cusps they change gradually to an increasingly oblique direction until they are almost vertical in the region of the edge or tip of the cusps. The arrangement of the rods in permanent teeth is similar in the occlusal two thirds of the crown. In the cervical region, however, the rods deviate from the horizontal in an apical direction (Fig. 3-12, *B*).

The rods are rarely, if ever, straight throughout. They follow a wavy course from the dentin to the enamel surface. The most significant deviations from a straight radial course can be described as follows. If the middle part of the crown is divided into thin horizontal discs, the rods in the adjacent discs bend in opposite directions. For instance, in one disc the rods start from the dentin in an oblique direction and bend more or less sharply to the left side (Fig. 3-13, *A*), whereas in the adjacent disc the rods bend toward the right (Fig. 3-13, *B*). This alternating clockwise and counterclockwise deviation of the rods from the radial direction can be observed at all levels of the crown if the discs are cut in the planes of the general rod direction.

If the discs are cut in an oblique plane, especially near the dentin in the region of the cusps or incisal edges, the rod arrangement appears to be further complicated—the bundles of rods seem to intertwine more irregularly. This optical appearance of enamel is called *gnarled enamel.*

The enamel rods forming the developmental fissures and pits, as on the occlusal surface of molar and premolars, converge in their outward course.

*Hunter-Schreger bands.* The more or less regular change in the direction of rods may be regarded as a functional adaptation, minimizing the risk of cleavage in the axial direction under the influence of occlusal masticatory forces. The change in the direction of rods is responsible for the appearance of the Hunter-Schreger bands. These are alternating dark and light strips of varying widths (Fig. 3-14, *A*) that can best be seen in a longitudinal ground section under oblique reflected light. They originate at the dentinoenamel border and pass outward, ending at some distance from the outer enamel surface. Some investigators claim that there are variations in calcification of the enamel that coincide with the distribution of the bands of Hunter-Schreger. Careful decalcification and staining of the enamel have provided further evidence that these structures may not be the result solely of an optical phenomenon but that they are composed of alternate zones having a slightly different permeabiilty and a different content of organic material (Fig. 3-14, *B*).

*Incremental lines of Retzius.* The incremental lines of Retzius appear as brownish bands in ground sections of the enamel. They illustrate the incremental pattern of the enamel, i.e., the successive apposition of layers of enamel during formation of the crown. In longitudinal sections they surround the tip

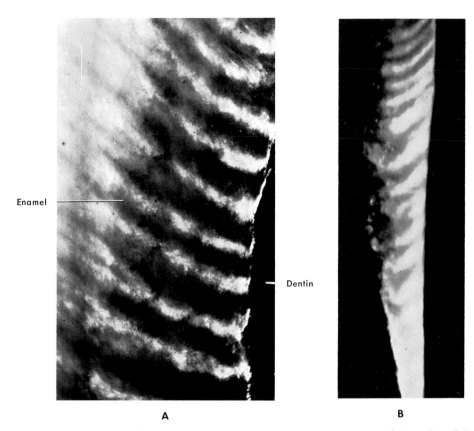

Enamel

Dentin

A                                    B

**Fig. 3-14. A,** Longitudinal ground section through enamel photographed by reflected light. Hunter-Schreger bands. **B,** Decalcified enamel, photographed by reflected light, showing Hunter-Schreger bands.

of the dentin (Fig. 3-15, *A*). In the cervical parts of the crown they run obliquely. From the dentinoenamel junction to the surface they deviate occlusally (Fig. 3-15, *B*). In transverse sections of a tooth the incremental lines of Retzius appear as concentric circles (Fig. 3-16). They may be compared to the growth rings in the cross section of a tree. The term "incremental lines" designates these structures appropriately, for they do, in fact, reflect variations in structure and mineralization, either hypomineralized or hypermineralized, that occur during growth of the enamel. The exact nature of these developmental changes is not known. The incremental lines have been attributed to periodic bending of the enamel rods, to variations in the basic organic structure (Fig. 3-17), or to a physiologic calcification rhythm.

The incremental lines of Retzius, if present in moderate intensity, are considered normal. However, the rhythmic alternation of periods of enamel matrix formation and of rest can be upset by metabolic disturbances, causing the rest periods to be unduly prolonged and close together. Such an abnormal condition

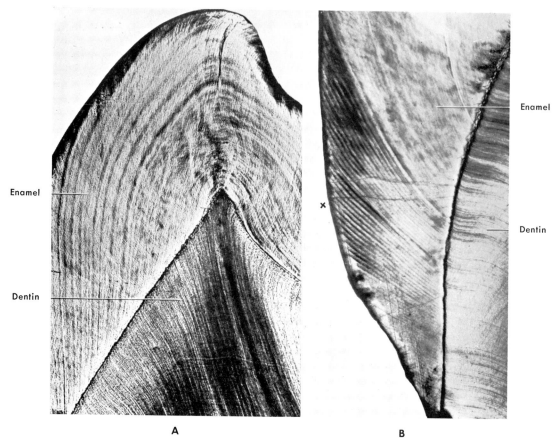

Enamel

Dentin

Enamel

Dentin

X

A

B

**Fig. 3-15.** Incremental lines of Retzius in Longitudinal ground sections. **A,** Cuspal region. **B,** Cervical region, X.

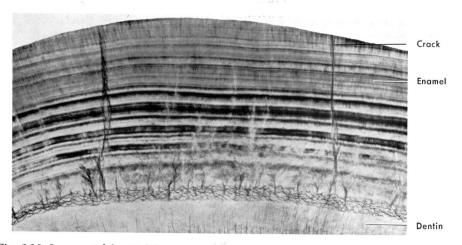

Crack

Enamel

Dentin

**Fig. 3-16.** Incremental lines of Retzius in transverse ground section, arranged concentrically.

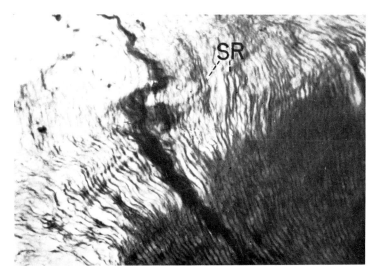

**Fig. 3-17.** Carefully decalcified section through enamel. Thickening of sheath substance, *SR*, in Retzius lines. (From Bodecker, C. F.: Dent. Rev. **20**:317, 1906.)

is responsible for the broadening of the incremental lines of Retzius, rendering them more prominent.

*Surface structures.* A relatively structureless layer of enamel, approximately 30 microns thick, has been described in 70% of permanent teeth and all deciduous teeth. This structureless enamel is found least often over the cusps tips and most commonly toward the cervical areas of the enamel surface. In this surface layer no prism outlines are visible, and all of the apatite crystals are parallel to one another and perpendicular to the striae of Retzius. It is also somewhat more heavily mineralized than the bulk of enamel beneath it (Fig. 3-18). Other microscopic details that have been observed on outer enamel surfaces of newly erupted teeth are perikymata, rod ends, and cracks (lamellae).

Perikymata are transverse, wavelike grooves, believed to be the external manifestations of the striae of Retzius. They are continuous around a tooth and usually lie parallel to each other and to the cementoenamel junction (Figs. 3-19 and 3-20). Ordinarily there are about thirty perikymata per millimeter in the region of the cementoenamel junction, and their concentration gradually decreases to about ten per millimeter near the occlusal or incisal edge of a surface. Their course usually is fairly regular, but in the cervical region it may be quite irregular.

The enamel rod ends are concave and vary in depth and shape. They are shallowest in the cervical regions of surfaces and deepest near the incisal or occlusal edges (Fig. 3-19, *B*).

The term "cracks" originally was used to describe the narrow, fissurelike structures that are seen on almost all surfaces (Fig. 3-20, *D*). It has since been demonstrated that they are actually the outer edges of lamellae (see discussion

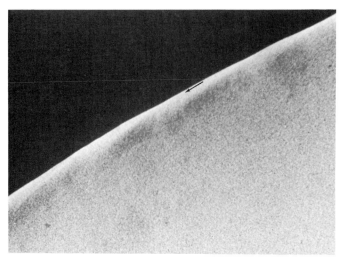

Fig. 3-18. Microradiograph of a ground section of sound human enamel. The relatively structureless surface layer *(arrow)* is more radiopaque than the bulk of the enamel below it. (Approximately ×200.) (Courtesy Dr. A. J. Gwinnett, Stony Brook, N.Y.)

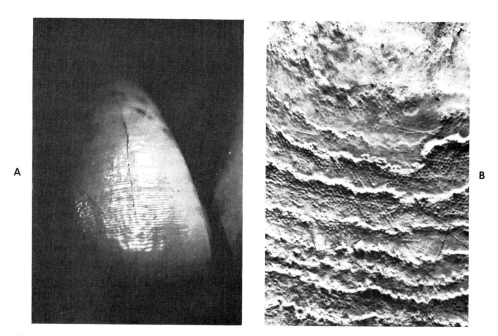

Fig. 3-19. **A,** Perikymata on lateral incisor. **B,** Shadowed replica of the surface of intact enamel (buccal surface of an upper left second molar showing the perikymata). (×1500.) (**B** from Scott, D. B., and Wyckoff, R. W. G.: Public Health Rep. **61:**1397, 1946.)

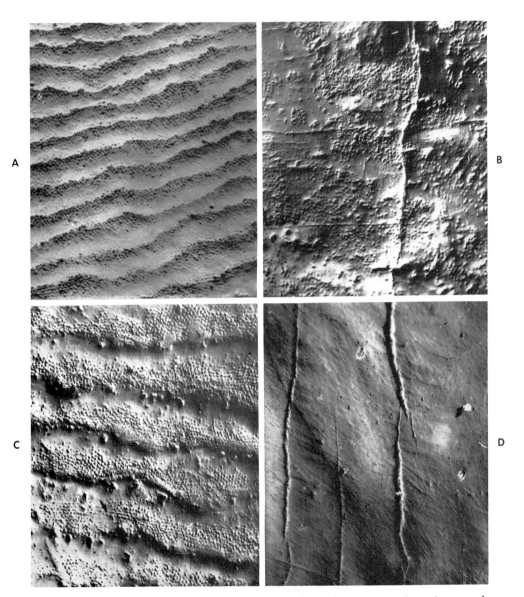

**Fig. 3-20.** Progressive loss of surface structure with advancing age. **A,** Surface of a recently erupted tooth showing pronounced enamel prism ends and perikymata. Patient 12 years of age. **B,** Early stage of structural loss that occurs during the first few years (wear is more rapid on anterior teeth than on posterior teeth and more rapid on facial or lingual surfaces than on proximal surfaces). Note small regions where prism ends are worn away. Patient 25 years of age. **C,** Later stage. Here the elevated parts between perikymata are worn smooth, while the structural detail in the depths of the grooves is still more or less intact. Eventually wearing proceeds to the point where all prism ends and perikymata disappear. Patient 52 years of age. (Since these are negative replicas, surface details appear inverted. Raised structures represent depressions in the actual surface.) **D,** Surface worn completely smooth and showing only "cracks," which actually represent the outer edges of lamellae. Patient 50 years of age. (All magnifications ×105.) (From Scott, D. B., and Wyckoff, R. W. G.: J. Am. Dent. Assoc. **39**:275, 1949.)

of enamel lamellae). They extend for varying distances along the surface, at right angles to the cementoenamel junction, from which they originate. Most of them are less than a millimeter in length, but some are longer, and a few reach the occlusal or incisal edge of a surface. They are fairly evenly spaced, but long lamellae appear thicker than short ones.

The enamel of the deciduous teeth develops partly before and partly after birth. The boundary between the two portions of enamel in the deciduous teeth is marked by an accentuated incremental line of Retzius, the *neonatal line* or *neonatal ring* (Fig. 3-21). It appears to be the result of the abrupt change in the

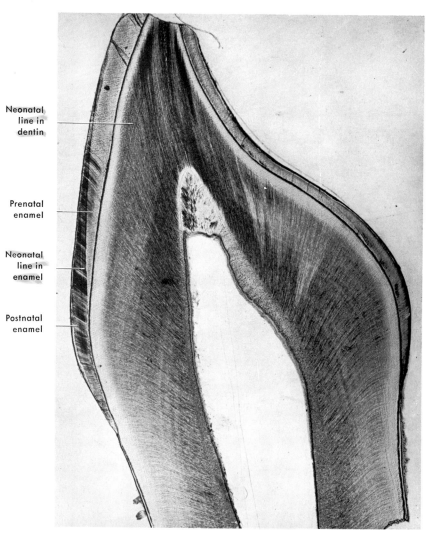

Neonatal
line in
dentin

Prenatal
enamel

Neonatal
line in
enamel

Postnatal
enamel

Fig. 3-21. Neonatal line in enamel. Longitudinal ground section of a deciduous canine. (From Schour, I.: J. Am. Dent. Assoc. **23:**1946, 1936.)

environment and nutrition of the newborn infant. The prenatal enamel usually is better developed than the postnatal enamel. This is explained by the fact that the fetus develops in a well-protected environment with an adequate supply of all the essential materials, even at the expense of the mother. Because of the undisturbed and even development of the enamel prior to birth, perikymata are absent in the occlusal parts of the deciduous teeth, whereas they are present in the postnatal cervical parts.

*Enamel cuticle.* A delicate membrane called *Nasmyth's membrane*, after its first investigator, or the *primary enamel cuticle* covers the entire crown of the newly erupted tooth but is probably soon removed by mastication. Electron microscope studies have indicated that this membrane is a typical basement membrane found beneath most epithelia (Fig. 3-22). It is probably visible with the light microscope because of it wavy course. This basement membrane is apparently secreted by the ameloblasts when enamel formation is completed. It is also been reported that the cervical area of the enamel is covered by afibrillar cementum, continuous with the cementum and probably of mesodermal origin (Fig. 3-23). This cuticle is apparently secreted after the epithelial enamel organ retracts from the cervical region during tooth development.

Finally, erupted enamel is normally covered by a *pellicle*, which is apparently a precipitate of salivary proteins (Fig. 3-24). This pellicle re-forms within hours after an enamel surface is mechanically cleaned. Within a day or two after the

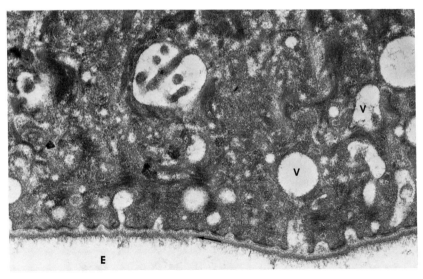

**Fig. 3-22.** Electron micrograph of reduced enamel epithelium covering surface of unerupted human tooth. Enamel has been removed by demineralization, *E.* Typical basement membrane separates enamel space from epithelium *(arrow).* Epithelial cells contain a number of intracytoplasmic vacuoles, *V.* (Approximately ×24,000.) (From Listgarten, M. A.: Arch. Oral Biol. **11:**999, 1966.)

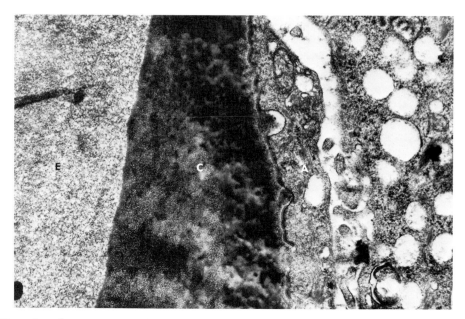

**Fig. 3-23.** Electron micrograph of gingival area of erupted human tooth. Remnants of enamel matrix appear at left, *E.* Cuticle, *C,* separates enamel matrix from epithelial cells of attached epithelial cuff, *A.* Inner layers of cuticle (afibrillar cementum) are deposited before eruption; the origin of the outer layers is not known. (Approximately ×37,000.) (From Listgarten, M. A.: Am. J. Anat. **119:**147, 1966.)

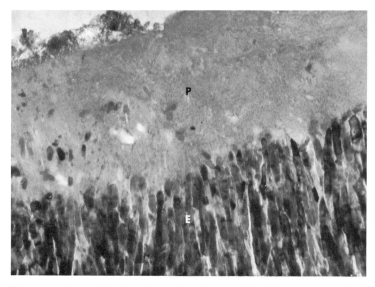

**Fig. 3-24.** Electron micrograph of surface of undemineralized human enamel. The enamel surface, *E,* is covered by a pellicle, *P.* Individual crystals can be seen in the enamel. (Approximately ×58,000.) (From Houver, G., and Frank, R. M.: Arch. Oral Biol. **12:**1209, 1967.)

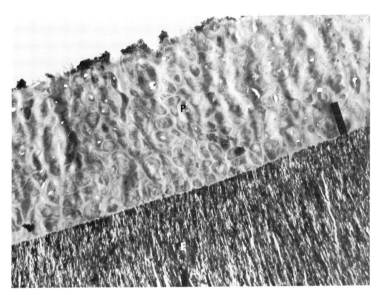

**Fig. 3-25.** Electron micrograph of undemineralized human enamel surface. Enamel, *E*, is covered by a bacterial plaque, *P*. *Black bar at right,* Thickness of pellicle seen in Fig. 3-24. (Approximately ×12,000.) (From Frank, R. M., and Brendel, A.: Arch. Oral Biol. **11**:883, 1966.)

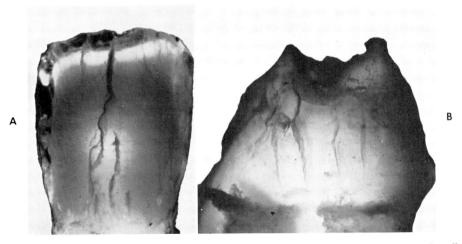

**Fig. 3-26. A,** Decalcified incisor with moderately severe mottled enamel. Numerous lamellae can be observed. (×8.) **B,** Maxillary first permanent molar of caries-free 2-year-old rhesus monkey. Numerous bands of organic matter, lamellae, can be seen after decalcification. (×8.) (**B** from Sognnaes, R. F.: J. Dent. Res. **29**:260, 1950.)

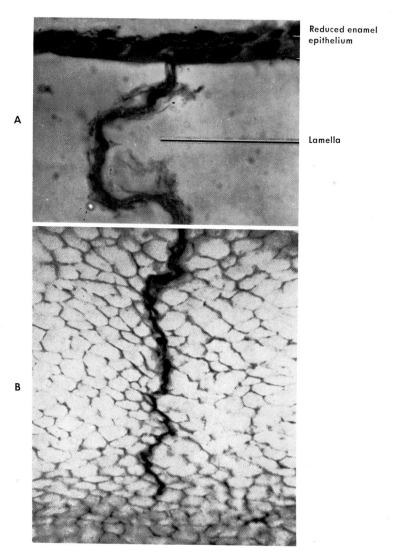

Reduced enamel
epithelium

Lamella

**Fig. 3-27. A,** Paraffin section through reduced enamel epithelium, enamel cuticle, and a lamella, isolated together by acid flotation from the surface of an unerupted human tooth. Note
intimate relationship between three elements. (Hematoxylin and eosin; ×1300.) **B,** Paraffin
section of decalcified enamel of human molar showing relation between a lamella and surrounding organic sheath substance. (Hematoxylin and eosin; ×1000.) (**A** from Ussing, M. J.:
Acta Odontol. Scand. **13:**23, 1955; reprinted in J. West. Soc. Periodont. **3:**71, 1955; **B** courtesy
Dr. R. F. Sognnaes, Los Angeles, Calif.)

pellicle has formed, it becomes colonized by microorganisms to form a bacterial plaque (Fig. 3-25).

***Enamel lamellae.*** Enamel lamellae are thin, leafllike structures that extend from the enamel surface toward the dentinoenamel junction (Fig. 3-26). They may extend to, and sometimes penetrate into, the dentin. They consist of organic material, with but little mineral content. In ground sections these structures may be confused with cracks caused by grinding of the specimen (Fig. 3-16). Careful decalcification of ground sections of enamel makes possible the distinction between cracks and enamel lamellae. The former disappear, whereas the later persist (Figs. 3-26, A, and 3-27).

Lamellae may develop in planes of tension. Where rods cross such a plane, a short segment of the rod may not fully calcify. If the disturbance is more severe, a crack may develop that is filled either by surrounding cells, if the crack occurred in the unerupted tooth, or by organic substances from the oral cavity, if the crack developed after eruption. Three types of lamellae can thus be differentiated: type A, lamellae composed of poorly calcified rod segments (Fig. 3-27, B); type B, lamellae consisting of degenerated cells; and type C, lamellae arising in erupted teeth where the cracks are filled with organic matter, presumably originating from saliva. The last type may be more common than formerly believed. Although lamellae of type A are restricted to the enamel, those of types B and C may reach into the dentin (Fig. 3-28). If cells from the enamel organ fill a crack in the enamel, those in the depth degenerate, whereas those close to the surface may remain vital for a time and produce a hornified cuticle in the cleft. In such cases the inner parts of the lamella consist of an organic cell detritus, the outer parts of a double layer of the cuticle. If connective tissue invades a crack in the enamel, cementum may be formed. In such cases lamellae consist entirely or partly of cementum.

Lamellae extend in the longitudinal and radial direction of the tooth, from the tip of the crown toward the cervical region (Fig. 3-26). This arrangement explains why they can be observed better in horizontal sections. It has been suggested that enamel lamellae may be a site of weakness in a tooth and may form a road of entry for bacteria that initiate caries.

***Enamel tufts.*** Enamel tufts (Fig. 3-29) arise at the dentinoenamel junction and reach into the enamel to about one fifth to one third of its thickness. They were so termed because they resemble tufts of grass when viewed in ground sections. This picture is erroneous. An enamel tuft does not spring from a single small area but is a narrow, ribbonlike structure, the inner end of which arises at the dentin. The impression of a tuft of grass is created by examining such structures in thick sections under low magnification. Under these circumstances the imperfections, lying in different planes and curving in different directions (Fig. 3-13), are projected into one plane (Fig. 3-29).

Tufts consist of hypocalcified enamel rods and interprismatic substance. Like the lamellae, they extend in the direction of the long axis of the crown. There-

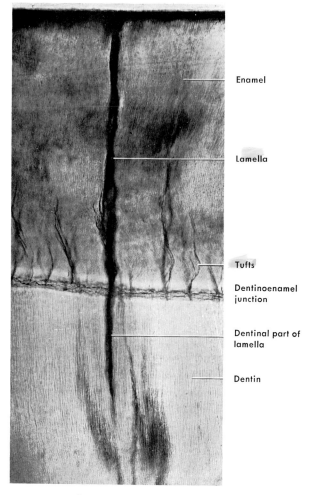

Enamel

Lamella

Tufts

Dentinoenamel junction

Dentinal part of lamella

Dentin

**Fig. 3-28.** Transverse ground section through lamella reaching from surface into dentin.

fore they are abundantly seen in horizontal, and rarely in longitudinal, sections. Their presence and their development are a consequence of, or an adaptation to, the spatial conditions in the enamel.

**Dentinoenamel junction.** The surface of the dentin at the dentinoenamel junctions is pitted. Into the shallow depressions of the dentin fit rounded projections of the enamel. This relation assures the firm hold of the enamel cap on the dentin. In sections, therefore, the dentinoenamel junction appears not as a straight but as a scalloped line (Figs. 3-29 and 3-30). The convexities of the scallops are directed toward the dentin. The pitted dentinoenamel junction is preformed even before the development of hard tissues and is evident in the

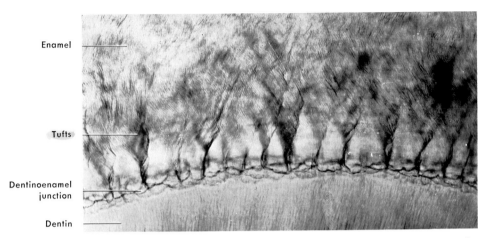

Enamel

Tufts

Dentinoenamel
junction

Dentin

**Fig. 3-29.** Transverse ground section through a tooth under low magnification. Numerous tufts extend from dentinoenamel junction into enamel.

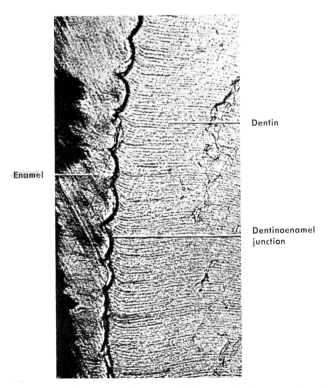

Dentin

Enamel

Dentinoenamel
junction

**Fig. 3-30.** Longitudinal ground section. Scalloped dentinoenamel junction.

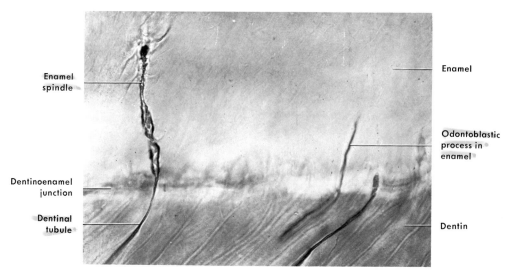

Fig. 3-31. Ground section. Odontoblastic processes extend into enamel as enamel spindles.

arrangement of the ameloblasts and the basement membrane of the dental papilla (Fig. 3-41).

In microradiographs of ground sections a hypermineralized zone about 30 microns thick can sometimes be demonstrated at the dentinoenamel junction. It is most prominent before mineralization is complete.

*Odontoblast processes and enamel spindles.* Occasionally odontoblast processes pass across the dentinoenamel junction into the enamel. Since many are thickened at their end (Fig. 3-31), they have been termed *enamel spindles.* They seem to originate from processes of odontoblasts that extended into the enamel epithelium before hard substances were formed. The direction of the odontoblastic processes and spindles in the enamel corresponds to the original direction of the ameloblasts—at right angles to the surface of the dentin. Since the enamel rods are formed at an angle to the axis of the ameloblasts, the direction of spindles and rods is divergent. In ground sections of dried teeth the organic content of the spindles disintegrates and is replaced by air, and the spaces appear dark in transmitted light.

### Age changes

The most apparent age change in enamel is attrition or wear of the occlusal surfaces and proximal contact points as a result of mastication. This is evidenced by a loss of vertical dimension of the crown and by a flattening of the proximal contour. In addition to these gross changes, the outer enamel surfaces themselves undergo posteruptive alterations in structure at the microscopic level. These result from environmental influences and occur with a regularity that can be related to age (Fig. 3-20).

The surfaces of unerupted and recently erupted teeth are covered completely with pronounced rod ends and perikymata. At the points of highest contour of the surfaces these structures soon begin to disappear. This is followed by a generalized loss of the rod ends and a much slower flattening of the perikymata. Finally, the perikymata disappear completely. The rate at which structure is lost depends on the location of the surface on the tooth and on the location of the tooth in the mouth. Facial and lingual surfaces lose their structure much more rapidly than do proximal surfaces, and anterior teeth lose their structure more rapidly than do posterior teeth.

Age changes within the enamel proper have been difficult to discern microscopically. The fact that alterations do occur has been demonstrated by chemical analysis, but the changes are not well understood. For example, the total amount of organic matrix is said by some to increase, by others to remain unchanged, and by still others to decrease. Localized increases of certain elements such as nitrogen and fluorine, however, have been found in the superficial enamel layers of older teeth. This suggests a continuous uptake, probably from the oral environment, during aging. As a result of age changes in the organic portion of enamel, presumably near the surface, the teeth may become darker, and their resistance to decay may be increased. Suggestive of an aging change is the greatly reduced permeability of older teeth to fluids. There is insufficient evidence to show that enamel becomes harder with age.

### Clinical considerations

The course of the enamel rods is of importance in cavity preparations. The choice of instruments depends upon the location of the cavity in the tooth. Generally the rods run at a right angle to the underlying dentin or tooth surface. Close to the cementoenamel junction the rods run in a more horizontal direction (Fig. 3-12, *B*). In preparing cavities, it is important that unsupported enamel rods are not left at the cavity margins because they would soon break and produce leakage. Bacteria would lodge in these spaces, inducing secondary dental caries. Enamel is brittle and does not withstand forces in thin layers or in areas where it is not supported by the underlying dentin (Fig. 3-32, *A*).

Deep enamel fissures predispose to caries. Although these deep clefts between adjoining cusps cannot be regarded as pathologic, they afford areas for retention of caries-producing agents. Caries penetrate the floor of fissures rapidly because the enamel in these areas is very thin (Fig. 3-32, *B*). As the destructive process reaches the dentin, it spreads along the dentinoenamel junction, undermining the enamel. An extensive area of dentin becomes carious without giving any warning to the patient because the entrance to the cavity is minute. Careful examination is necessary to discover such cavities because most enamel fissures are more minute than a single toothbrush bristle and cannot be detected with the dental probe.

Dental lamellae may also be predisposing locations for caries because they

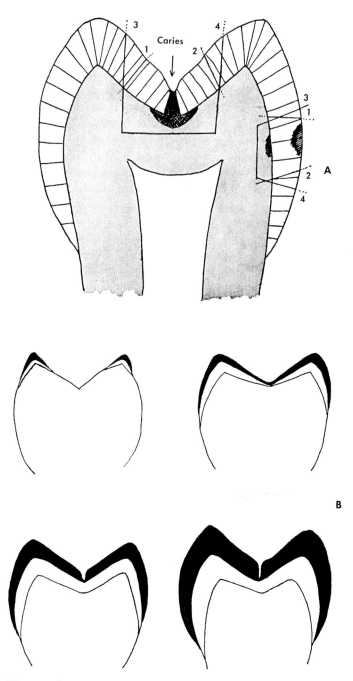

Fig. 3-32. **A,** Diagram of course of enamel rods in a molar in relation to cavity preparation. *1* and *2* indicate wrong preparation of cavity margins. *3* and *4* indicate correct preparation. **B,** Diagram of development of deep enamel fissure. Note thin enamel layer forming floor of fissure. (**B** from Kronfeld, R.: J. Am. Dent. Assoc. **22:**1131, 1935.)

contain much organic material. Primarily from the standpoint of protection against caries, the structure and reactions of the outer enamel surface are subject to much current research. In vitro tests have shown that the acid solubility of enamel can be greatly reduced by treatment with fluoride compounds. Clinical trials based on these studies have demonstrated reductions of 40% or more in the incidence of caries in children after topical applications of sodium or stannous fluoride. Incorporation of fluorides in dentifrices is now a well-accepted means of caries prevention. Fluorides containing mixtures such as stannous fluoride pastes, sodium fluoride rinses, and acidulated phosphate fluoride are also used by the dentist to alter the outer surface of the enamel in such a manner that it becomes more resistant to decay.

The most effective means for mass control of dental caries to date has been adjustment of the fluoride level in communal water supplies to 1 part per million. Epidemiologic studies in areas in which the drinking water contained natural fluoride revealed that the caries prevalence in both children and adults was about 65% lower than in nonfluoride areas, and long-term studies have demonstrated that the same order of protection is afforded through water fluoridation programs. The mechanisms of action are believed to be primarily a combination of changes in enamel resistance, brought about by incorporation of fluoride during calcification, and alterations in the environment of the teeth, particularly with respect to the oral bacterial flora.

The surface of the enamel in the cervical region should be kept smooth and well polished by proper home care and by regular cleansing by the dentist. If the surface of the cervical enamel becomes decalcified or otherwise roughened, food debris, bacterial plaques, etc. accumulate on this surface. The gingiva in contact with this roughened, debris-covered enamel surface undergoes inflammatory changes. The ensuing gingivitis, unless promptly treated, may lead to more serious periodontal disease.

One of the more recently developed techniques in operative dentistry consists of the use of composite resins. These materials can be mechanically "bonded" directly to the enamel surface. In this procedure the enamel surface is first etched with an acid (phosphoric acid 50%). This produces an uneven dissolution of the enamel rods and their "sheaths" or enamel "heads" and their "tails" so that a relatively smooth enamel surface becomes pitted and irregular. When a composite resin is put on this irregular surface, it can achieve mechanical bonding with the enamel. The same principle is used in coating the susceptible areas of the enamel with the so called pit and fissure sealants.

## DEVELOPMENT
### Epithelial enamel organ

The early development of the enamel organ and its differentiation have been discussed in Chapter 2. At the stage preceding the formation of hard structures (dentin and enamel) the enamel organ, originating from the stratified epithelium

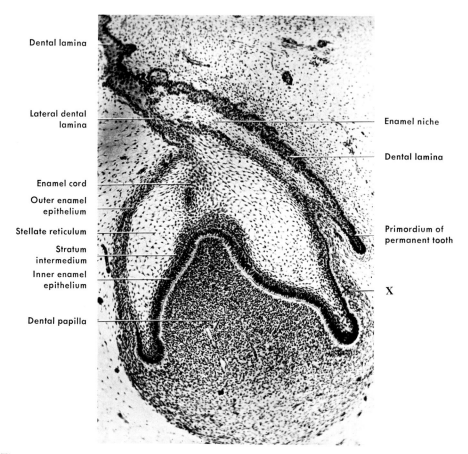

Dental lamina

Lateral dental lamina

Enamel cord

Outer enamel epithelium

Stellate reticulum

Stratum intermedium

Inner enamel epithelium

Dental papilla

Enamel niche

Dental lamina

Primordium of permanent tooth

X

**Fig. 3-33.** Tooth germ (deciduous lower incisor) of human embryo 105 mm., fourth month. Four layers of enamel organ. Area at X is shown at a higher magnification in Fig. 3-35.

of the primitive oral cavity, consists of four distinct layers: outer enamel epithelium, stellate reticulum, stratum intermedium, and inner enamel epithelium (ameloblastic layer) (Fig. 3-33). The borderline between the inner enamel epithelium and the connective tissue of the dental papilla is the subsequent dentinoenamel junction. Thus its outline determines the pattern of the occlusal or incisal part of the crown. At the border of the wide basal opening of the enamel organ, the inner enamel epithelium reflects onto the outer enamel epithelium. This is the *cervical loop*. The inner and outer enamel epithelia are elsewhere separated from each other by a large mass of cells differentiated into two distinct layers. The layer that is close to the inner enamel epithelium consists of two or three rows of flat polyhedral cells—the stratum intermedium. The other layer, which is more loosely arranged, constitutes the stellate reticulum.

The different layers of epithelial cells of the enamel organ are named according to their morphology, function, or location. The stellate reticulum derives its

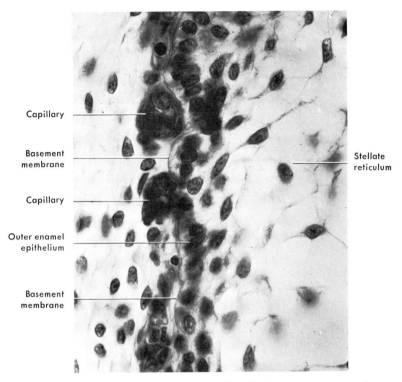

Capillary

Basement membrane

Capillary

Outer enamel epithelium

Basement membrane

Stellate reticulum

Fig. 3-34. Capillaries in contact with outer enamel epithelium. Basement membrane separates outer enamel epithelium from connective tissue.

name from the morphology of its cells. The outer enamel epithelium and the stratum intermedium are so named because of their location. The inner enamel epithelium is so named on the basis of its position. On the basis of function it is called the ameloblastic layer.

*Outer enamel epithelium.* In the early stages of development of the enamel organ the outer enamel epithelium consists of a single layer of cuboid cells, separated from the surrounding connective tissue of the dental sac by a delicate basement membrane (Fig. 3-34). Prior to the formation of hard structures, this regular arrangement of the outer enamel epithelium is maintained only in the cervical parts of the enamel organ. At the highest convexity of the organ (Fig. 3-33) the cells of the outer enamel epithelium become irregular in shape and cannot be distinguished easily from the outer portion of the stellate reticulum. The capillaries in the connective tissue surrounding the epithelial enamel organ proliferate and protrude toward it (Fig. 3-34). Immediately before enamel formation commences, capillaries may even indent the stellate reticulum. This increased vascularity ensures a rich metabolism when a plentiful supply of substances from the bloodstream to the inner enamel epithelium is required (Fig. 3-36).

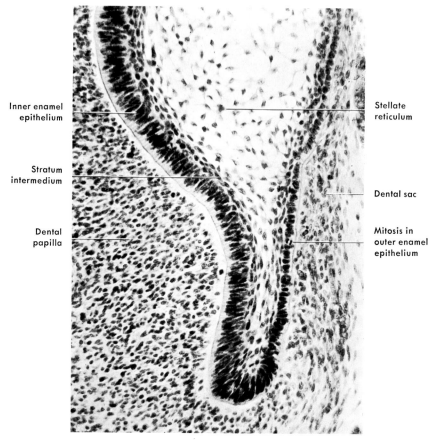

Fig. 3-35. Region of cervical loop (higher magnification of area x in Fig. 3-33). Transition of outer into inner enamel epithelium.

During enamel formation, cells of the outer enamel epithelium develop villi and cytoplasmic vesicles and large numbers of mitochondria, all indicating cell specialization for the active transport of materials. The capillaries in contact with the outer enamel epithelium also show areas with very thin walls, a structural modification also commonly found in areas of active transport.

*Stellate reticulum.* In the stellate reticulum, which forms the middle part of the enamel organ, the neighboring cells are separated by wide intercellular spaces filled by a large amount of intercellular substance. The cells are star shaped, with long processes reaching in all directions from a central body (Figs. 3-34 and 3-35). They are connected with each other and with the cells of the outer enamel epithelium and the stratum intermedium by desmosomes.

The structure of the stellate reticulum renders it resistant and elastic. Therefore it seems probable that it acts as a buffer against physical forces that might distort the conformation of the developing dentinoenamel junction, giving rise

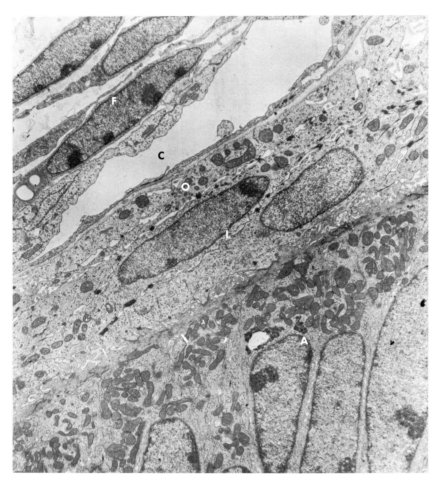

**Fig. 3-36.** Electron micrograph of epithelial enamel organ over area of rodent incisor in which enamel secretion is underway. From above downward are the fibroblasts of the dental sac, *F;* a capillary, *C;* cells of the outer enamel epithelium, *O;* cells of the stratum intermedium, *I;* and the proximal ends of the ameloblasts, *A.* (Approximately ×7000.) (Courtesy Dr. P. R. Garant, Stony Brook, N.Y.)

to gross morphologic changes. It seems to permit only a limited flow of nutritional elements from the outlying blood vessels to the formative cells. Indicative of this is the fact the stellate reticulum is noticeably reduced in thickness when the first layers of dentin are laid down, and the inner enamel epithelium is thereby cut off from the dental papilla, its original source of supply (Fig. 3-37). During involution of the stellate reticulum the cells apparently undergo a process that resembles the keratinization of surface epithelial cells.

**Stratum intermedium.** The cells of the stratum intermedium are situated between the stellate reticulum and the inner enamel epithelium. They are flat to cuboid in shape and are arranged in one to three layers. They are connected with each other and with the neighboring cells of the stellate reticulum and the inner enamel epithelium by desmosomes. Tonofibrils, with an orientation parallel to the surface of the developing enamel, are found in the cytoplasm. The function of the stratum intermedium is not understood, but it is believed to play a role in production of the enamel itself, either through control of fluid diffusion into and out of the ameloblasts or by the actual contribution of necessary formative elements or enzymes. The cells of the stratum intermedium show mitotic division even after the cells of the inner enamel epithelium cease to divide.

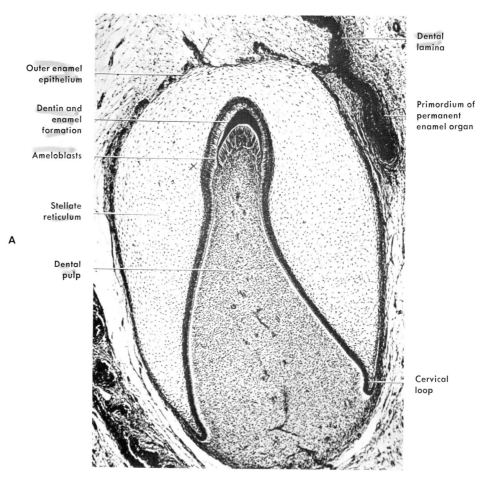

Fig. 3-37. **A,** Tooth germ (lower incisor) of human fetus (fifth month). Beginning of dentin and enamel formation. Stellate reticulum at tip of crown is reduced in thickness. **B,** High magnification of inner enamel epithelium from area X in **A.** In cervical region, cells are short, and outermost layer of pulp is cell free. Occlusally cells are long, and cell-free zone of pulp has disappeared. Ameloblasts are again shorter where dentin formation has begun and enamel formation is imminent. (**B** from Diamond, M., and Weinmann, J. P.: J. Dent. Res. **21:** 403, 1942.)

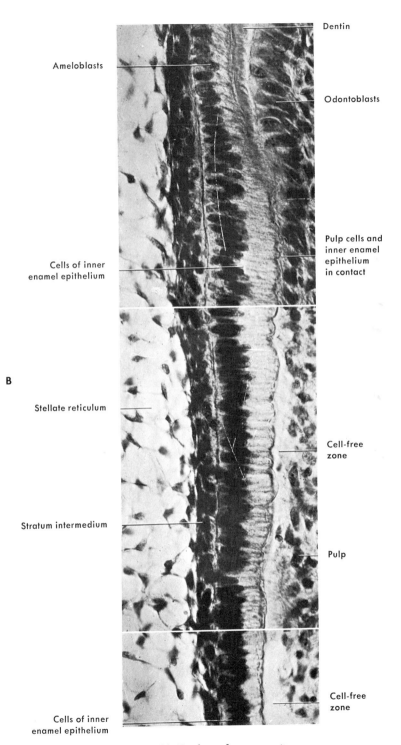

Dentin

Ameloblasts

Odontoblasts

Pulp cells and
inner enamel
epithelium
in contact

Cells of inner
enamel epithelium

B

Stellate reticulum

Cell-free
zone

Stratum intermedium

Pulp

Cell-free
zone

Cells of inner
enamel epithelium

Fig. 3-37, cont'd. For legend see opposite page.

*Inner enamel epithelium.* The cells of the inner enamel epithelium are derived from the basal cell layer of the oral epithelium. Before enamel formation begins, these cells assume a columnar form and differentiate into ameloblasts that produce the enamel matrix. The changes in shape and structure that the cells of the inner enamel epithelium undergo will be described in detail in the discussion of the life cycle of the ameloblasts. It should be mentioned, however, that cell differentiation occurs earlier in the region of the incisal edge or cusps than in the area of the cervical loop.

*Cervical loop.* At the free border of the enamel organ the outer and inner enamel epithelial layers are continuous and reflected into one another as the cervical loop (Figs. 3-33 and 3-35). In this zone of transition between the outer enamel epithelium and the inner enamel epithelium the cuboid cells gradually gain in length. When the crown has been formed, the cells of this portion give rise to Hertwig's epithelial root sheath (Chapter 2).

### Life cycle of the ameloblasts

According to their function, the life-span of the cells of the inner enamel epithelium can be divided into six stages: (1) morphogenic, (2) organizing, (3) formative, (4) maturative, (5) protective, and (6) desmolytic. Since the differentiation of ameloblasts is most advanced in the region of the incisal edge or tips of the cusps and least advanced in the region of the cervical loop, all or some stages of the developing ameloblasts can be observed in one tooth germ.

*Morphogenic stage.* Before the ameloblasts are fully differentiated and produce enamel, they interact with the adjacent mesenchymal cells, determining the shape of the dentinoenamel junction and the crown (Fig. 3-37, A). During this morphogenic stage the cells are short and columnar, with large oval nuclei that almost fill the cell body.

The Golgi apparatus and the centrioles are located in the proximal end of the cell,* whereas the mitochondria are evenly dispersed throughout the cytoplasm. During ameloblast differentiation, terminal bars appear concomitantly with the migration of the mitochondria to the basal region of the cell (Fig. 3-42). The terminal bars represent points of close contact between cells. They were previously believed to consist of dense intercelluar substance, but under the electron microscope it has been found that they comprise thickening of the opposing cell membranes, associated with condensations of the underlying cytoplasm.

The inner enamel epithelium is separated from the connective tissue of the dental papilla by a delicate basement membrane. The adjacent pulpal layer is a cell-free, narrow, light zone containing fine argyrophil fibers and the cytoplasmic processes of the superficial cells of the pulp (Figs. 3-37, B, and 3-38).

---

*In modern usage, to conform with the terminology applied to other secretory cells, the dentinal end of the ameloblast, at which enamel is formed, is called *distal,* and the end facing the stratum intermedium is called *basal* or *proximal.*

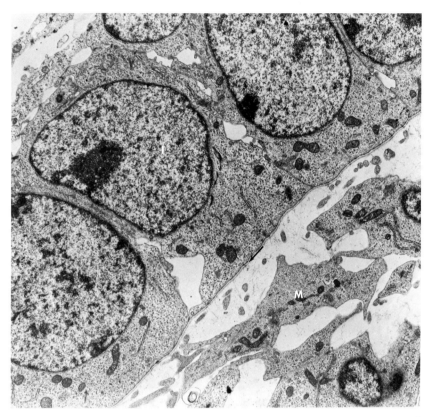

**Fig. 3-38.** Electron micrograph of inner enamel epithelium, *I*, and adjacent mesenchymal cells of dental papilla, *M*, at an early stage of tooth formation. Cytoplasm of cells of inner enamel epithelium is filled with mitochondria and free ribosomes. A typical basement membrane separates epithelium from mesenchyme *(arrow)*. Reticular fibers and cytoplasmic processes of mesenchymal cells appear between inner enamel epithelium and cells of dental papilla. (Approximately ×9000.) (Courtesy Dr. P. R. Garant, Stony Brook, N.Y.)

*Organizing stage.* In the organizing stage of development the inner enamel epithelium interacts with the adjacent connective tissue cells, which differentiate into odontoblasts. This stage is characterized by a change in the appearance of the cells of the inner enamel epithelium. They become longer, and the nucleus-free zones at the distal ends of the cells become almost as long as the proximal parts containing the nuclei (Fig. 3-37, *B*). In preparation for this development a reversal of the functional polarity of these cells takes place by the migration of the centrioles and Golgi regions from the proximal ends of the cells into their distal ends (Fig. 3-39).

Special staining methods reveal the presence of fine acidophil granules in the proximal part of the cell. Electron microscope studies have shown that these granules are actually the mitochondria, which have become concentrated in this part of the cell. At the same time the clear cell-free zone between the inner enamel epithelium and the dental papilla disappears (Fig. 3-37, *B*), probably

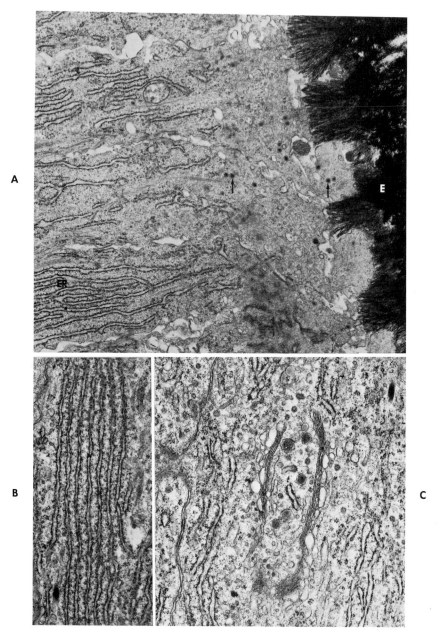

Fig. 3-39. **A,** Electron micrograph of secreting ends of ameloblasts. The electron-opaque, partially mineralized enamel matrix is at right, *E.* Ameloblasts contain an abundant endoplasmic reticulum at left, *ER,* and a number of secretory granules at right *(arrows).* (Approximately ×15,000.) **B,** Electron micrograph of an area of ameloblast cytoplasm between nucleus and secreting end of cell. Cytoplasm in this region is packed with rough-surfaced endoplasmic reticulum. (Approximately ×25,000.) **C,** Electron micrograph of region of ameloblast cytoplasm approximately halfway between nucleus and secreting end. In this region the rough-surfaced endoplasmic reticulum is displaced by the Golgi apparatus, which can be seen in the center of this figure. (Approximately ×25,000.) (**A** from Garant, P. R., and Nalbandian, J.: J. Ultrastruct. Res. **23:**427, 1968; **B** and **C** courtesy Dr. P. R. Garant, Stony Brook, N.Y.)

because of elongation of the epithelial cells toward the papilla. Thus the epithelial cells come into close contact with the connective tissue cells of the pulp, which differentiate into odontoblasts. During the terminal phase of the organizing stage the formation of the dentin by the odontoblasts begins (Fig. 3-37, *B*).

The first appearance of dentin seems to be a critical phase in the life cycle of the inner enamel epithelium. As long as it is in contact with the connective tissue of the dental papilla, it receives nutrient material from the blood vessels of this tissue. When dentin forms, however, it cuts off the ameloblasts from their original source of nourishment, and from then on they are supplied by the capillaries that surround and may even penetrate the outer enamel epithelium. This reversal of nutritional source is characterized by proliferation of capillaries of the dental sac and by reduction and gradual disappearance of the stellate reticulum (Figs. 3-36 and 3-37, *A*). Thus the distance between the capillaries and the stratum intermedium and the ameloblast layer is shortened. Experiments with vital stains demonstrate this reversal of the nutritional stream.

*Formative stage.* The ameloblasts enter their formative stage (Fig. 3-39) after the first layer of dentin has been formed. The presence of dentin seems to be necessary for the beginning of enamel matrix formation just as it was necessary for the epithelial cells to come into close contact with the connective tissue of the pulp during differentiation of the odontoblasts and the beginning of dentin formation. This mutual interaction between one group of cells and another is one of the fundamental laws of organogenesis and histodifferentiation.

During formation of the enamel matrix the ameloblasts retain approximately the same length and arrangement. Changes in the organization and number of cytoplasmic organelles and inclusions are related to the initiation of secretion of enamel matrix.

*Maturative stage.* Enamel maturation (full mineralization) occurs after most of the thickness of the enamel matrix has been formed in the occlusal or incisal area. In the cervical parts of the crown, enamel matrix formation is still progressing at this time. During enamel maturation the ameloblasts are slightly reduced in length and are closely attached to the enamel matrix. The cells of the stratum intermedium lose their cuboidal shape and regular arrangement and assume a spindle shape. It is certain that the ameloblasts also play a part in the maturation of the enamel. During maturation, ameloblasts display microvilli at their distal extremities, and cytoplasmic vacuoles containing material resembling enamel matrix are present (Figs. 3-48 to 3-50). These structures indicate an absorptive function of these cells.

*Protective stage.* When the enamel has completely developed and has fully calcified, the ameloblasts cease to be arranged in a well-defined layer and can no longer be differentiated from the cells of the stratum intermedium and outer enamel epithelium (Fig. 3-48). These cell layers then form a stratified epithelial covering of the enamel, the so-called reduced enamel epithelium. The function of the reduced enamel epithelium is that of protecting the mature enamel by separating it from the connective tissue until the tooth erupts. If connective tissue

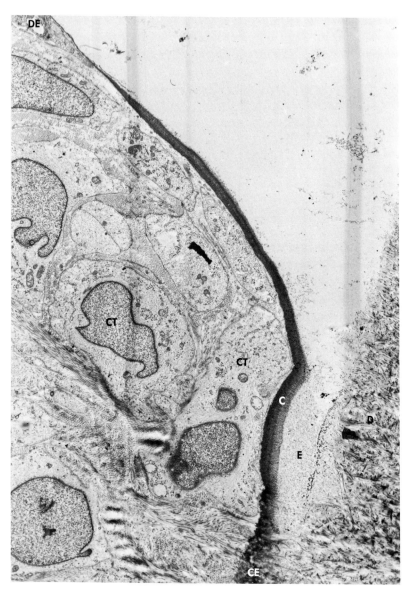

Fig. 3-40. Electron micrograph of cervical region of unerupted human tooth. Dentin matrix, *D*, and remnants of the demineralized enamel matrix, *E*, are at right. Afibrillar cementum, apparently of mesodermal origin, runs through center of figure, *C*, and is continuous with cementum, *CE*. Cells of adjacent connective tissue, *CT*, and retracted end of enamel organ, *DE*, are at left. (Approximately ×6500.) (From Listgarten, M. A.: Arch. Oral Biol. **11**:999, 1966.)

comes in contact with the enamel, anomalies may develop. Under such conditions the enamel may be either resorbed or covered by a layer of cementum.

During this phase of the life cycle of ameloblasts the epithelial enamel organ may retract from the cervical edge of the enamel. The adjacent mesenchymal cells may then deposit a cuticle (afibrillar cementum) on the enamel surface (Fig. 3-40).

*Desmolytic stage.* The reduced enamel epithelium proliferates and seems to induce atrophy of the connective tissue separating it from the oral epithelium, so that fusion of the two epithelia can occur (Chapter 9). It is probable that the epithelial cells elaborate enzymes that are able to destroy connective tissue fibers by desmolysis. Premature degeneration of the reduced enamel epithelium may prevent the eruption of a tooth.

## Amelogenesis

On the basis of ultrastructure and composition, two processes are involved in the development of enamel: organic matrix formation and mineralization. Although the inception of mineralization does not await the completion of matrix formation, the two processes will be treated separately.

### Formation of the enamel matrix

The ameloblasts begin their secretory activity when a small amount of dentin has been laid down. The first enamel matrix is deposited extracellularly by the ameloblasts in a thin layer along the dentin (Figs. 3-37, *B*, and 3-41). This has been termed the dentinoenamel membrane. Its presence accounts for the fact that the distal ends of the enamel rods are not in direct contact with the dentin.

*Development of Tomes' processes.* The surfaces of the ameloblasts facing the developing enamel are not smooth. There is an interdigitation of the cells and the enamel rods, which they produce (Fig. 3-43). This interdigitation is partly a result of the fact that the long axes of the ameloblasts are not parallel to the long axes of the rods (Figs. 3-44 and 3-45). The projections of the ameloblasts into the enamel matrix have been named Tomes' processes. It was once believed that these processes were transformed into enamel matrix, but more recent electron microscope studies have demonstrated that matrix synthesis and secretion by ameloblasts are very similar to the same processes occurring in other protein-secreting cells. Although Tomes' processes are partly delineated by incomplete septa (Fig. 3-44), they also contain typical secretion granules as well as rough endoplasmic reticulum and mitochondria (Figs. 3-39, 3-42, *B*, and 3-51, *B*).

Fig. 3-45 is a drawing derived from the electron micrograph in Fig. 3-44. It is clear from this sketch that at least two ameloblasts are involved in the synthesis of each enamel rod. If the surface of devolping enamel is examined in the scanning electron microscope, which permits a three-dimensional visualization of the surface, the depressions resulting from the presence of Tomes' processes

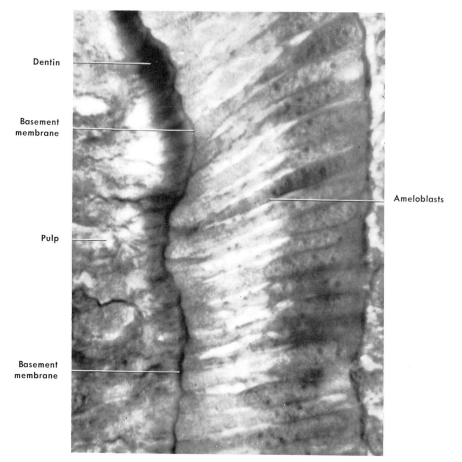

Dentin

Basement
membrane

Ameloblasts

Pulp

Basement
membrane

**Fig. 3-41.** Basement membrane of dental papilla can be followed on outer surface of dentin, forming the dentinoenamel membrane. (From Orban, B., Sicher, H., and Weinmann, J. P.: J. Am. Coll. Dent. **10:**13, 1943.)

are quite obvious (Fig. 3-46). One interpretation of the relationships between the keyhole-shaped enamel rods and the roughly hexagonal ameloblasts is indicated in Fig. 3-47. The bulk of the "head" of each rod is formed by one ameloblast, whereas three others contribute components to the "tail" of each rod. According to this interpretation, each rod is formed by four ameloblasts, and each ameloblast contributes to four different rods.

*Distal terminal bars.* At the time Tomes' processes begin to form, terminal bars appear at the distal ends of the ameloblasts, separating the Tomes' processes from the cell proper (Fig. 3-42, A). Structurally, they are localized condensations of cytoplasmic substance closely associated with thickened cell membranes. They are observed during the enamel-producing stage of the ameloblasts, but their exact function is not known.

*Ameloblasts covering maturing enamel.* At the light microscope level one can

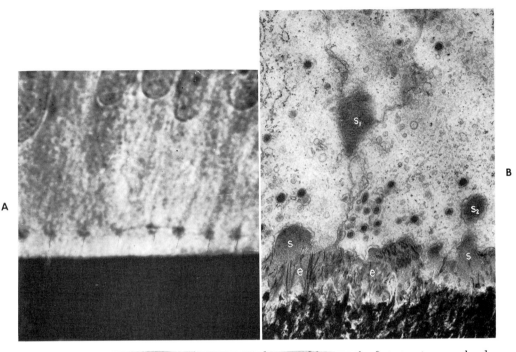

Fig. 3-42. **A,** Formation of Tomes' processes and terminal bars as the first step in enamel rod formation. Rat incisor. **B,** Electron photomicrograph showing an early stage in the formation of enamel in the lower incisor of the rat. At this stage, dentin (at bottom of photomicrograph) is well developed. Enamel, *e,* appears as a less dense layer on the surface of the dentin and consists of thin, ribbon-shaped elements running more or less perpendicular to the dentino-enamel junction and masses of a less dense stippled material, *s.* Separating the enamel from the cytoplasm of the ameloblasts, which occupies most of the upper part of the photomicrograph, is the ameloblast plasma membrane. Parts of three ameloblasts are shown. In the middle of the photomicrograph in a region bounded by the membranes of the three ameloblasts lies another mass of stippled material, $s_1$, while a second mass, $s_2$, lies at the right surrounded by membrane, but within the bounds of the ameloblast. Numerous small, membrane-bound granules lie within the cytoplasm. The contents of these have the same general consistency as the stippled material, but rather higher density. It is possible that these represent unsecreted granules of stippled material, which in turn is a precursor of enamel matrix. (×24,000.) (**A** from Orban, B., Sicher, H., and Weinmann, J. P.: J. Am. Coll. Dent. **10:**13, 1943; **B** from Watson, M. L.: J. Biophys. Biochem. Cytol. **7:**489, 1960.)

see that the ameloblasts over maturing enamel are considerably shorter than the ameloblasts over incompletely formed enamel (Fig. 3-48). These short ameloblasts have a villous surface near the enamel and the ends of the cells are packed with mitochondria (Figs. 3-49 and 3-50). This morphology is typical of absorptive cells, and it has been demonstrated that ameloblasts are apparently transporting organic components from the matrix. The fact that organic components as well as water are lost in mineralization is a striking difference between enamel and other mineralized tissues. Over 90% of the initially secreted protein is lost during enamel maturation, and that which remains forms envelopes around indi-

*Text continued on p. 92.*

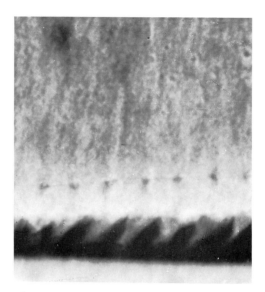

**Fig. 3-43.** "Picket fence" arrangement of Tomes' processes. Rods are at angle to ameloblasts and Tomes' processes. (From Orban, B., Sicher, H., and Weinmann, J. P.: J. Am. Coll. Dent. **10:**13, 1943.)

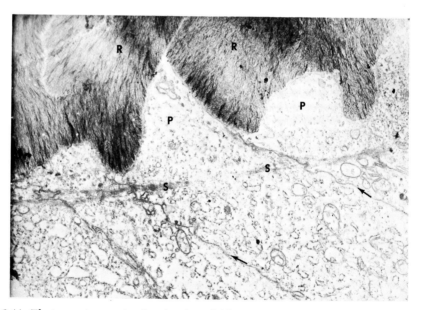

**Fig. 3-44.** Electron micrograph of ends of ameloblasts and adjacent enamel in a developing human deciduous tooth. Positions of ameloblast cell membranes *(arrows)* indicate that the cells are nearly perpendicular to long axes of rods, R. An incomplete septum, S, can be seen, indicating the approximate position of Tomes' processes, P. (Approximately ×16,000.) (From Rönnholm, E.: J. Ultrastruct. Res. 6:249, 1962.)

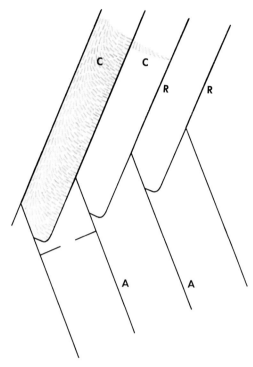

**Fig. 3-45.** Drawing derived from Fig. 3-44. *Dark lines* indicate rod boundaries, R, and amelo-blast cell surfaces, A, as well as the incomplete septum near distal end of ameloblast at left. *Gray lines* indicate approximate orientation of apatite crystals, C.

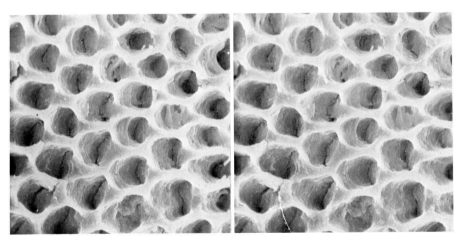

**Fig. 3-46.** Pair of stereographic scanning electron micrographs of the surface of developing human enamel. Great depth of focus of this instrument permits visualization of interdigitated nature of this surface. Depressions were occupied by Tomes' processes, which were stripped away with the epithelial enamel organ. (Courtesy Dr. A. R. Boyde, London, England.)

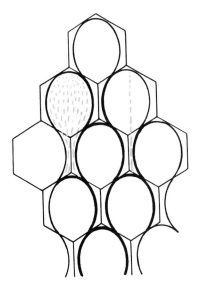

Fig. 3-47. Drawing illustrating one interpretation of relationships between enamel rods and ameloblasts. Cross sections of ameloblasts are indicated by the *thin lines* arranged in a regular hexagonal array. Enamel rods are indicated by the *thicker curved black lines*, outlining the keyhole- or paddle-shaped rods. *Gray lines* indicate approximate orientation of enamel crystals, which are parallel to the long axes of the rods in their "bodies" and approach a position perpendicular to the long axes in the "tails." One can see that each rod is formed by four ameloblasts and that each ameloblast contributes to four different rods. (Modified from Boyde, A.: In Stack, M. V., and Fearnhead, R. W., editors: Tooth enamel, Bristol, 1965, John Wright & Sons, Ltd.

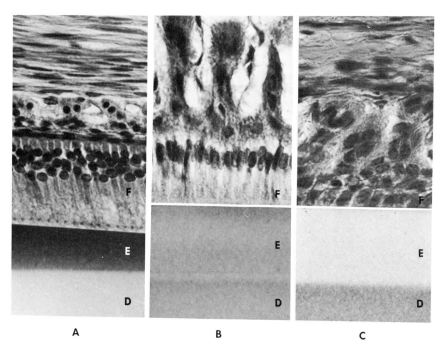

A          B          C

Fig. 3-48. Light micrographs of various stages in life cycle of ameloblasts, *F,* in rat incisor matched with microradiographs of corresponding adjacent enamel, *E,* and dentin, *D.* **A,** Ameloblasts are secreting enamel, which is incompletely formed. Enamel is less radiopaque than dentin, indicating that it is less mineralized. **B,** In area of enamel maturation ameloblasts are shorter, and enamel matrix is about as heavily mineralized as dentin. **C,** In area in which ameloblasts are in the protective stage the enamel is fully mineralized and is much more radiopaque than the underlying dentin. (All about ×260.)

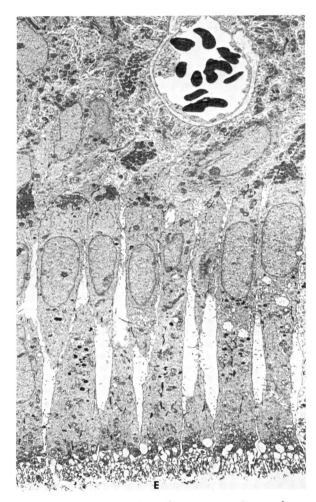

**Fig. 3-49.** Electron micrograph of ameloblasts during stage of enamel maturation. Enamel has been lost during demineralization. The cells are covered at their surfaces adjoining the enamel, *E*, and on their lateral surfaces by numerous microvilli. (Approximately ×3400.) (From Reith, E. J.: J. Biophys. Biochem. Cytol. **9:**825, 1961.)

vidual crystals (Fig. 3-10), although there may be a higher content of organic matter in the area of the prism sheath where the abrupt change in crystal orientation occurs. In the electron microscope, several substages can be identified in the transition of ameloblasts from the formative stage through the maturative stage (Fig. 3-51). Shifts are apparent in the cellular organelles from those associated with protein synthesis and secretion to those related to absorption. In

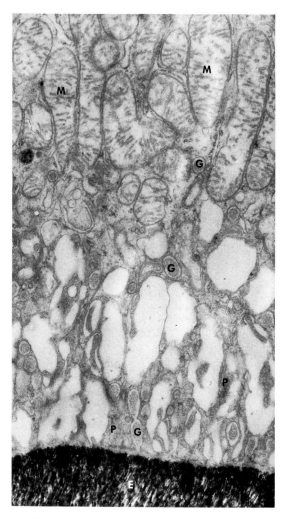

**Fig. 3-50.** Higher magnification of electron micrograph of the ends of ameloblasts during stage of enamel maturation. Adjacent to enamel, *E*, are elaborate cell processes of ameloblasts, *P*, as well as numerous mitochondria within ameloblast cytoplasm, *M*. Granular material, possibly being resorbed, is seen both between cell processes and within ameloblast cytoplasm, *G*. This structure is typical of resorptive cells. (Approximately ×36,000.) (From Reith, E. J.: J. Cell Biol. **18:**691, 1963.)

addition, a sequence of changes in cell-to-cell contacts and communications between cell layers occurs.

### Mineralization and maturation of the enamel matrix

Mineralization of the enamel matrix takes place in two stages, although the time interval between the two appears to be very small. In the first stage an immediate partial mineralization occurs in the matrix segments and the interprismatic substance as they are laid down. Chemical analyses indicate that the initial influx may amount to 25% to 30% of the eventual total mineral content. It has been shown recently by electron microscopy and diffraction that this first mineral actually is in the form of crystalline apatite (Fig. 3-54, *A*).

The second stage, or *maturation*, is characterized by the gradual completion of mineralization (Fig. 3-49). The process of maturation starts from the height of the crown and progresses cervically (Fig. 3-52). However, at each level, maturation seems to begin at the dentinal end of the rods. Thus there is an integration of two processes: each rod matures from the depth to the surface, and the sequence of maturing rods is from cusps or incisal edge toward the cervical line.

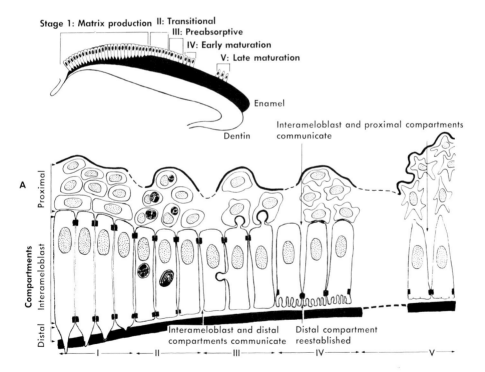

**Fig. 3-51.** Drawings of electron micrographs of enamel organ of rat incisor. Five substages have been identified from formative to maturative. **A,** Overview of enamel organ.

*Continued.*

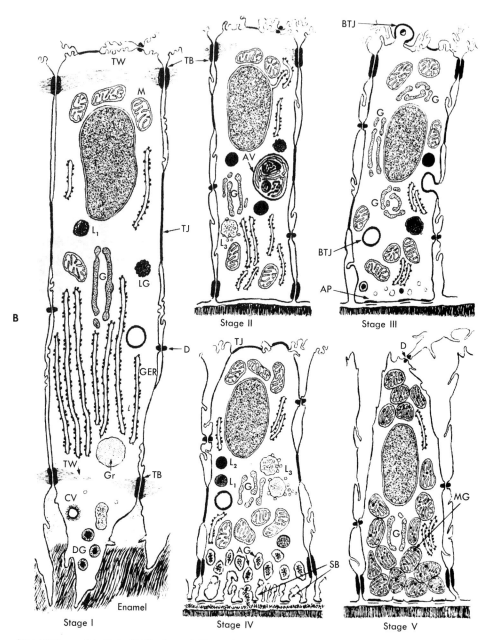

**Fig. 3-51, cont'd. B,** Individual ameloblasts from the five substages. Organelles: *AG,* absorption granules; *AP,* apical contact specializations (hemidesmosomes); *AV,* autophagic vacuoles (lysosomes); *BTJ,* bulb type of contacts; *CV,* coated (absorptive?) vesicles; *D,* desmosomes; *DG,* dense (secretory) granules; *G,* Golgi apparatus; *GER,* granular (rough) endoplasmic reticulum; *Gr,* pale (secretory?) granules; *L₁, L₂, L₃* lysosomes; *LG,* lipid granules; *M,* mitochondria; *MG,* mitochondrial granules; *SB,* striated border; *TB,* terminal bars; *TJ,* tight junctions; *TW,* terminal web. (From Reith, E. J.: J. Ultrastruct. Res. **30:**111, 1970.)

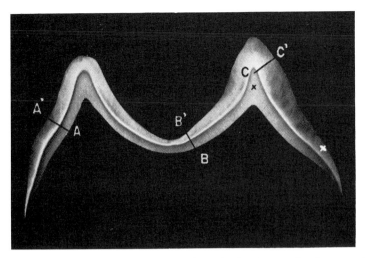

**Fig. 3-52.** Microradiograph of ground section through developing deciduous molar. From gradation in radiopacity, maturation can be seen to progress from dentinoenamel junction toward enamel surface. Mineralization is more advanced occlusally than in the cervical region. Lines *A, B,* and *C* indicate planes in which actual microdensitometric tracings were made. *Black* x, Cusp area. *White* x, Cervical area. (×15.) (From Hammarlund-Essler, E.: Trans. Roy. Schools Dent., Stockholm and Umea 4:15, 1958.)

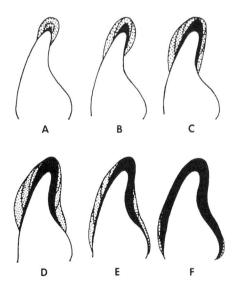

**Fig. 3-53.** Diagram showing pattern of mineralization of incisor tooth. *Stippled zones,* Consecutive layers of partly mineralized enamel matrix. *Black areas,* Advance of final mineralization during maturation. (From Crabb, H. S. M.: Proc. Roy. Soc. Med. **52:**118, 1959; and Crabb, H. S. M., and Darling, A. I.: Arch. Oral Biol. **2:**308, 1960.)

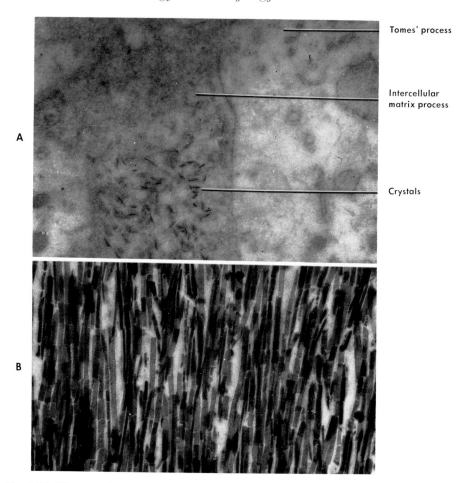

Tomes' process

Intercellular
matrix process

Crystals

**Fig. 3-54.** Electron photomicrographs illustrating difference between short, needlelike crystals laid down in newly deposited enamel matrix, **A**, and long, ribbonlike crystals seen in mature enamel, **B**. (×70,000.)

Maturation begins before the matrix has reached its full thickness. Thus it is going on in the inner, first-formed matrix at the same time as initial mineralization is taking place in the outer, recently formed matrix. The advancing front is at first parallel to the dentinoenamel junction and later to the outer enamel surface. Following this basic pattern, the incisal and occlusal regions reach maturity ahead of the cervical regions (Fig. 3-53).

At the ultrastructural level, maturation is characterized by growth of the crystals seen in the primary phase (Fig. 3-54, *A*). The original ribbon-shaped crystals increase in thickness more rapidly than in width (Fig. 3-55). Concomitantly the organic matrix gradually becomes thinned and more widely spaced to make room for the growing crystals. Chemical analysis shows that the loss in volume of the organic matrix is caused by withdrawal of a substantial amount of protein as well as water.

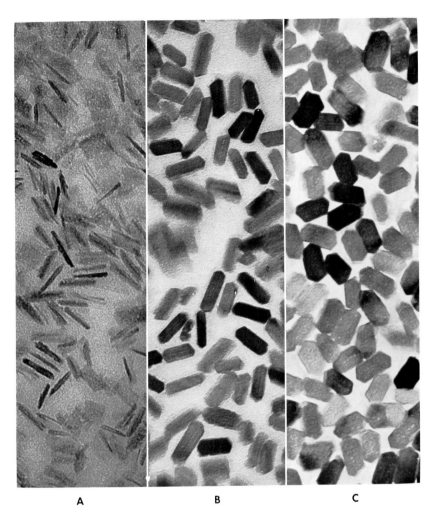

A                    B                    C

**Fig. 3-55.** Electron photomicrographs of transverse sections through enamel rods in rat incisor showing three stages in growth of apatite crystals during enamel maturation. From **A** (recently formed enamel) through **C** (more mature enamel) the crystals increase in thickness more rapidly than in width. Spaces between crystals will become even smaller as maturation is completed. (×240,000.) (Modified from Nylen, M. U., Eanes, E. D., and Omnell, K.-Å.: J. Cell Biol. **18:**109, 1963.)

## Clinical considerations

Clinical interest in amelogenesis is centered primarily on the perfection of enamel formation. Although there is relatively little the dentist can do directly to alter the course of events in amelogenesis, it may be possible to minimize certain of the factors believed to be associated with the etiology of defective enamel structure. The principal expressions of pathologic amelogenesis are hypoplasia, which is manifested by pitting, furrowing, or even total absence of the enamel, and hypocalcification, in the form of opaque or chalky areas on normally contoured enamel surfaces. The causes of such defective enamel formation can be generally classified as systemic, local, or genetic. The most common systemic influences are nutritional deficiencies, endocrinopathies, febrile diseases, and certain chemical intoxications. It thus stands to reason that the dentist should exert his influence to ensure sound nutritional practices and recommended immunization procedures during periods of gestation and postnatal amelogenesis. Chemical intoxication of the ameloblasts is not prevalent and is limited essentially to the ingestion of excessive amounts of water-borne fluoride. Where the drinking water contains fluoride in excess of 1.5 parts per million, chronic endemic fluorosis may occur as a result of continuous use throughout the period of amelogenesis. In such areas it is important to urge substitution of a water with levels of fluoride (about 1 part per million) well below the threshold for fluorosis, yet optimal with regard to protection against dental caries (see discussion of clinical considerations in section on histology).

Since it has been realized that enamel development occurs in two phases, i.e., matrix formation and maturation, developmental disturbances of the enamel can be understood more fully. If matrix formation is affected, enamel hypoplasia will ensue. If maturation is lacking or incomplete, hypocalcification of the enamel results. In the case of hypoplasia a defect of the enamel is found. In the case of hypocalcification a deficiency in the mineral content of the enamel is found. In the latter the enamel persists as enamel matrix and is therefore soft and acid insoluble in routine preparation after formalin fixation.

Hypoplasia as well as hypocalcification may be caused by systemic, local, or hereditary factors. Hypoplasia of systemic origin is termed chronologic hypoplasia because the lesion is found in the areas of those teeth where the enamel was formed during the systemic (metabolic) disturbance. Since the formation of enamel extends over a longer period and the systemic disturbance is, in most cases, of short duration, the defect is limited to a circumscribed area of the affected teeth. A single narrow zone of hypoplasia (smooth or pitted) may be indicative of a disturbance of enamel formation during a short period in which only those ameloblasts that at that time had just started enamel formation were affected. Multiple hypoplasia develops if enamel formation is interupted on more than one occasion.

No specific etiology of chronologic hypoplasia has been established as yet. Recent investigations have demonstrated that exanthematous diseases are not so frequently a cause of enamel hypoplasia as was heretofore commonly believed. The most frequent etiologic factors are said to be rickets and hypoparathyroidism, but hypoplasia cannot be predicted with any reliability even in the most severe forms of those diseases.

The systemic influences causing enamel hypoplasia are, in the majority of cases, active during the first year of life. Therefore the teeth most frequently affected are the incisors, canines, and first molars. The upper lateral incisor is sometimes found to be unaffected because its development starts later than that of the other teeth mentioned.

Local factors affect single teeth, in most cases only one tooth. If more than one tooth is affected by local hypoplasia, the location of the defects shows no relation to chronology of development. The cause of local hypoplasia may be an infection of the pulp with subsequent infection of the periapical tissues of a deciduous tooth if the irritation occurred during the period of enamel formation of its permanent successor.

The hereditary type of enamel hypoplasia is probably a generalized disturbance of the ameloblasts. Therefore the entire enamel of all the teeth, deciduous as well as permanent, is affected rather than merely a beltlike zone of the enamel of a group of teeth, as in systemic cases. The anomaly is transmitted as a mendelian dominant character. The enamel of such teeth is so thin that it cannot be noticed clinically or in radiographs. The crowns of the teeth of affected family members are yellow-brown, smooth, glossy, and hard, and their shape resembles teeth prepared for jacket crowns.

An example of systemic hypocalcification of the enamel is the so-called mottled enamel. A high fluoride content in the water is the cause of the deficiency in calcification. Fluoride hypocalcification is endemic; i.e., it is limited in its distribution to definite areas in which the drinking water contains more than 1 part of fluoride per 1 million parts of water. It has been demonstrated that a small amount of fluoride (about 1 to 1.2 parts per million) reduces susceptibility to dental caries without causing mottling. For this reason many communities are adding small quantities of fluoride to the community water supplies.

The same local causes that might affect the formation of the enamel can disturb maturation. If the injury occurs in the formative stage of enamel development, hypoplasia of the enamel will result. An injury during the maturation stage will cause a deficiency in calcification.

The hereditary type of hypocalcification is characterized by the formation of a normal amount of enamel matrix that, however, does not fully mature. Such teeth, if investigated before or shortly after eruption, show a normal shape. Their surfaces do not have the luster of normal enamel but appear dull. The enamel is opaque. The hypocalcified soft enamel matrix is soon discolored, abraded by mastication, or peeled off in layers. When parts of the soft enamel are lost, the teeth show an irregular, rough surface. When the enamel is altogether lost, the teeth are small and brown, and the exposed dentin is extremely sensitive. In a rare hereditary disturbance of the enamel organ called odontodysplasia, both the apposition and maturation of the enamel is disturbed. Such teeth have irregular, "moth-eaten," poorly calcified enamel.

The discoloration of enamel from administration of tetracyclines during childhood is a very common clinical problem. In some cases the discoloration can be severe and unsightly and may require the placement of porcelain jacket crowns. In mild cases, however, the use of some of the newly developed surface-binding restorative materials can produce good esthetic results.

## REFERENCES
### Structure

Arnold, F. A., Jr.: Grand Rapids fluoridation study—results pertaining to the eleventh year of fluoridation, Am. J. Public Health **47**:539, 1957.

Bartelstone, H. J., Mandel, I. D., Oshry, E., and Seidlin, S. M.: Use of radioactive iodine as a tracer in the study of the physiology of the teeth, Science **106**:132, 1947.

Bergman, G., Hammerlund-Essler, E., and Lysell, L.: Studies on mineralized dental tissues. XII. Microradiographic study of caries in deciduous teeth, Acta Odontol. Scand. **16**:113, 1958.

Beust, T.: Morphology and biology of the enamel tufts with remarks on their relation to caries, J. Am. Dent. Assoc. **19**:488, 1932.

Bhussry, B. R., and Bibby, B. G.: Surface changes in enamel, J. Dent. Res. **36**:409, 1957.

Bibby, B. G., and Van Huysen, G.: Changes in the enamel surfaces; a possible defense against caries, J. Am. Dent. Assoc. **20**:828, 1933.

Bodecker, C. F.: Enamel of the teeth decalcified by the celloidin decalcifying method and examined by ultraviolet light, Dent. Rev. **20**:317, 1906.

Bodecker, C. F.: The color of the teeth as an index of their resistance to decay, Int. J. Orthod. **19**:386, 1933.

Brabant, H., and Klees, L.: Histological contribution to the study of lamellae in human dental enamel, Int. Dent. J. **8**:539, 1958.

Brudevold, F., and Söremark, R.: Chemistry of the mineral phase of enamel. In Miles, A. E. W., editor: Structural and chemical organization of teeth. Vol. II, New York, 1967, Academic Press Inc.

Burgess, R. C., Nikiforuk, G., and Maclaren, C.: Chromatographic studies of carbohydrate components in enamel, Arch. Oral Biol. **1**:8, 1960.

Chase, S. W.: The number of enamel prisms in human teeth, J. Am. Dent. Assoc. **14**:1921, 1927.

Crabb, H. S., and Darling, A. I.: The pattern of progressive mineralisation in human dental enamel, Int. Ser. Monogr. Oral Biol. **2**:1, 1962.

Decker, J. D.: Fixation effects on the fine structure of enamel crystal-matrix relationships, J. Ultrastruct. Res. **44**:58, 1973.

Eastoe, J. E.: Organic matrix of tooth enamel, Nature **187**:411, 1960.

Eastoe, J. E.: In Stack, M. V., and Fearnhead, R. W., editors: Tooth enamel, Bristol, 1965, John Wright & Sons, Ltd., p. 91.

Eggert, F. M., Allen, G. A., and Burgess, R. C.: Amelogenins. Purification and partial characterization of proteins from developing bovine dental enamel, J. Biochem. **131**:471, 1973.

Engel, M. B.: Glycogen and carbohydrate-protein complex in developing teeth of the rat, J. Dent. Res. **27**:681, 1948.

Fincham, A. G., Burkland, G. A., and Shapiro, I. M.: Lipophilia of enamel matrix. A chemical investigation of the neutral lipids and lipophilic proteins of enamel, Calcif. Tissue Res. **9**:247, 1972.

Frank, R. M., and Brendel, A.: Ultrastructure of the approximal dental plaque and the underlying normal and carious enamel, Arch. Oral Biol. **11**:883, 1966.

Frank, R. M., Sognnaes, R. F., and Kern, R.: In Sognnaes, R. F., editor: Calcification in biological systems, Washington, D. C., 1960, American Association for the Advancement of Science.

Frazier, P. D.: Adult human enamel: an electron microscopic study of crystallite size and morphology, J. Ultrastruct. Res. **22**:1, 1968.

Glas, J. E., and Omnell, K. A.: Studies on the ultrastructure of dental enamel, J. Ultrastruct. Res. **3**:334, 1960.

Glimcher, M. J., Bonar, L. C., and Daniel, E. J.: The molecular structure of the protein matrix of bovine dental enamel, J. Mol. Biol. **3**:541, 1961.

Gottlieb, B.: Dental caries, Philadelphia, 1947, Lea & Febiger.

Gray, J. A., Schweizer, H. C., Rosevear, F. B., and Broge, R. W.: Electron microscopic observations of the differences in the effects of stannous fluoride and sodium fluoride on dental enamel, J. Dent. Res. **37**:638, 1958.

Gustafson, A.-G.: A morphologic investigation of certain variations in the structure and mineralization of human dental enamel, Odont. T. **67**:361, 1959.

Gustafson, G.: The structure of human dental enamel, Odontol. T. **53**(suppl.), 1945.

Gustafson, G., and Gustafson, A.-G.: Human

dental enamel in polarized light and contact micro-radiography, Acta Odontol. Scand. **19**:259, 1961.

Gustafson, G., and Gustafson, A.-G.: Microanatomy and histochemistry of enamel: In Miles, A. E. W., editor: Structural and chemical organization of teeth. Vol. II, New York, 1967, Academic Press Inc.

Gwinnett, A. J.: The ultrastructure of the "prismless" enamel of deciduous teeth, Arch. Oral Biol. **11**:1109, 1966.

Gwinnett, A. J.: The ultrastructure of the "prismless" enamel of permanent human teeth, Arch. Oral Biol. **12**:381, 1967.

Gwinnett, A. J.: Human prismless enamel and its influence on sealant penetration, Arch. Oral Biol. **18**:441, 1973.

Helmcke, J.-G.: Ultrastructure of enamel: In Miles, A. E. W., editor: Structural and chemical organization of teeth. Vol. II, New York, 1967, Academic Press Inc.

Hinrichsen, C. F. L., and Engel, M. B.: Fine structure of partially demineralized enamel, Arch. Oral Biol. **11**:65, 1966.

Hodson, J. J.: An investigation into the microscopic structure of the common forms of enamel lamellae with special reference to their origin and contents, Oral Surg. **6**: 305, 383, 495, 1953.

Houver, G., and Frank, R. M.: Ultrastructural significance of histochemical reactions on the enamel surface of erupted teeth, Arch. Oral Biol. **12**:1209, 1967.

Leach, S. A., and Saxton, C. A.: An electron microscopic study of the acquired pellicle and plaque formed on the enamel of human incisors, Arch. Oral Biol. **11**:1081, 1966.

Listgarten, M. A.: Phase-contrast and electron microscopic study of the junction between reduced enamel epithelium and enamel in unerupted human teeth, Arch. Oral Biol. **11**:999, 1966.

Listgarten, M. A.: Electron microscopic study of the gingivo-dental junction of man, Am. J. Anat. **119**:147, 1966.

Meckel, A. H.: The formation and properties of organic films on teeth, Arch. Oral Biol. **10**:585, 1965.

Meckel, A. H., Griebstein, W. J., and Neal, R. J.: Structure of mature human dental enamel as observed by electron microscopy, Arch. Oral Biol. **10**:775, 1965.

Muhler, J. C.: Present status of topical fluoride therapy, J. Dent. Child. **26**:173, 1959.

Muhler, J. C., and Radike, A. W.: Effect of a dentifrice containing stannous fluoride on adults. II. Results at the end of two years of unsupervised use, J. Am. Dent. Assoc. **55**:196, 1957.

Nikiforuk, G., and Sognnaes, R. F.: Dental enamel, Clin. Orthop. **47**:229, 1966.

Orban, B.: Histology of enamel lamellae and tufts, J. Am. Dent. Assoc. **15**:305, 1928.

Osborn, J. W.: Three-dimensional reconstructions of enamel prisms, J. Dent. Res. **46**: 1412, 1967.

Osborn, J. W.: Directions and interrelationship of prisms in cuspal and cervical enamel of human teeth, J. Dent. Res. **47**: 395, 1968.

Osborn, J. W.: A relationship between the striae of Retzius and prism directions in the transverse plane of the human tooth, Arch. Oral Biol. **16**:1061, 1971.

Pautard, F. G. E.: An x-ray diffraction pattern from human enamel matrix, Arch. Oral Biol. **3**:217, 1961.

Piez, K. A.: The nature of the protein matrix of human enamel, J. Dent. Res. **39**:712, 1960.

Piez, K. A., and Likins, R. C.: The nature of collagen. II. Vertebrate collagens. In Sognnaes, R. F., editor: Calcification in biological systems, Washington, D.C., 1960, American Association for the Advancement of Science, p. 411.

Ripa, L. W., Gwinnett, A. J., and Buonocore, M. G.: The "prismless" outer layer of deciduous and permanent enamel, Arch. Oral Biol. **11**:41, 1966.

Robinson, C., Weatherell, J. A., and Hallsworth, S. A.: Variation in composition of dental enamel within thin ground tooth sections, Caries Res. **5**:44, 1971.

Rönnholm, E.: The amelogenesis of human teeth as revealed by electron microscopy. II. The development of the enamel crystallites, J. Ultrastruct. Res. **6**:249, 1962.

Rushton, M. A.: On the fine contour lines of the enamel of milk teeth, Dent. Rec. **53**: 170, 1933.

Schmidt, W. J., and Keil, A.: Die gesunden und die erkrankten Zahngewebe des Menschen und der Wirbeltiere im Polarisationsmikroskop [Normal and pathological tooth structure of humans and vertebrates in the polarization microscope], München, 1958, Carl Hanser Verlag.

Schour, I.: The neonatal line in the enamel and dentin of the human deciduous teeth and first permanent molar, J. Am. Dent. Assoc. **23**:1946, 1936.

Schour, I., and Hoffman, M. M.: Studies in tooth development. I. The 16 microns rhythm in the enamel and dentin from fish to man, J. Dent. Res. **18**:91, 1939.

Scott, D. B.: The electron microscopy of enamel and dentin, J. New York Acad. Sci. **60**:575, 1955.

Scott, D. B.: The crystalline component of dental enamel, Fourth International Conference on Electron Microscopy, Berlin, 1960, Springer Verlag.

Scott, D. B., and Wyckoff, R. W. G.: Typical structures on replicas of apparently intact tooth surfaces, Public Health Rep. **61**: 1397, 1946.

Scott, D. B., and Wyckoff, R. W. G.: Studies of tooth surface structure by optical and electron microscopy, J. Am. Dent. Assoc. **39**:275, 1949.

Scott, D. B., Kaplan, H., and Wyckoff, R. W. G.: Replica studies of changes in tooth surfaces with age, J. Dent. Res. **28**:31, 1949.

Scott, D. B., Ussing, M. J., Sognnaes, R. F., and Wyckoff, R. W. G.: Electron microscopy of mature human enamel, J. Dent. Res. **31**:74, 1952.

Selvig, K. A.: The crystal structure of hydroxyapatite in dental enamel as seen with the electron microscope, J. Ultrastruct. Res. **41**:369, 1972.

Shaw, J. H.: Fluoridation as a public health measure, Washington, D.C., 1954, American Association for the Advancement of Science.

Skillen, W. C.: The permeability of enamel in relation to stain, J. Am. Dent. Assoc. **11**:402, 1924.

Sognnaes, R. F.: The organic elements of the enamel. III. The pattern of the organic framework in the region of the neonatal and other incremental lines of the enamel, J. Dent. Res. **28**:558, 1949.

Sognnaes, R. F.: The organic elements of the enamel. IV. The gross morphology and the histological relationship of the lamellae to the organic framework of the enamel, J. Dent. Res. **29**:260, 1950.

Sognnaes, R. F.: Microstructure and histochemical characteristics of the mineralized tissues, J. New York Acad. Sci. **60**:545, 1955.

Sognnaes, R. F., Shaw, J. H., and Bogoroch, R.: Radiotracer studies of bone, cementum, dentin and enamel of rhesus monkeys, Am. J. Physiol. **180**:408, 1955.

Spiers, R. L.: The nature of surface enamel, Br. Dent. J. **107**:209, 1959.

Stack, M. V.: Organic constituents of enamel, J. Am. Dent. Assoc. **48**:297, 1954.

Stack, M. V.: Chemical organization of the organic matrix of enamel. In Miles, A. E. W., editor: Structural and chemical organization of teeth. Vol. II, New York, 1967, Academic Press Inc.

Swancar, J. R., Scott, D. B., and Njemirovskij, Z.: Studies on the structure of human enamel by the replica method, J. Dent. Res. **49**:1025, 1970.

Wainwright, W. W., and Lemoine, F. A.: Rapid diffuse penetration of intact enamel and dentin by carbon[14]-labeled urea, J. Am. Dent. Assoc. **41**:135, 1950.

Warshawsky, H.: A light and electron microscopic study of the nearly mature enamel of rat incisors, Anat. Rec. **169**:559, 1971.

Watson, M. L.: The extracellular nature of enamel in the rat, J. Biophys. Biochem. Cytol. **7**:489, 1960.

Yoon, S. H., Brudwold, F., Gardner, D. E., and Smith, F. A.: Distribution of fluoride in teeth from areas with different levels of fluoride in the water supply, J. Dent. Res. **39**:845, 1960.

**Development**

Allan, J. H.: Investigations into the mineralization pattern of human dental enamel, J. Dent. Res. **38**:1096, 1959.

Allan, J. H.: Maturation of enamel. In Miles, A. E. W., editor: Structural and chemical organization of teeth. Vol. I, New York, 1967, Academic Press Inc.

Angmar-Månsson, B.: A quantitative microradiographic study on the organic matrix of developing human enamel in relation to the mineral content, Arch. Oral Biol. **16**: 135, 1971.

Boyde, A.: The structure of developing mammalian dental enamel. In Stack, M. V., and Fearnhead, R. W., editors: Tooth enamel, Bristol, 1965, John Wright & Sons, Ltd.

Crabb, H. S. M.: The pattern of mineralization of human dental enamel, Proc. Roy. Soc. Med. **52**:118, 1959.

Crabb, H. S. M., and Darling, A. I.: The

gradient of mineralization in developing enamel, Arch. Oral Biol. **2**:308, 1960.

Deakins, M.: Changes in the ash, water, and organic content of pig enamel during calcification, J. Dent. Res. **21**:429, 1942.

Deakins, M., and Burt, R. L.: The deposition of calcium, phosphorus, and carbon dioxide in calcifying dental enamel, J. Biol. Chem. **156**:77, 1944.

Dean, H. T.: Chronic endemic dental fluorosis, J.A.M.A. **107**:1269, 1936.

Decker, J. D.: The development of a vascular supply to the rat molar enamel organ, Arch. Oral Biol. **12**:453, 1967.

Engel, M. B.: Some changes in the connective tissue ground substance associated with the eruption of the teeth, J. Dent. Res. **30**:322, 1951.

Fosse, G.: A quantitative analysis of the numerical density and distributional pattern of prisms and ameloblasts in dental enamel and tooth germs. VII. The numbers of cross-sectioned ameloblasts and prisms per unit area in tooth germs, Acta Odontol. Scand. **26**:573, 1968.

Frank, R. M., and Nalbandian, J.: Ultrastructure of amelogenesis. In Miles, A. E. W., editor: Structural and chemical organization of teeth. Vol. I, New York, 1967, Academic Press Inc.

Fearnhead, R. W.: Mineralization of rat enamel, Nature **189**:509, 1960.

Garant, P. R., and Nalbandian, J.: The fine structure of the papillary region of the mouse enamel organ, Arch. Oral Biol. **13**:1167, 1968.

Garant, P. R., and Nalbandian, J.: Observations on the ultrastructure of ameloblasts with special reference to the Golgi complex and related components, J. Ultrastruct. Res. **23**:427, 1968.

Garant, P. R., and Gillespie, R.: The presence of fenestrated capillaries in the papillary layer of the enamel organ, Anat. Rec. **163**:71, 1969.

Glick, P. L., and Eisenmann, D. R.: Electron microscopic and microradiographic investigation of a morphologic basis for the mineralization pattern in rat incisor enamel, Anat. Rec. **176**:289, 1973.

Glimcher, M. J., Friberg, V. A., and Levine, P. T.: The isolation and amino acid composition of the enamel proteins of erupted bovine teeth, Biochem. J. **93**:202, 1964.

Gustafson, A.-G.: A morphologic investigation of certain variations in the structure

and mineralization of human dental enamel, Odont. T. **67**:361, 1959.

Hals, E.: Fluorescence microscopy of developing and adult teeth, Oslo, 1953, Norwegian Academic Press.

Hammarlund-Essler, E.: A microradiographic, microphotometric and x-ray diffraction study of human developing enamel, Trans. Roy. Schools Dent., Stockholm and Umea **4**:15, 1958.

Irving, J. T.: The pattern of sudanophilia in developing rat molar enamel, Arch. Oral Biol. **18**:137, 1973.

Kallenbach, E.: Fine structure of rat incisor ameloblasts during enamel maturation, J. Ultrastruct. Res. **22**:90, 1968.

Kallenbach, E.: The fine structure of Tomes' process of rat incisor ameloblasts and its relationship to the elaboration of enamel, Tissue and Cell **5**:501, 1973.

Kallenbach, E.: Fine structure of rat incisor ameloblasts in transition between enamel secretion and maturation stages, Tissue and Cell **6**:173, 1974.

Kreshover, S. J., and Hancock, J. A., Jr.: The pathogenesis of abnormal enamel formation in rabbits inoculated with vaccinia, J. Dent. Res. **35**:685, 1936.

Listgarten, M. A.: Phase-contrast and electron microscopic study of the junction between reduced enamel epithelium and enamel in unerupted human teeth, Arch. Oral Biol. **11**:99, 1966.

Matthiessen, M. E., and Møllgard, K.: Cell junctions of the human enamel organ, Z. Zellforsch. Mikrosk. Anat. **146**:69, 1973.

Morningstar, C. H.: Effect of infection of the deciduous molar on the permanent tooth germ, J. Am. Dent. Assoc. **24**:786, 1937.

Nylen, M. U., and Scott, D. B.: An electron microscopic study of the early stages of dentinogenesis, Pub. 613, U.S. Public Health Service, Washington, D.C., 1958, U.S. Government Printing Office.

Nylen, M. U., and Scott, D. B.: Electron microscopic studies of odontogenesis, J. Indiana State Dent. Assoc. **39**:406, 1960.

Nylen, M. U., Eanes, E. D., and Omnell, K.-Å.: Crystal growth in rat enamel, J. Cell. Biol. **18**:109, 1963.

Orban, B., Sicher, H., and Weinmann, J. P.: Amelogenesis (a critique and a new concept), J. Am. Coll. Dent. **10**:13, 1943.

Osborn, J. W.: The mechanism of ameloblast

movement: A hypothesis, Calc. Tissue Res. 5:344, 1970.

Pannese, E.: Observations on the ultrastructure of the enamel organ. I. Stellate reticulum and stratum intermedium, J. Ultrastruct. Res. 4:372, 1960.

Pannese, E.: Observations on the ultrastructure of the enamel organ. II. Involution of the stellate reticulum, J. Ultrastruct. Res. 5:328, 1961.

Pannese, E.: Observations on the ultrastructure of the enamel organ. III. Internal and external enamel epithelial, J. Ultrastruct. Res. 6:186, 1962.

Reith, E. J.: The ultrastructure of ameloblasts during matrix formation and the maturation of enamel, J. Biophys. Biochem. Cytol. 9: 825, 1961.

Reith, E. J.: The ultrastructure of ameloblasts during early stages of maturation of enamel, J. Cell. Biol. 18:691, 1963.

Reith, E. J., and Butcher, E. O.: Microanatomy and histochemistry of amelogenesis. In Miles, A. E. W., editor: Structural and chemical organization of teeth. Vol. I, New York, 1967, Academic Press Inc.

Reith, E. J., and Cotty, V. F.: The absorptive activity of ameloblasts during the maturation of enamel, Anat. Rec. 157:577, 1967.

Reith, E. J., and Ross, M. H.: Morphological evidence for the presence of contractile elements in secretory ameloblasts of the rat, Arch. Oral Biol. 18:445, 1973.

Rönnholm, E.: An electron microscopic study of the amelogenesis in human teeth. I. The fine structure of the ameloblasts, J. Ultrastruct. Res. 6:229, 1962.

Rönnholm, E.: The amelogenesis of human teeth as revealed by electron microscopy. II. The development of the enamel crystallites, J. Ultrastruct. Res. 6:249, 1962.

Rönnholm, E.: The amelogenesis of human teeth as revealed by electron microscopy. III. The structure of the organic stroma of human enamel during amelogenesis, J. Ultrastruct. Res. 6:368, 1962.

Sarnat, B. G., and Schour, I.: Enamel hypoplasia (chronologic enamel aplasia) in relation to systemic disease, J. Am. Dent. Assoc. 28:1989, 1941; 29:67, 1942.

Scott, D. B., and Nylen, M. U.: Changing concepts in dental histology, Ann. New York Acad. Sci. 85:133, 1960.

Scott, D. B., and Nylen, M. U.: Organic-inorganic interrelationships in enamel and dentin—a possible key to the mechanism of caries, Int. Dent. J. 12:417, 1962.

Scott, D. B., Nylen, M. U., and Takuma, S.: Electron microscopy of developing and mature calcified tissues, Rev. Belg. Sci. Dent. 14:329, 1959.

Suga, S.: Amelogenesis—some histological and histochemical observations, Int. Dent. J. 9:394, 1959.

Travis, D. F., and Glimcher, M. J.: The structure and organization of and the relationship between the organic matrix and the inorganic crystals of embryonic bovine enamel, J. Cell. Biol. 23:447, 1964.

Ussing, M. J.: The development of the epithelial attachment, Acta Odontol. Scand. 13:123, 1955; reprinted in J. West. Soc. Periodont. 3:71, 1955.

Wasserman, F.: Analysis of the enamel formation in the continuously growing teeth of normal and vitamin C deficient guinea pigs. J. Dent. Res. 23:463, 1944.

Watson, M. L., and Avery, J. K.: The development of the hamster lower incisor as observed by electron microscopy, Am. J. Anat. 95:109, 1954.

Watson, M. L.: The extracellular nature of enamel in the rat, J. Biophys. Biochem. Cytol. 7:489, 1960.

Weber, D. F., and Eisenmann, D. R.: Microscopy of the neonatal line in developing human enamel, Am. J. Anat. 132:375, 1971.

Weinmann, J. P.: Developmental disturbances of the enamel, Bur 43:20, 1943.

Weinmann, J. P., Wessinger, G. D., and Reed, G.: Correlation of chemical and histological investigations on developing enamel, J. Dent. Res. 21:171, 1942.

Weinmann, J. P., Svoboda, J. F., and Woods, R. W.: Hereditary disturbances of enamel formation and calcification, J. Am. Dent. Assoc. 32:397, 1945.

Weinstock, A.: Matrix development in mineralizing tissues as shown by radioautography: Formation of enamel and dentin. In Slavkin, H. C., and Bavetta, L. A., editors: Developmental aspects of oral biology, New York, 1972, Academic Press Inc.

Weinstock, A., and Leblond, C. P.: Elaboration of the matrix glycoprotein of enamel by the secretory ameloblasts of the rat incisor as revealed by radioautography after galactose-[3]H injection, J. Cell Biol. 51:26, 1971.

# 4 Dentin

The dentin constitutes the bulk of the tooth. As a living tissue it consists of specialized cells, the odontoblasts, and an intercellular substance. Although the bodies of the odontoblasts are arranged on the pulpal surface of the dentin, the entire cell biologically and morphologically has to be considered the cell of the dentin. In its physical and chemical qualities the dentin closely resembles bone. The main morphologic difference between bone and dentin is that some of the osteoblasts that formed the bone become enclosed in the intercelluar substance as osteocytes, whereas the dentin contains only cytoplasmic processes of the odontoblasts.

## PHYSICAL PROPERTIES

In the teeth of young individuals the dentin usually is light yellowish in color. Unlike enamel, which is very hard and brittle, dentin is subject to slight deformation and is highly elastic. It is somewhat harder than bone but is considerably softer than enamel. The smaller content of mineral salts in dentin renders it more radiolucent than enamel.

Under polarized light, dentin exhibits a slight positive birefringence. Actually, the organic matrix fibrils are optically positive, and the inorganic crystals are optically negative. The observed birefringence represents a net effect.

## CHEMICAL COMPOSITION

Dentin consists of 30% organic matter and water and 70% inorganic material. The organic substance consists of collagenous fibrils and a ground substance of mucopolysaccharides. The inorganic component has been shown by roentgen-ray diffraction to consist of hydroxyapatite, as in bone, cementum, and enamel. Each hydroxyapatite crystal is composed of several thousand unit cells. The unit cells have a formula of $3Ca_3(PO_4)_2 \cdot Ca(OH)_2$. The crystals are described as plate shaped and are much smaller than the hydroxyapatite crystals in enamel. Dentin also contains small amounts of phosphates, carbonates, and sulfates. Organic and inorganic substances can be separated by decalcification or incineration. In the process of decalcification the organic constituents can be retained and maintain the shape of the dentin. Incineration removes the organic constitutents. The inorganic substances shrink but retain the shape of the organ and become very brittle and porous.

## STRUCTURE

Dentin is composed of a matrix of collagen fibers that are arranged in a random network. As dentin calcifies, the hydroxyapatite crystals mask the individual collagen fibers.

As indicated earlier, the bodies of the odontoblasts are arranged in a layer on the pulpal surface of the dentin, and only their cytoplasmic processes are embedded in the mineralized matrix. Each cell gives rise to one process, which

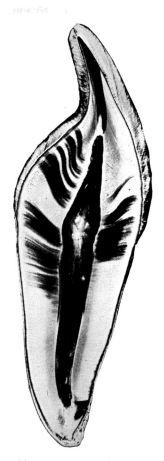

**Fig. 4-1.** Ground section of human incisor. Observe course of dentinal tubules.

traverses the predentin and calcified dentin to terminate in a branching network at the junction with enamel or cementum. Tubules are found throughout normal dentin and are therefore a characteristic of it.

**Dentinal tubules.** The course of the dentinal tubules is somewhat curved and resembles an S in shape (Fig. 4-1). Starting at right angles from the pulpal surface, the first convexity of this doubly curved course is directed toward the apex of the tooth. In the root and in the area of incisal edges and cusps the tubules are almost straight. Over their entire lengths the tubules exhibit minute, relatively regular secondary curvatures that are sinusoid in shape.

The ratio between surface areas at the outside and inside of the dentin is about 5:1. Accordingly, the tubules are farther apart in the peripheral layers and are more closely packed near the pulp (Fig. 4-4). In addition, they are wider near the pulpal cavity (3 to 4 microns) and became narrower at their outer ends (1 micron). The ratio between the numbers of tubules per unit area on the pulpal and outer surfaces of the dentin is about 4:1. Near the pulpal surface of the dentin the number per square millimeter is said to vary between 30,000 and

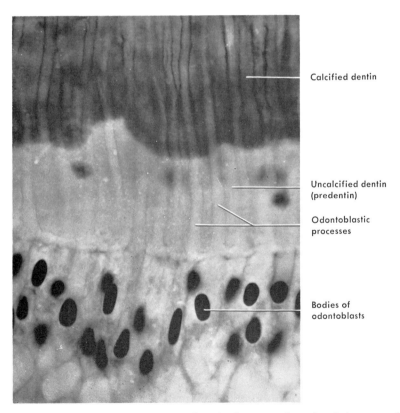

Calcified dentin

Uncalcified dentin (predentin)

Odontoblastic processes

Bodies of odontoblasts

**Fig. 4-2.** Odontoblastic processes (Tomes' fibers), lying in detinal tubules, extend from perikaryon of odontoblasts into dentin.

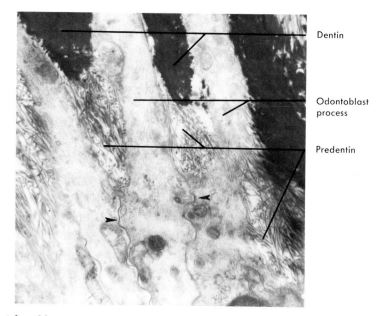

Dentin

Odontoblast
process

Predentin

**Fig. 4-3.** Odontoblast processes coursing from odontoblasts below through the predentin into the dentin above. Observe the fine filaments that comprise cytoskeleton of processes. Tight junctions join adjacent odontoblasts. *Arrows*, Tight junctions. (×12,000.)

75,000. There are more tubules per unit area in the crown than in the root. The dentinal tubules have lateral branches throughout dentin, which are termed canaliculi. These canaliculi are 1 micron or less in diameter and originate more or less at right angles to the main tubule (Fig. 4-6).

*Odontoblastic processes.* The odontoblastic processes are cytoplasmic extensions of the odontoblasts (Figs. 4-2 and 4-3) occupying a space in the dentin matrix known as the dentinal tubules (Fig. 4-4). The processes are larger near the junction with the cell body of the odontoblast (Fig. 4-3). The cytoplasmic contents of the process are sparse; the predominant structures include microtubules of 200 to 250 Å diameter and filaments of 50 to 75 Å diameter (Fig. 4-3). Other contents include an occasional mitochondrion, some dense bodies resembling lysosomes, coated vesicles that may open to the extracellular space, and microvesicles. There is a conspicuous absence of ribosomes and endoplasmic reticulum.

The odontoblastic processes divide near their ends near the dentinoenamel junction into several terminal branches (Fig. 4-5). Along their course from the pulp to the periphery they send out thin secondary processes enclosed in fine tubules, which seem to unite with similar lateral extensions from neighboring odontoblastic processes (Fig. 4-6). These may be compared to the anastomosing processes of osteocytes. Some terminal branches of the odontoblastic processes extend a short distance into the enamel (Chapter 3). Occasionally a process splits

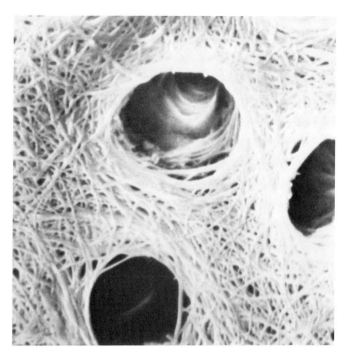

**Fig. 4-4.** Scanning electron microscope picture of pulpal surface of dentin illustrating random arrangement of calcifying collagen fibers of matrix and surrounding dentinal tubules. Organic material removed by ethylene diamine treatment. (×15,000.) (Courtesy A. Boyde, London, England.)

into two almost equally thick branches. This division can occur at any distance from the pulp (Fig. 4-7). In reality, all these divisions of the cell processes are developed during dentinogenesis, as the odontoblasts recede from the dentino-enamel or dentinocemental junction. In electron micrographs, the branches of the odontoblastic processes can be readily seen (Fig. 4-10).

*Peritubular dentin.* The structural interrelations in dentin are visualized best in cross sections. When undemineralized ground sections are observed by transmitted light, a ring-shaped transparent zone surrounding the odontoblastic process can be differentiated from the remaining darker matrix (Fig. 4-8, *A*). This transparent zone, which forms the wall of the dentinal tubule, has been termed peritubular dentin, and the regions external to it, intertubular dentin. Studies with soft roentgen rays and with the electron microscope have shown convincingly that the peritubular dentin is more highly mineralized than the intertubular dentin (Figs. 4-8, *B*, and 4-10). A very delicate organic matrix has been demonstrated in the peritubular dentin (Fig. 4-8, *B*), but this usually is lost in demineralized sections, and then the odontoblastic process appears to be surrounded by an empty space.

The interface between the peritubular and the intertubular dentin stands out

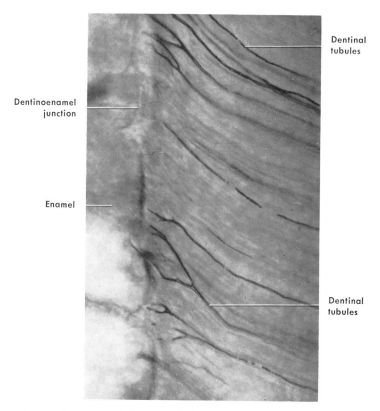

Fig. 4-5. Branching of dentinal tubules close to dentinoenamel junction.

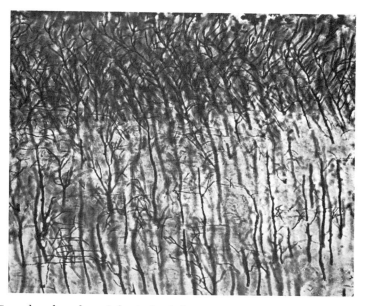

Fig. 4-6. Secondary branches of dentinal tubules anastomosing with those of neighboring as well as distant tubules. (Courtesy Dr. Gerrit Bevelander, Houston, Texas.)

Enamel

Terminal branches
of dentinal
tubules

Splitting of
dentinal
tubules

Splitting of
dentinal
tubules

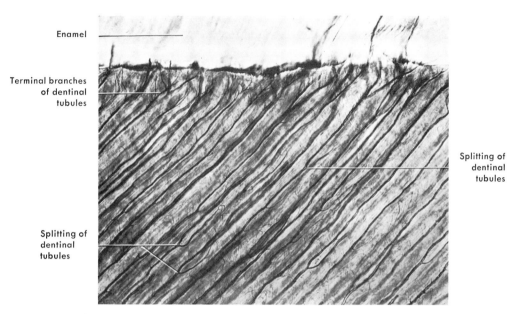

**Fig. 4-7.** Splitting of dentinal tubules into branches. (Courtesy Dr. Gerrit Bevelander, Houston, Texas.)

Peritubular
dentin
Odontoblastic
process

Peritubular
dentin

Odontoblastic
process

A

B

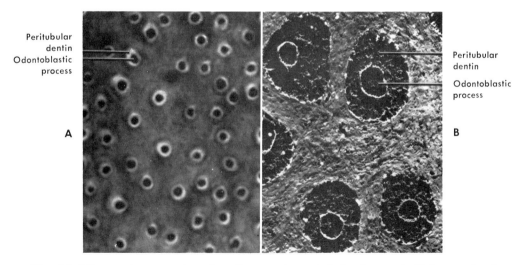

**Fig. 4-8.** Microscopic preparations that illustrate the peritubular dentin. **A,** Undemineralized ground section photographed by transmitted light. Peritubular zone appears translucent. **B,** Electron photomicrograph of demineralized section of dentin. Organic matrix in peritubular zone is comparatively sparse. (**A,** ×1000; **B,** ×5000.)

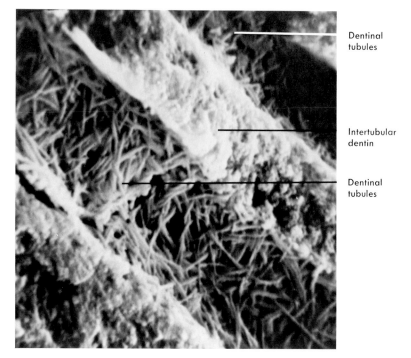

Dentinal
tubules

Intertubular
dentin

Dentinal
tubules

**Fig. 4-9.** Dentinal tubule representative of young dentin as revealed by scanning electron microscope. Collagen fibers are evident, composing the walls of dentin tubules. (×18,000.) (Courtesy A. Boyde, London, England. From Beitr. Elektromikroskop Direktabb. Oberfl. 1[S]:213-222, 1968, Münster, Germany.)

very clearly in ground sections (Fig. 4-8, *A*), and in earlier years investigators believed that this sharply defined boundary was attributable to a special structure known as the sheath of Neumann. Electron microscopic studies have so far failed to confirm the presence of such a sheath. On the contrary, the organic fibrils of the peritubular dentin appear to intermix with the fibrils of the intertubular dentin (Fig. 4-9). Differences in staining reactions between the boundary area and the dentin on either side indicate, however, that this boundary area does have special properties, although its true nature is not understood.

*Intertubular dentin.* The main body of the dentin is composed of intertubular dentin. Although it is highly mineralized, over one half of its volume is taken up by the organic matrix. This matrix consists of large numbers of collagen fibrils enveloped in an amorphous ground substance (Figs. 4-11 and 4-12, *A*). The fibrils are from 0.05 to 0.2 micron in diameter, and they show the crossbanding at 640 Å intervals, which is typical of collagen (Fig. 4-12, *B*). They are quite densely packed together, often in the form of bundles, and they run in random fashion to the dentin surface and around the tubules (Figs. 4-11 and 4-12, *A*). The external, first-formed portions of the dentin beneath both the enamel and the cementum contain variable amounts of coarse fibril bundles, which are arranged

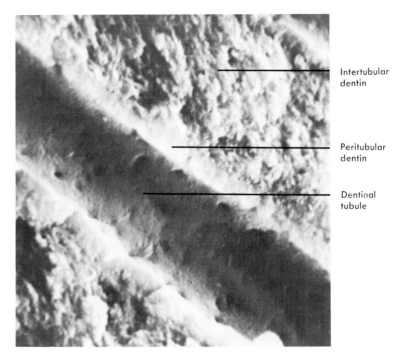

Intertubular
dentin

Peritubular
dentin

Dentinal
tubule

**Fig. 4-10.** Dentinal tubule in calcified dentin viewed by scanning electron microscope. Collagen fibers in tubule wall are masked. Observe the numerous side branches (canaliculi) of dentinal tubule. (×15,000.) (Courtesy A. Boyde, London, England. From Beitr. Elektromikroskop Direktabb. Oberfl. 1[S]:213-222, 1968, Münster, Germany.)

at right angles to the dentinal surface and give the layer a different microscopic appearance. This is called *mantle dentin.* The subsequently formed main portion is known as *circumpulpal dentin.*

*Mineral component.* Roentgen-ray diffraction studies have shown that the apatite crystals that comprise the mineral component of dentin have average lengths of about 0.04 micron. Because of their minuteness and the masking effect of the organic elements, microscopically, the crystals have been very difficult to discern in mature dentin. When they have been observed under the electron microscope, they have appeared as flat platelets up to 0.1 micron long.

The orientation of dentin crystallites appears to follow the collagen fibers. In areas of calcification defects such as those seen in dentinogenesis imperfecta, the collagen matrix is clearly discernible within the calcified dentin (Fig. 4-13).

The apatite crystals of dentin resemble those found in bone and cementum. They are considerably different from the enamel crystallites only in size (Fig. 4-14).

Polarized light studies have shown that the mineralization of dentin is largely the result of crystallization within and between the collagen fibrils. Electron microscopic investigations have shown that the fibrils themselves mineralize.

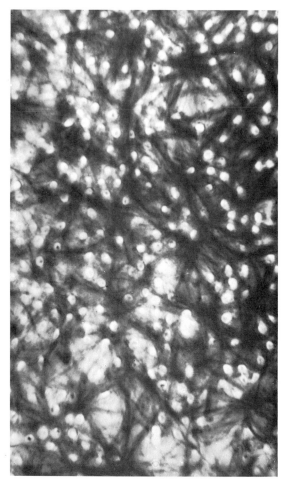

**Fig. 4-11.** Collagenous fibrils of dentin (decalcified transverse section; Mallory-Azan). (From Orban, B.: J. Am. Dent. Assoc. **16:**1547, 1929.)

Within and around individual collagen fibrils, the crystals appear to be oriented with their long axes paralleling the fibril direction. Since the fibrils form a network, the overall distribution pattern of the crystals in dentin is far more complex than in enamel.

*Incremental lines.* The imbrication or incremental lines of von Ebner appear as fine lines, which in cross sections run at right angles to the dentinal tubules (Fig. 4-15). They correspond to the Retzius lines in the enamel and likewise reflect variations in structure and mineralization during formation of the dentin. The course of the lines indicates the growth pattern of the dentin. The distance between the lines corresponds to the daily rate of apposition. In the crown it varies from 4 to 8 microns and becomes decreasingly less in the root (Fig. 4-16).

Occasionally some of the incremental lines are accentuated because of distur-

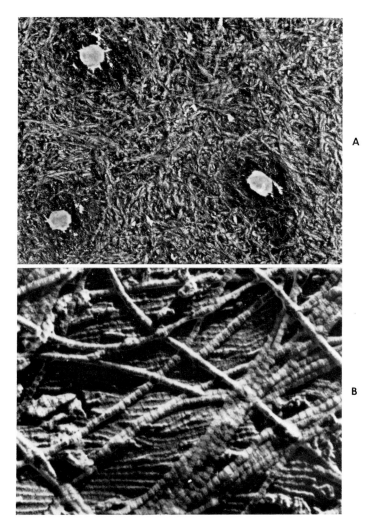

**Fig. 4-12. A,** Cross section of undecalcified human dentin showing crisscross arrangement of collagenous matrix fibrils. Also note densely calcified peritubular dentin. (Electron photomicrograph; ×9000.) **B,** Fibrils of intertubular matrix at higher magnification showing typical crossbanding of collagen. (Electron photomicrograph; ×40,000.)

bances in the mineralization process. Such lines, readily demonstrated in ground sections, are known as the contour lines of Owen (Fig. 4-17). Studies with soft roentgen rays have shown that these lines represent hypocalcified bands.

In the deciduous teeth and in the first permanent molars, where the dentin is formed partly before and partly after birth, the prenatal and postnatal dentins are separated by an accentuated contour line, the so-called *neonatal line* (Fig. 4-18). This line is the result of incomplete calcification and represents the abrupt changes in environment and nutrition that occur at birth.

***Interglobular dentin.*** Mineralization of the dentin sometimes begins in small

*Text continued on p. 120.*

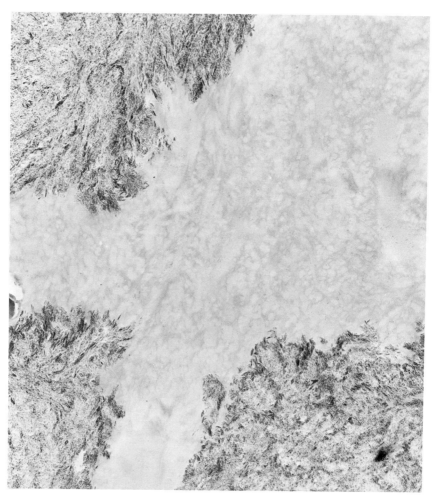

**Fig. 4-13.** Globular area in dentin of a patient with dentinogenesis imperfecta. Collagen fibers are seen in central area and are surrounded by fully calcified dentin. (Electron photomicrograph; ×20,000.)

Enamel

Dentin

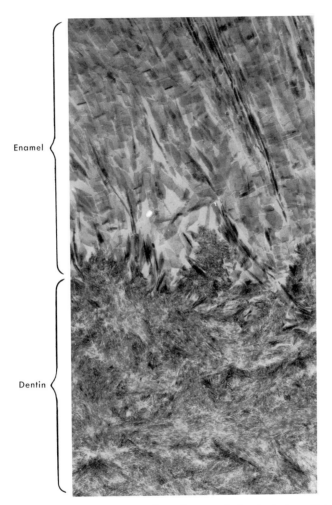

**Fig. 4-14.** Dentinoenamel junction. Enamel is above and dentin below. Note difference in size and orientation between crystallites of enamel and dentin. (Electron microphotograph; ×35,000.)

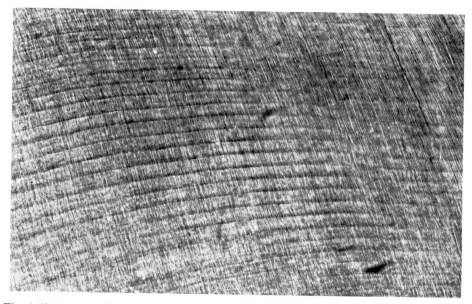

**Fig. 4-15.** Incremental lines in dentin. Imbrication or incremental lines of von Ebner. Ground section.

**Fig. 4-16.** Diagram of incremental, appositional pattern (upper deciduous central incisor). *5 m.i.u.* 5 months in utero. (From Schour, I., and Massler, M.: J. Am. Dent. Assoc. **23:**1946, 1936.)

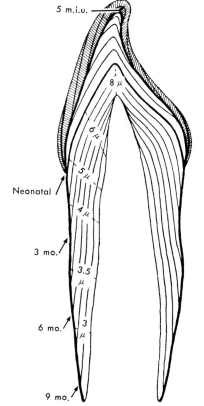

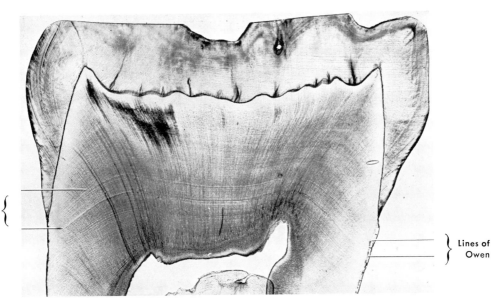

Lines of
Owen {

} Lines of
Owen

Fig. 4-17. Accentuated incremental lines in dentin: contour lines of Owen.

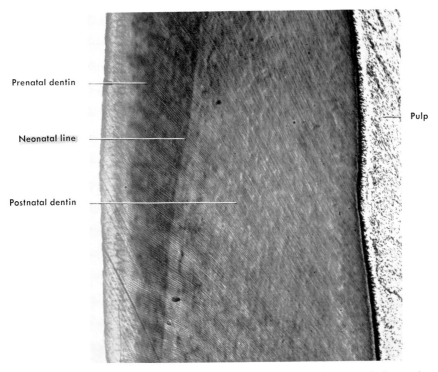

Prenatal dentin

Neonatal line

Postnatal dentin

Pulp

Fig. 4-18. Postnatally formed dentin is separated from prenatally formed dentin by accentuated incremental line, the neonatal line. (From Schour, I., and Poncher, H. G.: Am. J. Dis. Child. **54**:757, 1937.)

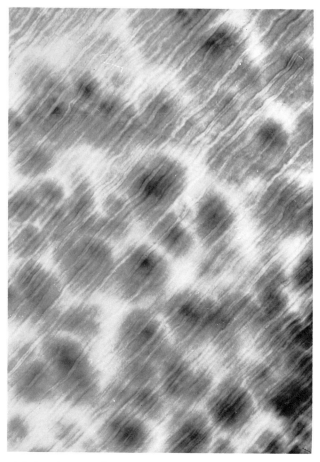

Fig. 4-19. Interglobular dentin (decalcified section). Dentinal tubules pass uninterrupted through uncalcified and hypocalcified areas.

globular areas that normally fuse to form a uniformly calcified dentin layer (see discussion of dentinogenesis). If fusion does not take place, unmineralized or hypomineralized regions remain between the globules. These are termed interglobular dentin. The dentinal tubules pass uninterrupted through the uncalcified areas (Fig. 4-19). Interglobular dentin is found chiefly in the crown, near the dentinoenamel junction, and it follows the incremental pattern of the tooth.

In dry ground sections the interglobular dentin is sometimes lost and replaced by air. Then the interglobular "spaces" appear black (Fig. 4-20).

*Tomes' granular layer.* In the ground sections a thin layer of dentin adjacent to the cementum almost invariably appears granular (Fig. 4-21). This is known as Tomes' granular layer, and it is believed to be made up of minute areas of interglobular dentin. The configuration is found only in the root, and it does not follow the incremental pattern. It is believed to represent an interference with

Dentinoenamel
junction      Enamel

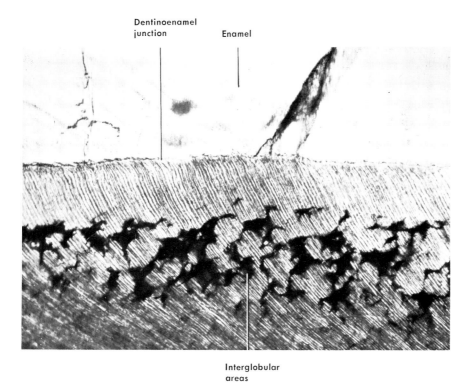

Interglobular
areas

**Fig. 4-20.** Interglobular dentin as seen in dry ground section. Interglobular areas are filled with air and appear black in transmitted light. (Courtesy Dr. Gerrit Bevelander, Houston, Texas.)

mineralization of the entire surface layer of the root dentin prior to the beginning of cementum formation. Recent evidence indicates that the granular layer of dentin underlying the cementum may result from the looping of the terminal portions of the dentinal tubules. This would be the result of a slightly different orientation of the odontoblast process in the initial stages of root dentin formation as compared to that adjacent to the enamel.

## INNERVATION

Despite the obvious clinical observation that dentin is highly sensitive to a diversity of stimuli, the anatomic basis for this sensitivity is still controversial. The literature contains many accounts of the presence of nerve fibers and nerve endings in the dentinal tubules. Most nerve endings in the dentin are found in the tubules of the predentin and inner dentin. None have been found at the dentinoenamel junction. Pain perceived at this location must be explained on another basis than nerve endings. Either movement of the odontoblast process activating the endings in inner dentin or conduction by the odontoblast processes to these endings have both been presented as possible explanations of pain trans-

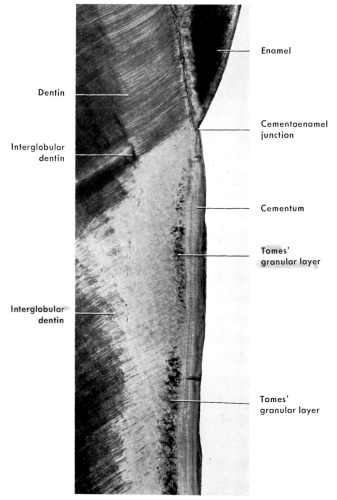

Fig. 4-21. Tomes' granular layer lies in the peripheral zone of the root dentin. Ground section.

mission in dentin. The endings in the tubules appear as oval or elongated bodies containing vesicles and mitochondria (Fig. 4-22).

The pulp contains numerous unmyelinated and myelinated nerve fibers. Some of the former end on pulpal blood vessels, but they both can be followed into the subodontoblastic layer. Here they lose their myelin sheath and can be followed into the odontoblastic layer itself. In this layer many of the fibers apparently end in contact with the cell body or perikaryon of the odontoblasts. Some of the nerve fibers or endings are found in the predentin or the dentin tubules. Some of the small unmyelinated nerve fibers or terminals found in close contact with the odontoblastic process may be adrenergic in nature. It is theorized that these may function in reparative dentin formation and not in pain transmission. Most end-

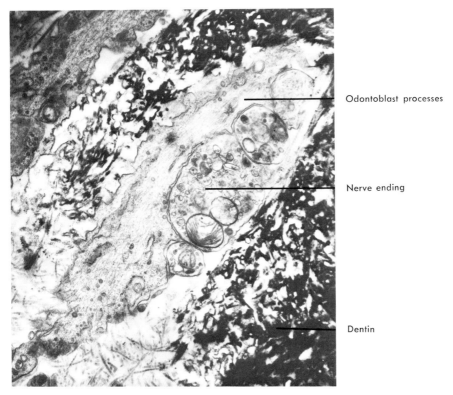

Odontoblast processes

Nerve ending

Dentin

**Fig. 4-22.** Nerve ending in dentinal tubule. This vesiculated ending is located at the pre-dentin-dentin junction. Vesicles contain neurotransmitter substance. Mitochondria are also seen in these terminals. (×18,000.)

ings are likely terminal processes of the myelinated nerve fibers of the dental pulp concerned with pain sensation in the dentin. The myelinated nerve fibers of the pulp continue as small unmyelinated branches and terminate adjacent to the cell bodies of the odontoblasts (Chapter 5).

## AGE AND FUNCTIONAL CHANGES

*Vitality of dentin.* Since the odontoblast, as well as its process, is an integral part of the dentin, there is no doubt that dentin is a vital tissue. Also, if vitality is understood to be the capacity of the tissue to react to physiologic and patho-logic stimuli, dentin must be considered a vital tissue. Dentin is laid down throughout life, although after the teeth have erupted and have been in function for a short time, dentinogenesis slows and further dentin formation is at a much slower pace. Some authors describe this later-formed dentin as *secondary dentin* (Fig. 4-23).

Pathologic effects of dental caries abrasion, attrition, or cutting of dentin by operative procedures causes changes in dentin. These are described as develop-

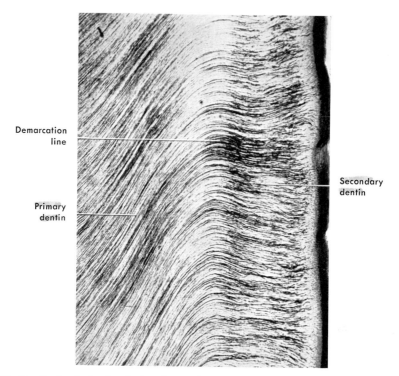

Demarcation
line

Secondary
dentin

Primary
dentin

**Fig. 4-23.** Dentinal tubules bend sharply as they pass from primary into secondary dentin. Dentinal tubules are somewhat irregular in secondary dentin. Ground section. Pulpal surface at right.

ment of *dead tracts, sclerosis,* or addition of *reparative dentin.* The formation of reparative dentin pulpally underlying an area of injured odontoblast processes can be explained on the basis of increased dentinogenic activity of the odontoblasts. The mechanisms by which dentin is altered by means of dead tracts or sclerosis are not fully understood. These will now be discussed.

*Secondary dentin.* Under normal conditions, the odontoblasts are active and formation of dentin may continue throughout life. Frequently the dentin formed in later life is separated from that previously formed by a darkly stained line. In such cases the dentinal tubules bend more or less sharply at this line (Fig. 4-23). In other cases the newly formed dentin shows irregularities of varying degree. The tubules are often wavy and less numerous for a unit area of the dentin. The dentin, forming pulpward of the line of demarcation, is called secondary dentin. This dentin is deposited on the entire pulpal surface of the dentin. However, its formation does not proceed at an even rate in all areas. This is observed best in premolars and molars, where more secondary dentin is produced on the floor and on the roof of the pulpal chamber than on the side walls (Chapter 5).

The change in the structure from primary to secondary dentin may be caused

Dentin

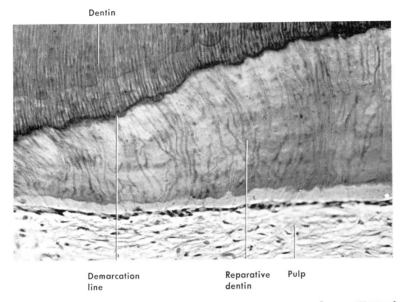

Demarcation       Reparative   Pulp
line               dentin

**Fig. 4-24.** Reparative dentin stimulated by penetration of caries into dentin. Dentinal tubules are irregular and less numerous than in regular dentin. Decalcified section.

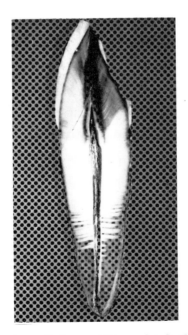

**Fig. 4-25.** Root transparency in tooth from middle-aged individual. Note glasslike character of apical dentin, which permits almost unobstructed visualization of the underlying grid. (Courtesy Dr. A. E. W. Miles.)

by the progressive crowding of the odontoblasts, which finally leads to the elimination of some and to the rearrangement of the remaining odontoblasts.

*Reparative dentin.* If, by extensive wear, erosion, caries, or operative procedures, odontoblastic processes are exposed or cut, the entire cell is more or less severely damaged. Such damaged odontoblasts may either continue to form a hard substance or may degenerate. In the latter case they are replaced by migration to the dentinal surface of undifferentiated cells from the deeper layers of the pulp. Damaged or newly differentiated odontoblasts are stimulated to a defense reaction whereby hard tissue seals off the area of injury. This hard tissue is best called *reparative* dentin. Here the course of the tubules is frequently twisted, and their number is greatly reduced (Fig. 4-24). Some areas of reparative dentin contain few or no tubules. Dentin-forming cells are often included in the

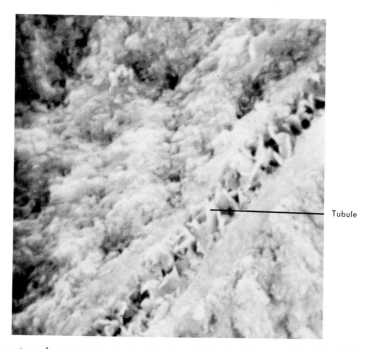

Tubule

Fig. 4-26. Scanning electron micrograph of sclerosed dentin showing thin plate-like crystals forming a delicate meshwork occluding the tubule lumen. (×9700.) (Courtesy Lester and A. Boyde. Reprinted with permission from Virchows Arch. [Zellpathol.] 344:196-212, 1968.)

Fig. 4-27. Transparent dentin under carious area viewed by, **A**, transmitted light, **B**, reflected light, and **C**, grenz rays. Normal dentinal tubules are filled with air in dried ground sections and appear dark in transmitted light, **A**, and white in reflected light, **B**. Transparent dentin shows opposite behavior because tubules are filled with calcium salts. In a grenz-ray film, **C**, transparent dentin appears more white because of its higher degree of radiopacity. (**C** courtesy Dr. E. Applebaum, New York.)

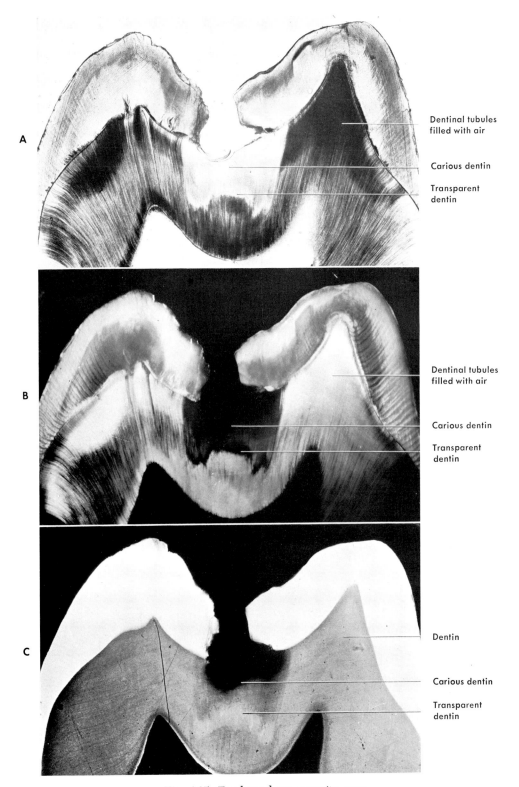

A

Dentinal tubules
filled with air

Carious dentin

Transparent
dentin

B

Dentinal tubules
filled with air

Carious dentin

Transparent
dentin

C

Dentin

Carious dentin

Transparent
dentin

Fig. 4-27. For legend see opposite page.

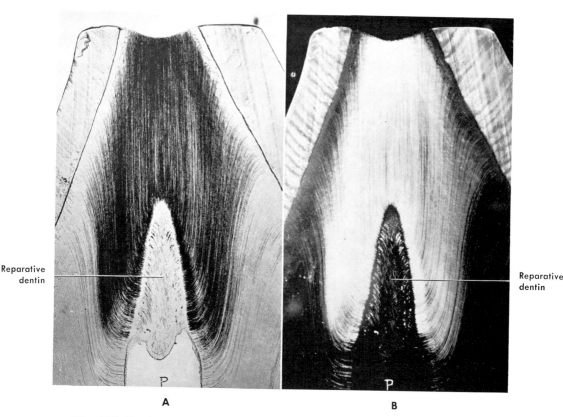

Reparative dentin

Reparative dentin

A

B

Fig. 4-28. Dead tracts in the dentin of a vital tooth caused by attrition and exposure of a group of dentinal tubules. Corresponding to the dead tract is reparative dentin formation. *P*, Pulp. Dead tracts appear dark in transmitted light, **A**, and white in reflected light, **B**.

rapidly produced intercellular substance. Such cells degenerate and vacate the spaces that they formerly occupied. Frequently reparative dentin is separated from primary or secondary dentin by a deeply staining line.

*Transparent (sclerotic) dentin.* Stimuli of a different nature not only induce additional formation of reparative dentin but also lead to changes in the dentin itself. Calcium salts may be deposited in or around degenerating odontoblastic processes and may obliterate the tubules. The refractive indices of dentin in which the tubules are occluded are equalized, and such areas become transparent. Transparent dentin can be observed in the teeth of elderly people, especially in the roots (Fig. 4-25). On the other hand, zones of transparent dentin develop around the dentinal part of type B enamel lamellae (see Fig. 3-28) and under slowly progressing caries (Fig. 4-27). In such cases the blocking of the tubules may be considered a defensive reaction of the dentin. Roentgen-ray absorption tests and permeability studies have shown that such areas are denser, and hardness tests have demonstrated that they are harder than normal dentin.

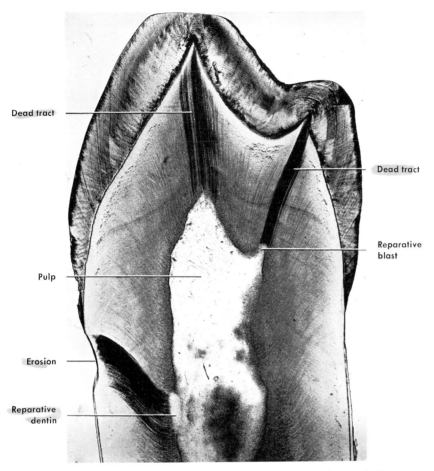

Fig. 4-29. Dead tracts in dentin of a vital tooth caused by crowding and degeneration of odontoblasts in narrow pulpal horns and exposure of dentinal tubules in erosion.

Transparent dentin can be demonstrated in ground sections or scanning electron micrographs (Fig. 4-26). It appears light in transmitted (Fig. 4-27, *A*) and dark in reflected light (Fig. 4-27, *B*) because the light passes through the transparent dentin but is reflected from the normal dentin. Dentin decalcified by caries, normal dentin, and transparent dentin can be differentiated by the examination of ground sections with soft roentgen rays—grenz rays (Fig. 4-27, *C*).

*Dead tracts.* In dried ground sections of normal dentin the odontoblastic processes disintegrate, and the empty tubules are filled with air. They appear black in transmitted and white in reflected light (Fig. 4-28). Disintergration of odontoblastic processes may also occur in teeth containing a vital pulp as a result of such injuries as caries, attrition, abrasion, cavity preparation, or erosion (Figs. 4-28 and 4-29). Their degeneration is often observed in the narrow pulpal horns (Fig. 4-29) because of crowding of odontoblasts. Reparative dentin seals these tubules at their pulpal end. In all these cases dentinal tubules are filled with gaseous substances. In ground sections such groups of tubules appear black in transmitted and white in reflected light. Dentin areas characterized by degenerated odontoblastic processes have been called dead tracts. These areas demonstrate decreased sensitivity.

## DEVELOPMENT

*Life cycle of odontoblasts.* The odontoblasts, which have been described previously in this chapter as integral parts of mature dentin structure, are highly specialized connective tissue cells that differentiate from the peripheral cellular layer of the dental papilla. Prior to differentiation of the odontoblasts, the inner enamel epithelium is separated from the dental papilla by a very thin, continuous basement membrane. The cells of the papilla are spindle shaped, relatively uniform in size, and generally separated by rather large intercellular spaces. Some of the cells, however, come into contact with each other and with the basement membrane. At the beginning of differentiation, which takes place only in the presence of the inner enamel epithelium, the peripheral cells of the dental papilla assume a short columnar shape and become aligned in a single layer along the basement membrane. The nuclei are already basally situated at this early stage in odontoblast formation, and they remain in this position permanently. The distal ends of the cells are villose, and several projections from each cell extend to the basement membrane. As differentiation progresses, the cells grow to several times their original length, appearing columnar in shape, whereas their width remains quite constant. Concomitantly, pronounced changes occur in the cytoplasm of the odontoblasts. These take the form of sharp increases in the concentration of organelles, granular components, and globular elements (Fig. 4-30). It is currently believed that such cytoplasmic alterations reflect a rise in cellular activity. This is taken as evidence that the odontoblasts participate actively in the formation of the dentinal matrix, a concept that has found additional support in histochemical and isotope studies.

With the use of radiolabeled proline and electron microscopy, protein synthesis has been demonstrated to occur in these cells. Proline first appeared in the endoplasmic reticulum and Golgi apparatus of the odontoblasts. It then appeared to migrate from the Golgi zone to the odontoblastic process in the form of dense granules, which then emptied into the extracellular collagenous matrix.

The odontoblasts begin to recede from the basement membrane with the formation of the first dentin layer, and their distal ends become funnel shaped. As more dentin is laid down, the cells continue to draw back, so that they are always located in a layer along the pulpal surface of the most recently formed predentin. As a cell recedes, it leaves behind a single extension, the odontoblastic process, which becomes enclosed in a tubule. As matrix formation continues, the odontoblast process lengthens, as does the dentinal tubule.

The fully differentiated odontoblast cell bodies decrease slightly in size dur-

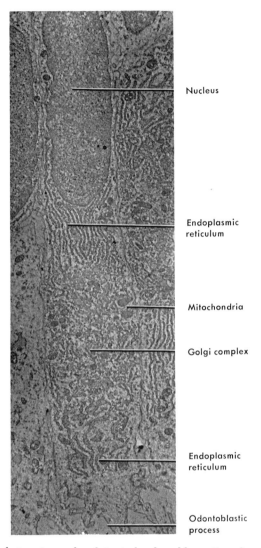

Nucleus

Endoplasmic
reticulum

Mitochondria

Golgi complex

Endoplasmic
reticulum

Odontoblastic
process

**Fig. 4-30.** Electron photomcirograph of typical odontoblast. Cytoplasm resembles that of ameloblasts, except that mitochondria are scattered throughout cell and there are fewer granules and vacuoles. (×7000.)

ing further dentin formation but otherwise retain their structural characteristics throughout life. The cell process continues to lengthen as long as dentin matrix is formed. At this point the odontoblasts enter a quiescent state. Unless they are stimulated by external influences to produce reparative dentin, their activity is restricted to an ordinary very slow formation of secondary dentin.

*Dentinogenesis.* Dentinogenesis takes place in a two-phase sequence, the first of which is the elaboration of an uncalcified organic matrix called predentin. The second phase, mineralization, does not begin until a fairly wide band of predentin has been laid down. Mineralization proceeds at a rate that roughly

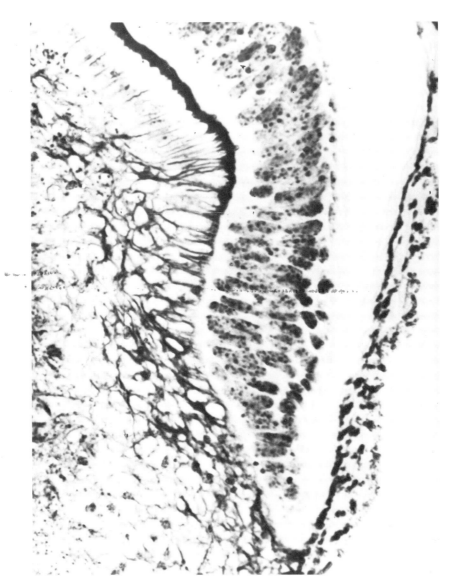

**Fig. 4-31.** Cervical loop region showing presence and distribution of Korff's fibers. In the area of odontoblast differentiation below and in early dentinogenesis, fanning of the silver-stained collagen fibers is seen. As dentinogenesis proceeds above, the intercellular location of collagen fibers decreases. (Bulk impregnated with silver and Epon-embedded; ×1050.) (Courtesy Ten Cate, A. R., Melcher, A. H., Pudy, G., and Wagner, D.: Anat. Rec. 168[4]: 491-523, 1970.)

parallels that of matrix formation. Thus, until the matrix is completed, the width of the predentin layer remains relatively constant.

The formation and calcification of dentin begin at the tips of the cusps or incisal edges and proceed inward by a rhythmic apposition of conic layers, one within the other. When the dentin of the crown has been laid down, the apical layers assume the shape of elongated, truncated cones (Fig. 4-16). With completion of the root dentin, primary dentin formation comes to an end.

*Predentin formation.* The first sign of predentin development is the appearance of bundles of fibrils between the differentiating odontoblasts (Figs. 4-31 and 4-32). Near the basement membrane, where the cells are now funnel shaped, the fibrils diverge in a fanlike arrangement (Figs. 4-31 and 4-32, *A*). These fibrillar bundles are known as Korff's fibers, and their origin and role in dentinogenesis have been the subject of much discussion. Because they stain black with silver (argyrophil reaction), it was concluded that they are precollagenous, but more recent studies with the electron microscope have revealed that at their first appearance the fibrils already demonstrate all the structural characteristics of collagen itself (Fig. 4-32, *B*). Collagen first appears as straight fibers, 200 Å wide, between odontoblast cell bodies and processes. In more mature regions of the predentin the larger diameter collagen exhibiting the typical 640 Å crossbanding is seen.

Korff's fibers are a major constituent of the first-formed matrix because of the fanlike arrangement of the fibrils near the basement membrane. This relatively narrow layer comprises the mantle predentin. In addition to Korff's fibers, with

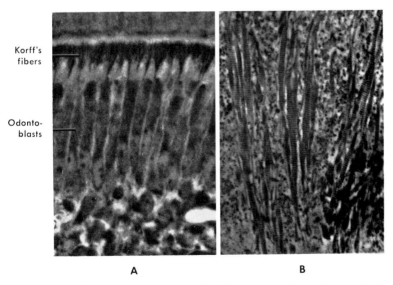

Korff's
fibers

Odonto-
blasts

**A**                    **B**

Fig. 4-32. **A**, Fanlike arrangement of Korff's fibers in mantle predentin. **B**, Electron photomicrograph showing at higher magnification the fibrils making up Korff's fibers. Note crossbandings that identify these fibrils as collagen. (×10,000.)

fibrils from 0.1 to 0.2 micron in diameter, the remainder of the mantel predentin is made up of smaller collagen fibrils, around 0.05 micron in diameter. The latter fibrils, which form a network, predominate throughout all the succeeding circumpulpal predentin layers, whereas Korff's fibers, now compact bundles of parallel fibrils, become a minor component (Fig. 4-33, *B*).

Electron microscope studies have shown that the smaller collagen fibrils of

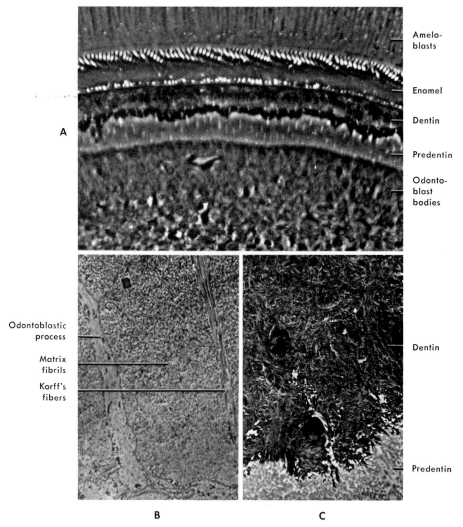

Fig. 4-33. **A,** Predentin and dentin layers in a developing rodent tooth, as seen by phase contrast. Observe the relations of all the layers of the odontogenic complex, from amelobasts to odontoblasts. (×350.) **B,** Circumpulpal predentin layer, as seen under electron microscope. Note odontoblastic process, compact Korff's fiber bundles, and network of fine matrix fibrils. (×6000.) **C,** Dentin layer, as seen under electron microscope. Note the increased density in contrast to the predentin as a result of mineralization. (×6000.)

the predentin are formed in the immediate vicinity of the distal ends of the odontoblasts. This finding is in agreement with the general concept that collagen fibril synthesis in connective tissues takes place through the extracellular aggregation of molecules secreted by fibril-forming cells.

*Mineralization.* After several microns of predentin have been laid down, mineralization of the layers closest to the dentinoenamel junction begins in small islands that subsequently fuse and form a continuous, calcified layer. With further predentin formation, mineralization usually advances pulpward as a linear front roughly paralleling the odontoblastic layer (Fig. 4-33, *A* and *C*). Sometimes advancing mineralization occurs, however, in globular areas that subsequently fuse (Fig. 4-34).

Inception and advance of mineralization are accompanied by a number of changes in the ground substance of the organic matrix. Histochemical and radioautographic investigations show that a mucopolysaccharide is present in the matrix and that it beomes especially prominent in the peritubular areas.

The phenomena actually involved in mineralization within collagenous matrices are still under investigation. There seems to be little doubt that the muco-

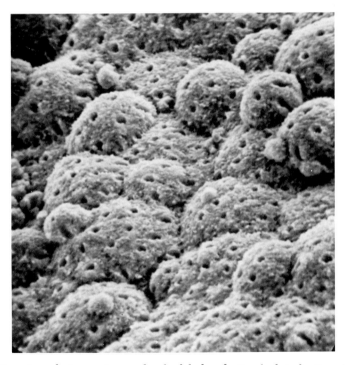

**Fig. 4-34.** Scanning electron micrograph of globular dentin (calcospherite mineralization) formation at predentin-forming front. Later-forming dentin may be linear, causing interglobular spaces to appear among earlier-formed globular dentin. Treated with ethylene diamine to remove organic material. (Courtesy A. Boyde, London, England.)

polysaccharide ground substane plays a most important part in mineralization, but it has not yet been determined if it serves to initiate or promote the process or rather to regulate it. It is likewise quite evident that the molecular configurations of the collagen fibrils influence the geometric distribution of the crystals that are laid down.

The basic mineralization sequence in dentin appears to be as follows. The earliest crystal deposition is in the form of very fine plates of hydroxyapatite on the surfaces of the collagen fibrils and in the ground substance. Subsequently, crystals seem to be laid down within the fibrils themselves. The crystals associated with the collagen fibrils are arranged in an orderly fashion, with their long axes paralleling the fibril axes, and in rows conforming to the 640 Å striation pattern. Within the globular islands of mineralization, crystal deposition appears to take place radially from common centers, in a so-called spherulite form.

The general calcification process is gradual, but the peritubular region becomes highly mineralized at a very early stage (Fig. 4-10). Although there is obviously some crystal growth as dentin matures, the ultimate crystal size remains very small, with the greatest length being on the order of 0.1 micron.

## CLINICAL CONSIDERATIONS

The cells of the exposed dentin should not be insulted by strong drugs, undue operative trauma, unnecessary thermal changes, or irritating filling materials. One should bear in mind that when 1 mm.$^2$ of dentin is exposed, about 30,000 odontoblastic processes are exposed and thus 30,000 living cells are damaged. It is advisable to cover the exposed dentin surface with a nonirritating insulating substance.

The rapid penetration and spreading of caries in the dentin are the result of the high content of organic substances in the dentin matrix. The enamel may be undermined at the dentinoenamel junction, even when caries in the enamel are confined to a small area. The dentinal tubules form a passage for invading bacteria that may thus reach the pulp through a thick dentinal layer.

Electron micrographs of carious dentin show regions of massive bacterial invasion of dentinal tubules (Fig. 4-35). The tubules appear enlarged by presence of the microorganisms. The sensitivity of the dentin varies considerably in different layers. In most cases it is greater close to the outer surface of the dentin  and diminishes in the deeper layers. The sensitivity of the dentin therefore is not a warning signal to avoid exposure of the pulp. Operations in the dentin can be rendered less painful by avoiding heat and pressure and by the use of coolants and of sharp instruments. Undue trauma from operative instruments may damage the odontoblasts. Air-driven cutting instruments and the use of air coolant cause dislodgement of the odontoblasts from the periphery of the pulp and their "aspiration" a great distance within the dentinal tubule. This may not, however, hinder the subsequent repair and secondary dentin formation, since repair prob-

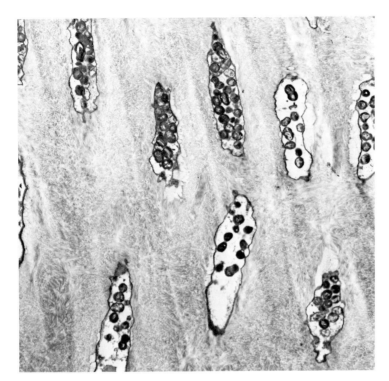

**Fig. 4-35.** Electron micrograph of dentin underlying carious lesion. Bacteria are seen filling many of the tubules. (×10,000.)

ably only requires the participation of deeper pulpal cells through mitosis and cytodifferentiation.

The sensitivity of the dentin has been explained by the hypothesis that any injury or alteration of the odontoblast leads to changes in the surface charges of the cell body and that these changes stimulate the nerve endings on these cells (Fig. 4-22 and p. 163). If this hypothesis is correct, then the greater sensitivity of the dentin near the dentinoenamel junction could be related to the branching of the odontoblastic processes in this zone and therefore to the larger surface area of exposed cytoplasm of each cell.

Because of the ability of the dentin to form throughout the life of a tooth, it is now possible to save teeth that previously were either extracted or treated by endodontic therapy. Thus teeth with deep carious lesions are treated by only partial removal of carious dentin and insertion of a "dressing" containing calcium hydroxide or zinc oxide for a period of a few weeks or months. During this period the odontoblasts form a new dentin on the pulpal side of the carious lesion and the dentist can now reopen the cavity and remove the remaining decay without endangering the pulp.

During operative procedures on the dentin, one must remember that it is a living connective tissue and therefore its dehydration must be avoided.

## REFERENCES

Anderson, D. J., and Ronning, G. A.: Dye diffusion in human dentine, Arch. Oral Biol. 7:505, 1962.

Anderson, D. J., and Ronning, G. A.: Osmotic excitants of pain in human dentine, Arch. Oral Biol. 7:513, 1962.

Applebaum, E., Hollander, F., and Bodecker, C. F.: Normal and pathological variations in calcification of teeth as shown by the use of soft x-rays, Dent. Cosmos 75:1097, 1933.

Arwill, T.: Innervation of the teeth, Stockholm, 1958, Ivar Haeggströms Boktryckeri AB.

Battistone, G. C., and Burnett, G. W.: The amino acid composition of human dentinal protein, J. Dent. Res. 35:255, 1956.

Bergman, G., and Engfeldt, B.: Studies on mineralized dental tissues. II. Microradiography as a method for studying dental tissue and its application to the study of caries, Acta Odontol. Scand. 12:99, 1954.

Bergman, G., and Engfeldt, B.: Studies on mineralized dental tissues. VI. The distribution of mineral salts in the dentine with special reference to the dentinal tubules, Acta Odontol. Scand. 13:1, 1955.

Bernick, S.: Innervation of the human tooth, Anat. Rec. 101:81, 1948.

Bevelander, G.: The development and structure of the fiber system of dentin, Anat. Rec. 81:79, 1941.

Bevelander, G., and Amler, M. H.: Radioactive phosphate absorption by dentin and enamel, J. Dent. Res. 24:45, 1944.

Bhaskar, S. N., and Lilly, G. E.: Intrapulpal temperature during cavity preparation, J. Dent. Res. 44:644, 1965.

Blake, G. C.: The peritubular translucent zones in human dentine, Br. Dent. J. 104:57, 1958.

Boyde, A., and Lester, K. S.: An electron microscope study of fractured dentinal surfaces, Calcif. Tissue Res. 1:122, 1967.

Bradford, E. W.: The interpretation of decalcified sections of human dentine, Br. Dent. J. 98:153, 1955.

Bradford, E. W.: The maturation of the dentine, Br. Dent. J. 105:212, 1958.

Bradford, E. W.: The dentine, a barrier to caries, Br. Dent. J. 109:387, 1960.

Cape, A. T., and Kitchin, P. C.: Histologic phenomena of tooth tissues as observed under polarized light, J. Am. Dent. Assoc. 17:193, 1930.

Ebner, V. von: Ueber die Entwicklung der leimgebenden Fibrillen im Zahnbein [Development of collagenous fibrils in the dentin], Sitzungsber. Akad. Wissensch. Vienna 115:281, 1906; Anat. Anz. 29:137, 1906.

Fearnhead, R. W.: Histological evidence for the innervation of human dentine, J. Anat. 91:267, 1957.

Frank, R. M.: Electron microscopy of undecalcified sections of human adult dentine, Arch. Oral Biol. 1:29, 1959.

Frank, R. M.: Étude au microscope électronique de l'odontoblaste et du canalicule dentinaire humain, Arch. Oral Biol. 11:179, 1966.

Furseth, R., and Mjör, I.: Electron microscopy of human coronal dentine. A methological study with emphasis on the "aspiration" of odontoblast nuclei, Acta Odontol. Scand. 27:577, 1969.

Harcourt, J. K.: Further observations on the peritubular translucent zone in human dentine, Aust. Dent. J. 9:387, 1964.

Hess, W. C., Leo, D. Y., and Peckham, S. C.: The lipid content of enamel and dentin, J. Dent. Res. 35:273, 1956.

Johansen, E., and Parks, H. F.: Electron microscopic observations on the three dimensional morphology of apatite crystallites of human dentine and bone, J. Biophys. Biochem. Cytol. 7:743, 1960.

Kerébel, B., and Grimbert, L.: Rôle des odontoblastes [Role of the odontoblasts], Rev. Mensuelle Suisse Odont. 68:729, 1958.

Korff, K. von: Die Entwicklung der Zahnbein Grundsubstanz der Säugetiere [The development of the dentin matrix in mammals], Arch. Mikrosk. Anat. 67:1, 1905.

Korff, K. von: Wachstum der Dentingrundsubstanz verschiedener Wirbeltiere [Growth of the dentin matrix of different vertebrates], Z. Mikrosk. Anat. Forsch. 22:445, 1930.

Kramer, I. R. H.: The distribution of collagen fibrils in the dentine matrix, Br. Dent. J. 91:1, 1951.

Jessen, H.: The ultrastructure of odontoblasts in perfusion fixed, demineralized incisors of adult rats, Acta Odontol. Scand. 25:491, 1967.

Lenz, H.: Elektronenmikroskopische Untersuchungen der Dentinentwicklung [Electron microscopic studies of dentin development], Dtsch. Zahn. Mund. Kieferheilkd. 30:367, 1959.

Lester, K. S., and Boyde, A.: Electron microscopy of predentinal surfaces, Calcif. Tissue Res. 1:44, 1967.

Lester, K. S., and Boyde, A.: Some preliminary observations on caries ("remineralization") crystals in enamel and dentine by surface electron microscopy, Virchows Arch. [Pathol. Anat.] 344:196-212, 1968.

Losee, F. L., Leopold, R. F., and Hess, W. C.: Dentinal protein, J. Dent. Res. 30:565, 1951.

Martens, P. J., Bradford, E. W., and Frank, R. M.: Tissue changes in dentine, Int. Dent. J. 9:330, 1959.

Miller, J.: The micro-radiographic appearance of dentine, Br. Dent. J. 97:72, 1954.

Muntz, J. A., Dorfman, A., and Stephan, R. M.: In vitro studies on sterilization of carious dentin, J. Am. Dent. Assoc. 30: 1893, 1943.

Nalbandian, J., Gonzales, F., and Sognnaes, R. F.: Sclerotic age changes in root dentin of human teeth as observed by optical, electron, and x-ray microscopy, J. Dent. Res. 39:598, 1960.

Noble, H., Carmichael, A., and Rankine, D.: Electron microscopy of human developing dentine, Arch. Oral Biol. 7:399, 1962.

Nylen, M. U., and Scott, D. B.: An electron microscopic study of the early stages of dentinogenesis, Pub. 613, U.S. Public Health Service, Washington, D.C., 1958, U.S. Government Printing Office.

Nylen, M. U., and Scott, D. B.: Basic studies in calcification, J. Dent. Med. 15:80, 1960.

Orban, B.: The development of the dentin, J. Am. Dent. Assoc. 16:1547, 1929.

Piez, K. A., and Likens, R. C.: The nature of collagen. II. Vertebrate collagens. In Sognnaes, R. F., editor: Calcification in biological systems, Washington, D.C., 1960, American Association for the Advancement of Science.

Powers, M. M.: The staining of nerve fibers in teeth, J. Dent. Res. 31:383, 1952.

Schmidt, W. J., and Keil, A.: Die gesunden und die erkrankten Zahngewebe des Menschen und der Wirbeltiere im Polarisationsmikroskop [Normal and pathological tooth structure of humans and vertebrates in the polarization microscope], München, 1958, Carl Hanser Verlag.

Schour, I., and Massler, M.: The neonatal line in enamel and dentin of the human deciduous teeth and first permanent molar, J. Am. Dent. Assoc. 23:1946, 1936.

Schour, I., and Poncher, H. G.: The rate of apposition of human enamel and dentin as measured by the effects of acute fluorosis, Am. J. Dis. Child. 54:757, 1937.

Schour, I., and Hoffman, M. M.: The rate of apposition of enamel and dentin in man and other animals, J. Dent. Res. 18:161, 1939.

Schour, I., and Massler, M.: Studies in tooth development: The growth pattern of the human teeth, J. Am. Dent. Assoc. 27:1778, 1918, 1940.

Scott, D. B., and Wyckoff, R. W. G.: Electron microscopy of human dentin, J. Dent. Res. 29:556, 1950.

Scott, D. B.: Recent contributions in dental histology by the use of the electron microscope, Int. Dent. J. 4:64, 1953.

Scott, D. B.: The electron microscopy of enamel and dentin, J. New York Acad. Sci. 60:575, 1955.

Scott, D. B., and Nylen, M. U.: Changing concepts in dental histology, Ann. New York Acad. Sci. 85:133, 1960.

Scott, D. B., Nylen, M. U., and Takuma, S.: Electron microscopy of developing and mature calcified tissues, Rev. Belg. Sci. Dent. 14:329, 1959.

Selvig, K. A.: Ultrastructural changes in human dentine exposed to a weak acid, Arch. Oral Biol. 13:719, 1968.

Shroff, F. R., Williamson, K. I., and Bertaud, W. S.: Electron microscope studies of dentin, Oral Surg. 7:662, 1954.

Shroff, F. R.: Further electron microscope studies on dentin: The nature of the odontoblast process, Oral Surg. 9:432, 1956.

Sicher, H.: The biology of dentin, Bur 46: 121, 1946.

Sognnaes, R. F.: Microstructure and histochemical characteristics of the mineralized tissues, J. New York Acad. Sci. 60:545, 1955.

Sognnaes, R. F., Shaw, J. H., and Bogoroch, R.: Radiotracer studies on bone, cementum, dentin, and enamel of rhesus monkeys, Am. J. Physiol. 180:408, 1955.

Stanley, H. R., Jr., and Swerdlow, H.: Reaction of the human pulp to cavity preparation: Results produced by eight different grinding techniques, J. Am. Dent. Assoc. 58:49, 1959.

Sundstrom, B., Takuma, S., and Nagai, N.: Ultrastructural aspects of human dentin decalcified with chromium sulfate, Calcif. Tissue Res. 4:305, 1970.

Takuma, S.: Preliminary report on the mineralization of human dentin, J. Dent. Res. **39**:964, 1960.

Takuma, S.: Electron microscopy of the structure around the dentinal tubule, J. Dent. Res. **39**:973, 1960.

Takuma, S., and Kurahashi, Y.: Electron microscopy of various zones in the carious lesion in human dentine, Arch. Oral Biol. **7**:439, 1962.

Ten Cate, A. R., Melcher, A. H., Pudy, G., and Wagner, D.: The non-fibrous nature of the von Korff fibers in developing dentine. A light and electron microscope study, Anat. Rec. **168**(4):491-523, 1970.

Ten Cate, A. R.: An analysis of Tomes' granular layer, Anat. Rec. **172**(2):137-148, Feb. 1972.

Wasserman, F.: The innervation of teeth, J. Am. Dent. Assoc. **26**:1097, 1939.

Watson, M. L., and Avery, J. K.: The development of the hamster lower incisor as observed by electron microscopy, Am. J. Anat. **95**:109, 1954.

Weider, F. R., Schour, I., and Mohammed, C. I.: Reparative dentin following cavity preparation and fillings in the rat molars, Oral Surg. **9**:221, 1956.

Wislocki, G. B., and Sognnaes, R. E.: Histochemical reactions of normal teeth, Am. J. Anat. **87**:239, 1950.

# 5 Pulp

## ANATOMY

*General features.* Every person normally has a total of 52 pulp organs, 32 in the permanent and 20 in the primary teeth. Each of these organs has a shape that conforms to that of the respective tooth. They have a number of morphologic characteristics that are similar. Each pulp organ resides in a pulp chamber surrounded by dentin containing the peripheral extensions of the cells that formed it. The total volumes of all the permanent teeth pulp organs is 0.38 cc. and the mean volume of a single adult human pulp is 0.02 cc. Molar pulps are three to four times larger than incisors (Fig. 5-1). Table 2 gives the variation in the size of pulp organ in different permanent teeth.

**Table 2.** Pulp volumes for the permanent human teeth from a preliminary investigation on a total of 160 teeth*

|  | Maxillary (cubic centimeters) | Mandibular (cubic centimeters) |
|---|---|---|
| Central incisor | 0.012 | 0.006 |
| Lateral incisor | 0.011 | 0.007 |
| Canine | 0.015 | 0.014 |
| First premolar | 0.018 | 0.015 |
| Second premolar | 0.017 | 0.015 |
| First molar | 0.068 | 0.053 |
| Second molar | 0.044 | 0.032 |
| Third molar | 0.023 | 0.031 |

*Figures for volumes from Fanibunda, K. B.: Personal communication. University of Newcastle upon Tyne, Department of Oral Surgery, Newcastle upon Tyne, England.

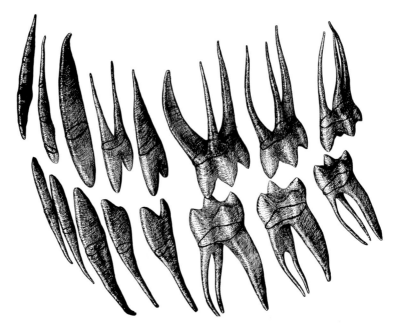

**Fig. 5-1.** Pulp organs of permanent human teeth. *Upper row,* Maxillary arch; left central incisor through third molar. *Lower row,* Mandibular arch; left central incisor through third molar.

The gross description of the pulps of the maxillary and the mandibular teeth is as follows.

### MAXILLARY TEETH

CENTRAL INCISOR
It is somewhat shovel shaped coronally with three short horns on the coronal roof, tapering down to a triangle root in cross section, with the point of the triangle pointing lingually.

LABIAL INCISOR
It has a small spoon shape coronally going to a round evenly tapering root to the apex.

CUSPID
It is the longest pulp with an elliptical cross section buccolingually and a distally inclined apex.

FIRST PREMOLAR
It has a large occlusocervical pulp chamber with a mesial concavity from the root surface onto the cervical third of the chamber. The chamber divides into two smooth funnel-shaped roots.

SECOND PREMOLAR
It is similar coronally to the first premolar, except only one root, which begins to taper at about its midpoint.

MOLARS
The molars are generally all similar, having a roughly rectangular cervical cross section with the greatest dimension buccolingually and also demonstrating mesiobuccal prominence; there are three roots; the lingual is longest and the distobuccal is shortest and straight, whereas the mesiobuccal is curved and flattened buccolingually with its convex surface mesially. From the first to third molars the crowns get smaller and the roots get closer together.

## MANDIBULAR TEETH

CENTRAL INCISOR
It is one of the smallest pulps in the dentition and is long and narrow with a flattened elliptical shape in cross section buccolingually.

LATERAL INCISOR
It is the same as the central incisor, only smaller in all dimensions.

CUSPID
It is similar to, but shorter, than the maxillary canine, and its root begins tapering at about its midpoint, ending in a distally inclined apex.

FIRST BICUSPID
It looks like a small mandibular canine with an insignificant or missing lingual pulp horn.

SECOND BICUSPID
The lingual horn is much smaller than the buccal horn and is about the dimension of the mandibular canine. In cervical section it is often roundly triangular or sometimes rectangular.

MOLARS
The mandibular molars are all similar. The coronal cross section is usually rectangular with the mesiodistal dimension greatest, and it also displays a mesiobuccal prominence. The horn height from highest to lowest are mesiobuccal, mesiolingual, distobuccal, distolingual. There are two roots, the distal being shorter and straighter and singular whereas the mesial is longer, curved, and often double. From first to third, the roots get smaller and closer together.

*Coronal pulp.* Each pulp organ is composed of a coronal pulp located centrally in the crowns of teeth and the root or radicular pulp. The coronal pulp in young individuals resembles the shape of the outer surface of the crown dentin. The coronal pulp has six surfaces: the occlusal, the mesial, the distal, the buccal, the lingual, and the floor. It has pulp horns, which are protrusions that extend into the cusp of each tooth. The number of these horns thus depends on the cuspal number. The cervical region of the organs constrict as does the contour of the crown, and at this zone the coronal pulp joins the radicular pulp (Fig. 5-1). Because of continuous deposition of dentin, the pulp becomes smaller with age. This is not uniform through the coronal pulp, but progresses faster on the floor than on the roof or side walls.

*Radicular pulp.* The radicular pulp is that pulp extending from the cervical region of the crown to the root apex. In the anterior teeth the radicular pulps are single and in posterior ones multiple. They are not always straight and vary in size, shape, and number. The radicular portions of the pulp organs are continuous with the periapical connective tissues through the apical foramen or foramina. The dentinal walls taper and the shape of the radicular pulp is tubular. During root formation the apical root end is a wide opening limited to an epithelial diaphragm (Fig. 5-2, A). As growth proceeds, more dentin is formed, so that when the root of the tooth has matured, the radicular pulp is narrower. The apical pulp canal is made smaller also because of apical cementum deposition (Fig. 5-2, B).

*Apical foramen.* The average size of the apical foramen of the maxillary teeth in the adult is 0.4 mm. The mandibular teeth are slightly smaller, being 0.3 mm. in diameter.

The location and shape of the apical foramen may undergo changes as a re-

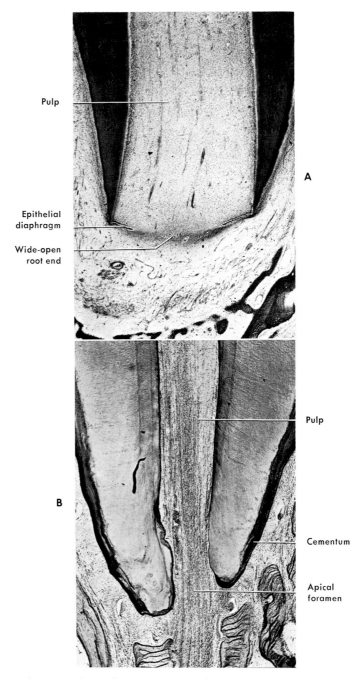

Fig. 5-2. Development of apical foramen. **A,** Undeveloped root end. Wide opening at end of root, partly limited by epithelial diaphragm. **B,** Apical foramen fully formed. Root canal straight. Apical foramen surrounded by cementum. (From Coolidge, E. D.: J. Am. Dent. Assoc. **16:**1456, 1929.)

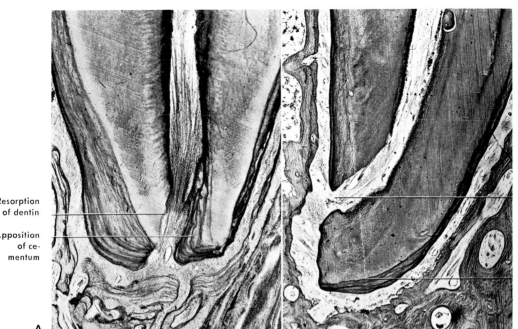

Resorption
of dentin

Apposition
of ce-
mentum

Apical
foramen

Apex

A

B

**Fig. 5-3.** Variations of apical foramen. **A,** Shift of apical foramen by resorption of dentin and cementum on one surface and apposition of cementum on the other. **B,** Apical foramen on the side of apex. (From Coolidge, E. D.: J. Am. Dent. Assoc. **16:**1456, 1929.)

sult of functional influences upon the teeth. A tooth may be tipped from horizontal pressure, or it may migrate mesially, causing the apex to tilt in the opposite direction. Under these conditions the tissues entering the pulp through the apical foramen may exert pressure on one wall of the foramen, causing resorption. At the same time, cementum is laid down on the opposite side of the apical root canal, resulting in a relocation of the original foramen (Fig. 5-3).

Sometimes the apical opening is found on the lateral side of the apex (Fig. 5-3), although the root itself is not curved. Frequently, there are two or more foramina separated by a portion of dentin and cementum, or cementum only.

*Accessory canals.* Accessory canals leading from the radicular pulp laterally through the root dentin to the periodontal tissue may be seen anywhere along the root, but are particularly numerous in the apical third of the root (Fig. 5-4). The mechanism by which they are formed is not known, but it is likely that they occur in areas where the developing root encounters a blood vessel. If the vessel is located in the area where the dentin is forming, it is possible the hard tissue will form around it, making a lateral canal or canals from the radicular pulp.

## DEVELOPMENT

The tooth pulp is initially called the dental papilla. This tissue is designated as "pulp" only after dentin forms around it. The dental papilla controls early

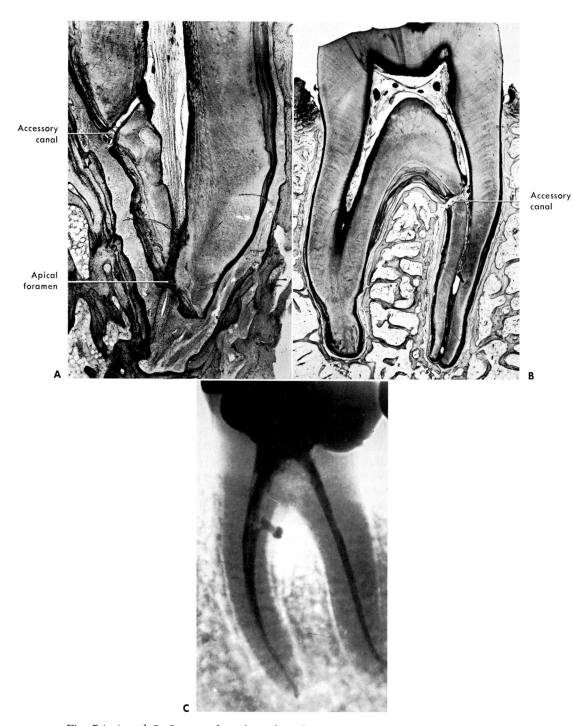

**Fig. 5-4. A** and **B**, Sections through teeth with accessory canals. **A**, Close to the apex. **B**, Close to the bifurcation. **C**, Roentgenogram of lower molar with accessory canal filled. (**C** from Johnston, H. B., and Orban, B.: J. Endodont. 3:21, 1948.)

tooth formation. In the earliest stages the papilla causes the oral epithelium to invaginate and form the enamel organs. The dental papilla further controls whether the forming enamel organ is to be an incisor or a molar. At the location of the future incisor the development of the dental pulp begins at about the eighth week of embryonic life in the human. Soon thereafter, the more posterior

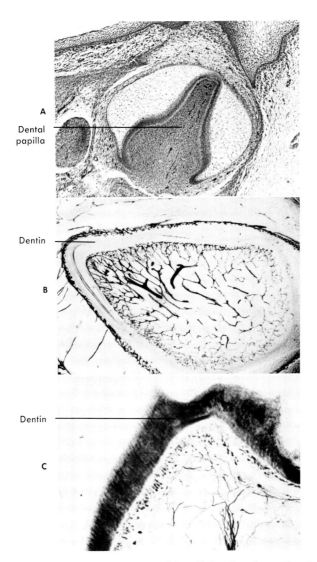

A

Dental papilla

Dentin

B

Dentin

C

Fig. 5-5. A, Young tooth bud exhibiting highly cellular dental papilla. Compare cell population to adjacent connective tissue. B, Young tooth with blood vessels injected with india ink to demonstrate extent of vascularity of pulp. Pulp surrounded by dentin and enamel. C, Young tooth stained with silver to demonstrate neural elements. Myelinated nerves appear in pulp horn only after considerable dentin is formed.

tooth organs begin differentiating. The cell density of the dental papilla is great as a result of proliferation of the cells within it (Fig. 5-5, *A*). The young dental papilla is highly vascularized and a well-organized network of vessels appears by the time dentin formation begins (Fig. 5-5, *B*). Capillaries crowd among the odontoblasts during this period of active dentinogenesis. The cells of the dental papilla appear as undifferentiated mesenchymal cells. Gradually these cells appear as stellate fibroblasts. After the inner enamel organ cells differentiate into ameloblasts, the odontoblasts then differentiate from the peripheral cells of the dental papilla and dentin production begins. As this occurs, the tissue is no

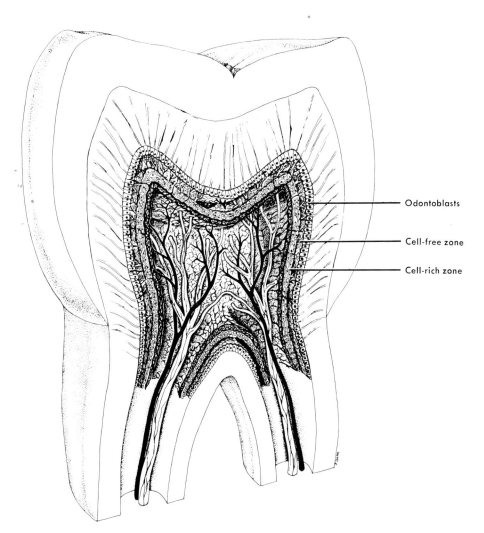

Odontoblasts

Cell-free zone

Cell-rich zone

**Fig. 5-6.** Diagram of pulp organ, illustrating architecture of large central nerve trunks *(dark)* and vessels *(light)* and the peripheral cell-rich, cell-free, and odontoblast rows. Observe small nerves on blood vessels.

longer called dental papilla but is now designated the pulp organ. Few large myelinated nerves are found in the pulp until the dentin of the crown is well advanced (Fig. 5-5, C). At that time nerves reach the odontogenic zone in the pulp horns. The sympathetic nerves, however, follow the blood vessels into the pulp before this time.

## STRUCTURAL ELEMENTS

The central region of the pulp contains large nerve trunks and blood vessels. Peripherally, the pulp is circumscribed by the specialized odontogenic region composed of the dentin-forming cells, the odontoblasts, the cell-free zone (Weil's zone), and the cell-rich zone (Fig. 5-6). Some believe that the cell-free zone is the area of mobilization and replacement of odontoblasts, and this may be why this zone is inconspicuous during early stages of rapid dentinogenesis. The cell-rich layer is composed principally of fibroblasts and undifferentiated mesenchymal cells. The latter are distinctive because they lack a ribosome-studded endoplasmic reticulum and have mitochondria with readily discernable cristae. During that time there are also many young collagen fibers in this zone.

*Intercellular substance.* The intercellular substance is dense and gel-like in nature and varies in appearance from finely granular to fibrillar and has clumps in some areas, with clear spaces left between various aggregates. It is composed of both acid mucopolysaccharides and protein polysaccharide compounds. During early development, the presence of chondroitin A, chondroitin B, and hyaluronic acid have been demonstrated in abundance. Glycoproteins are also

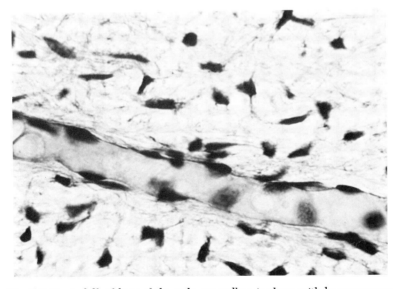

**Fig. 5-7.** Typical fibroblasts of the pulp are stellate in shape with long processes.

present in the ground substance. The aging pulp contains less of all of these substances.

*Fibroblasts and fibers.* The pulp organ is said to consist of specialized connective tissue because it lacks elastic fibers. Fibroblasts are the most numerous cell type in the pulp. As their name implies, they function in collagen fiber formation. They have the typical stellate shape and extensive processes that contact

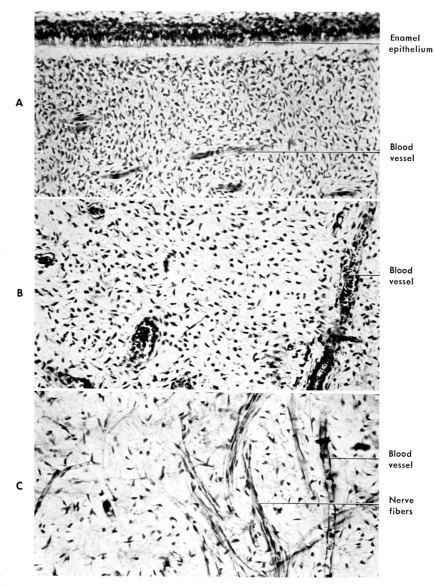

Fig. 5-8. Age changes of dental pulp. Cellular elements decrease and fibrous intercellular substance increases with advancing age. **A,** Newborn infant. **B,** Infant 9 months of age. **C,** Adult.

and are joined by intercellular junctions to the processes of other fibroblasts (Fig. 5-7). Under the light microscope the fibroblast nuclei stain deeply with basic dyes, and their cytoplasm is lighter stained and appears homogeneous. Electron micrographs reveal abundant rough-surfaced endoplasmic reticulum, mitochondria, and other organelles in the fibroblast cytoplasm. This indicates these cells are active in pulpal collagen production. There is some difference in appearance of these cells depending on the age of the pulp organ. In the young pulp the cells divide and are active in protein synthesis, but in the older pulp they are rounded, or with short processes, and appear less active with fewer intracellular organelles. They are then termed *fibrocytes*. In the course of development the relative number of cellular elements in the dental pulp decreases, whereas the fiber population increases (Fig. 5-8). In the embryonic and immature pulp the cellular elements predominate. In the mature tooth the fibrous components predominate.

Two types of fibers are found in the pulp organs, *collagenous* and *fine fibers*. Bundles of collagen fibers exhibiting cross-striations at 640 Å intervals appear in the pulp organ and range in length from 10 to 100 microns or more. The individual collagen fibers are composed of fibrils varying in diameter from 400 to 700 Å or more. In the young pulp predominantly fine fibers are found throughout the pulp and gradually the bundles increase in size with advancing age. The fine fibers measure 100 to 120 Å in diameter. The appearance of two patterns of collagen distibution can be seen in the older pulp—one is a diffuse collagen network with no definite orientation; the other is bundles of collagen.

Microscopic examination of the pulp, stained with hematoxylin and eosin does not present a complete picture of the structure of the pulp because not all of the elements are stained by this method (Fig. 5-9, *A*). The majority of the fine collagen fibrils are revealed by silver impregnation (Fig. 5-9, *B*). They stain black with silver and are therefore termed *argyrophilic fibers*. Many of these fibers originate from the pulp fibroblasts and may function in the formation of the predentin.

*Odontoblasts.* Odontoblasts, the second most prominent cell in the pulp, reside adjacent to the predentin with cell bodies in the pulp and cell processes in the dentinal tubules. They are approximately 5 to 7 microns in diameter and 25 to 40 microns in length. They have a constant location in what is termed the odontogenic zone of the pulp. The cell bodies of the odontoblasts are columnar in appearance with large oval nuclei, which fill the basal part of the cell (Fig. 5-10). Immediately adjacent to the nucleus basally is rough-surfaced endoplasmic reticulum and the Golgi apparatus. The cells in the odontoblastic row lie very close to each other and the plasma membrane of adjacent cells exhibit junctional complexes. Further toward the apex of the cell appears an abundance of rough-surfaced endoplasmic reticulum. Near the pulpal-predentin junction the cell cytoplasm is devoid of organelles. The clear terminal part of the cell body and the adjacent intercellular junction is described by some as the terminal bar apparatus

A

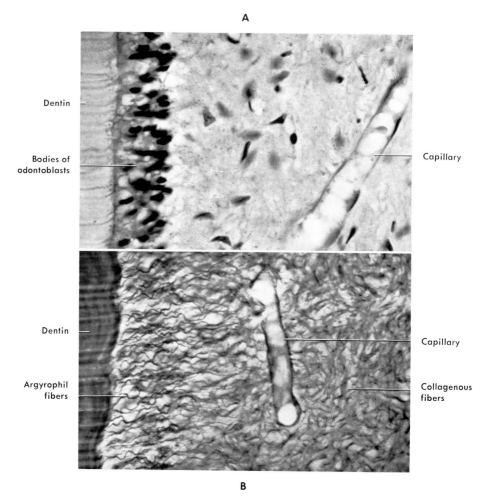

Dentin

Bodies of
odontoblasts

Capillary

Dentin

Capillary

Argyrophil
fibers

Collagenous
fibers

B

Fig. 5-9. Cellular and fibrous elements in pulp. **A,** Cellular elements stained with hematoxylin and eosin. **B,** Fibrous elements stained by silver impregnation. Both specimens are from the same tooth.

of the odontoblast. At this zone the cell constricts to a diameter of 3 to 4 microns, and the cell process enters the predentin tubule. The process of the cell contains no endoplasmic reticulum but during the early period of active dentinogenesis it does contain occasional mitochondria and vesicles. During the later stages of dentinogenesis these are infrequently seen. There is also a striking difference in the cytoplasm of the young cell body, active in dentinogenesis, and the older cell. During this early active phase the Golgi apparatus is more prominent. The rough-surfaced endoplasmic reticulum is more abundant, and numerous mitochondria appear throughout the odontoblast and its process. A great number of vesicles are seen along the periphery of the process where there is evidence of protein synthesis along the tubule wall. The cell actually increases in

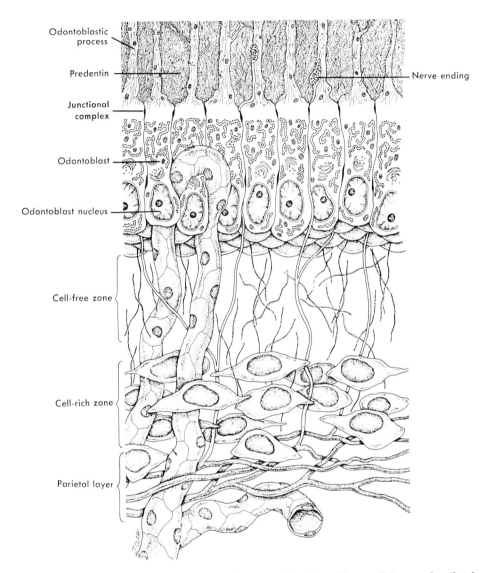

**Fig. 5-10.** Diagram of odontogenic zone illustrating the odontoblast, cell-free, and cell-rich zones, with blood vessels and nonmyelinated nerves among the odontoblasts.

size as its processes lengthens during dentin formation. When the cell process becomes 2 mm. long, it is then many times greater in volume than the cell body. The form and arrangement of the bodies of the odontoblasts are not uniform throughout the pulp. They are more cylindric and longer (tall columnar) in the crown (Fig. 5-11, *A*) and more cuboid in the middle of the root (Fig. 5-11, *B*). Close to the apex of an adult tooth the odontoblasts are flat and spindle shaped and can be recognized as odontoblasts only by their extensions into the dentin. In areas close to the apical foramen the dentin is irregular (Fig. 5-11, *C*).

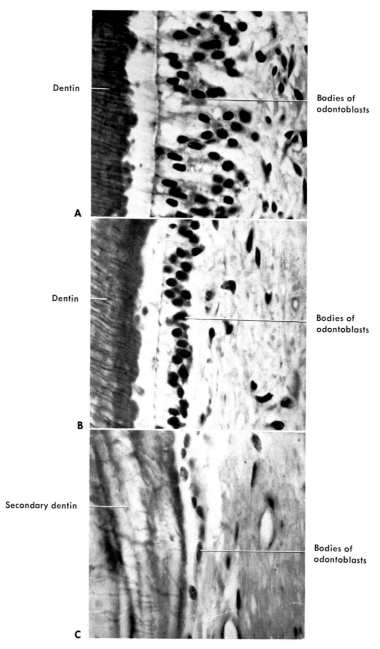

**Fig. 5-11.** Variation of odontoblasts in different regions of one tooth. **A,** High columnar odontoblasts in pulp chamber. **B,** Low columnar odontoblasts in root canal. **C,** Flat odontoblasts in apical region.

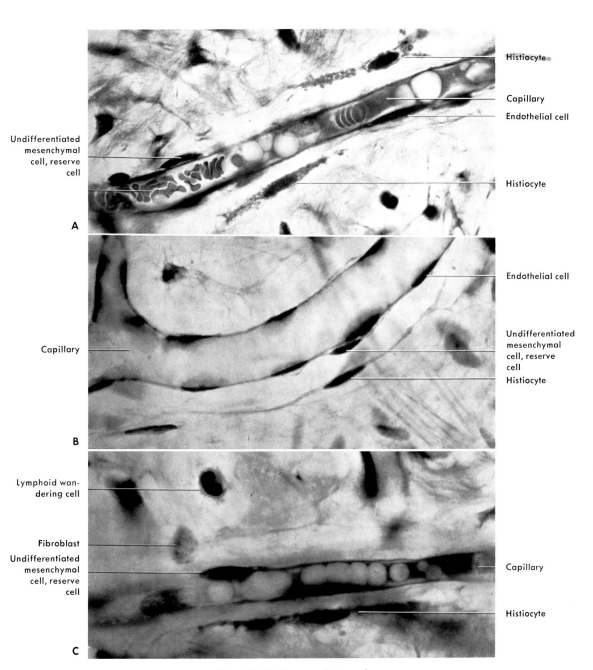

Histiocyte

Capillary

Endothelial cell

Undifferentiated
mesenchymal
cell, reserve
cell

Histiocyte

A

Endothelial cell

Capillary

Undifferentiated
mesenchymal
cell, reserve
cell

Histiocyte

B

Lymphoid wan-
dering cell

Fibroblast

Undifferentiated
mesenchymal
cell, reserve
cell

Capillary

Histiocyte

C

**Fig. 5-12.** Defense cells in pulp.

*Defense cells.* In addition to fibroblasts, odontoblasts, and the cells that are a part of the neural and vascular systems of the pulp, there are cells important to the defense of the pulp. These are histiocytes or macrophages, small lymphocytes, eosinophils, mast cells, and plasma cells.

The histiocyte, or macrophage, is an irregularly shaped cell with short blunt processes (Fig. 5-12). In the light microscope the nucleus is somewhat smaller, more rounded, and darker staining than that of fibroblasts, and exhibits granular cytoplasm. When the macrophages are inactive and not in the process of injesting foreign materials, one has difficulty distinguishing them from fibroblasts. In the

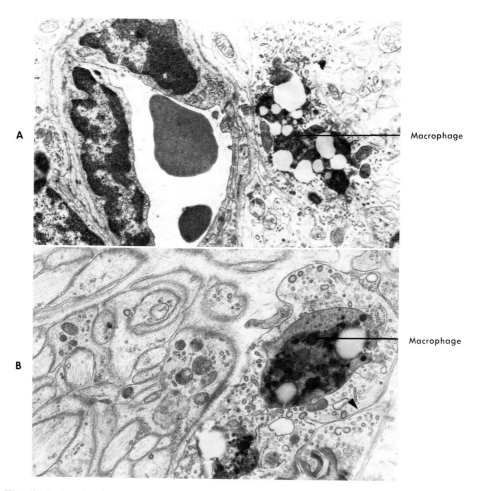

**Fig. 5-13. A,** This histiocyte or macrophage is located adjacent to a capillary in peripheral pulp. Characteristic aggregation of vesicles, vacuoles, and dense bodies phagocytized is seen to *right* of capillary wall. **B,** Multivesiculated body characteristic of macrophage. Note typical invagination of cell plasma membrane *(arrow).* This cell is located adjacent to a group of nonmyelinated nerve fibers seen on *left.*

case of a pulpal inflammation these cells exhibit granules and vacuoles in their cytoplasm, and their nuclei increase in size and exhibit a prominent nucleolus. Their presence is disclosed by intravital dyes such as trypan blue. These cells are usually associated with small blood vesels and capillaries. Ultrastructurally the macrophage exhibits a rounded outline with short blunt processes. Invaginations of the plasma membrane are noted, as are mitochondria, rough-surfaced endoplasmic reticulum, free ribosomes, and also a moderately dense nucleus. The distinguishing feature of macrophages is aggregates of vesicles, vacuoles, and phagocytized dense irregular bodies ( Fig. 5-13 ).

Both lymphocytes and eosinophils are found in the normal pulp (Fig. 5-14), but during inflammation they increase noticeably. Mast cells are seen along ves-

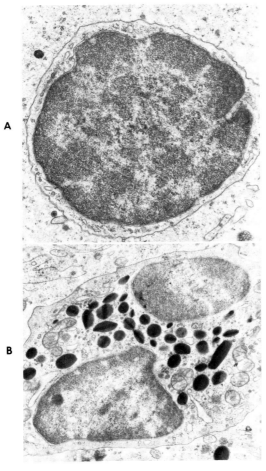

Fig. 5-14. **A,** Small lymphocyte located in pulp. Cytoplasm forms a narrow rim around large oval-to-round nucleus. **B,** Eosinophil in extravascular location in pulp organ. Nucleus is polymorphic, and granules in cytoplasm are characteristically banded.

sels in the coronal pulp. They have a round nucleus and contain many granules in the cytoplasm. Their number increases during inflammation.

The plasma cells are seen during inflammation of the pulp (Fig. 5-15). With the light microscope the plasma cell nucleus is small and appears concentric in the cytoplasm. The chromatin of the nucleus is adherent to the nuclear membrane and gives the cell a cartwheel appearance. The cytoplasm of this cell is basophilic with a light-stained Golgi zone adjacent to the nucleus. Under the electron microscope these cells have a densely packed rough-surfaced endoplasmic reticulum. Both immature and mature cells may be found. The mature type exhibits a typical small eccentric nucleus and more abundant cytoplasm. The plasma cells are known to produce antibodies.

*Blood vessels.* The pulp organ is extensively vascularized. It is known that the blood vessels of both the pulp and the periodontium arise from the same artery and drain by the same veins in both the mandibular and maxillary region. The communication of the vessels of the pulp with the periodontium in addition to the apical connections is further enhanced by connections through the accessory canals. These relationships are of considerable clinical significance in the event of a potential pathologic condition in the periodontium or the pulp, as it

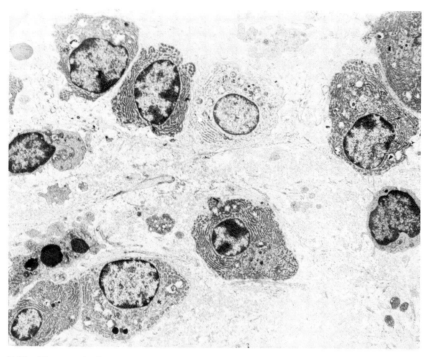

**Fig. 5-15.** Cluster of plasma cells in a pulp with early caries pulpitis. Observe dense peripheral nuclear chromatin and cytoplasm with cisternae of rough endoplasmic reticulum. (Courtesy C. Torneck, University of Toronto Dental School.)

has a potential to spread through these canals. Although branches of the alveolar arteries supply both the tooth and its supporting tissues, those entering the pulp are different in structure from the branches to the periodontium. As the vessels enter the tooth their walls become considerably thinner than those surrounding the tooth.

Small arteries and arterioles enter the apical canal and pursue a direct route to the coronal pulp. Along their course they give off numerous branches in the root pulp that pass peripherally to form a plexus in the odontogenic region (Fig. 5-16). Pulpal blood flow is more rapid than in most areas of the body. The flow of blood in arterioles is 0.3 to 1 mm. per second, in venules approximately 0.15 mm. per second, and in capillaries about 0.08 mm. per second. This is perhaps attributable to the fact that the pulpal pressure is among the highest of body tissues. The largest arteries in the human pulp are 50 to 100 microns in diameter, thus equaling in size arterioles found in most areas of the body. These vessels

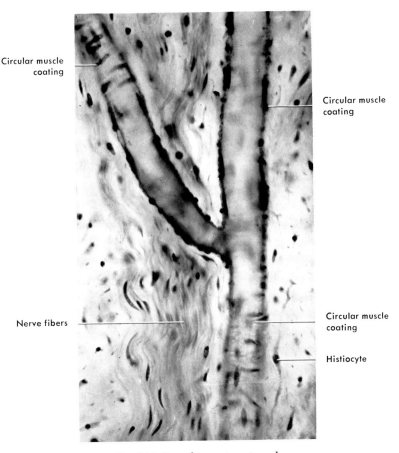

Fig. 5-16. Branching artery in pulp.

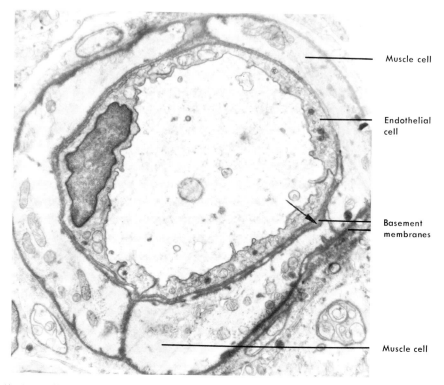

Muscle cell

Endothelial cell

Basement membranes

Muscle cell

**Fig. 5-17.** Small arteriole near central pulp exhibiting relatively thick layer of muscle cells. *Arrow,* Dense basement membrane interspersed between endothelial and muscle cells.

possess three layers. The first, the tunica intima consists of squamous or cuboid endothelial cells surrounded by a closely associated basal lamina. Where the endothelial cells contact, they appear overlapped to varying degrees. The second layer, the tunica media is approximately 5 microns thick and consists of one to three layers of smooth muscle cells (Figs. 5-16 and 5-17). A basal lamina surrounds and passes between these muscle cells and separates the muscle cell layer from the intima. Occasionally the endothelial cell wall is in contact with the muscle cells. This is termed a myoendothelial junction. The third and outer layer, the tunica adventitia is made up of a few collagen fibers forming a loose network around the larger arteries. This layer becomes more conspicuous in vessels in older pulps. Arterioles with diameters of 20 to 30 microns with one or occasionally two layers of smooth muscle cells are common throughout the coronal pulp (Fig. 5-17). The tunica adventitia blends with the fibers of the surrounding intercellular tissue. Terminal arterioles with diameters of 10 to 15 microns appear peripherally in the pulp. The endothelial cells of these vessels contain numerous micropinocytotic vesicles, which function in transendothelial fluid movement. A single layer of smooth muscle cells surrounds these small vessels. Occasionally a fibroblast or pericyte lies on the surface of these vessels. Pericytes are capillary-

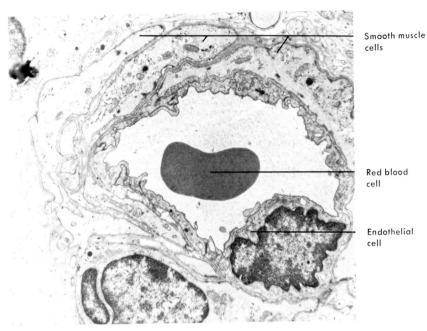

Smooth muscle cells

Red blood cell

Endothelial cell

**Fig. 5-18.** Peripheral pulp and small arteriole or precapillary exhibiting two thin layers of smooth muscle cells surrounding endothelial cell lining. The vessel contains a red blood cell. Nucleus at bottom of figure belongs to a pericyte.

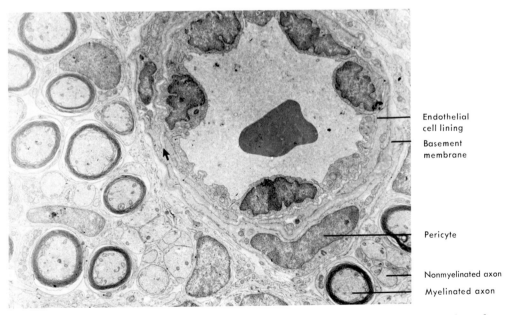

Endothelial cell lining

Basement membrane

Pericyte

Nonmyelinated axon

Myelinated axon

**Fig. 5-19.** Area near subodontoblastic plexus showing both myelinated and nonmyelinated axons adjacent to a large capillary or precapillary. Endothelial cell lining is surrounded by a basement membrane and pericytes.

associated fibroblasts, and their nuclei can be distinguished as round or slightly oval bodies closely associated with the outer surface of the terminal arterioles or precapillaries (Figs. 5-18 and 5-19). Some authors call the smaller diameter arterioles "precapillaries." They are slightly larger than the terminal capillaries and exhibit a complete or incomplete single layer of muscle cells surrounding the endothelial lining. These range in size from 8 to 12 microns.

Veins and venules that are larger than the arteries also appear in the central region of the root pulp. They measure 100 to 150 microns in diameter, and their walls appear less regular than those of the arteries because of bends and irregularities along their course. The microscopic appearance of the veins is similar to the arteries except that they have much thinner walls in relation to the size of the lumen. The endothelial cells appear more flattened and their cytoplasm does not project into the lumen. Less intracytoplasmic filaments appear in these cells than in the arterioles. The tunica media consists of a single layer or two of thin smooth muscle cells that wrap around the endothelial cells and appears discontinuous or absent in the smaller venules. The basement membranes of these vessels are thin and less distinct than those of arterioles. The adventitia is lacking or appears as fibroblasts and fibers continuous with the surrounding pulp tissue.

Blood capillaries, which appear as endothelium-lined tubules, are 8 to 10 microns in diameter. The nuclei of these cells may be lobulated and have cytoplasmic projections into the luminal surface. A few capillaries have fenestrations in the endothelial plasma membranes of the odontogenic zone. These pores are found in the thin part of the capillary wall and are spanned only by the thin diaphragm composed of the inner and outer membranes of the endothelial cells

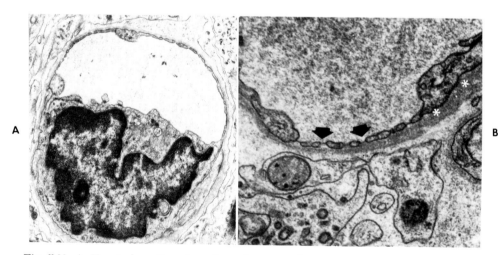

A                                                                                    B

**Fig. 5-20. A,** Terminal capillary loops located among odontoblasts may be fenestrated. These capillaries have both thick and thin segments in their walls. **B,** The endothelial cell wall bridges the pores *(arrows)* and is supported only by the basement membrane (° °).

(Fig. 5-20). These fenestrated capillaries may be involved in rapid transport of metabolites, when these are needed for both predentinal matrix formation and the subsequent process of calcification of dentin. Both fenestrated and non-fenestrated terminal capillaries are found in the odontogenic region. During active dentinogenesis capillaries appear among the odontoblasts adjacent to the predentin (Fig. 5-20). Later, after the teeth have reached occlusion and dentino-genesis slows down, these vessels usually retreat pulpally.

*Lymph vessels.* The presence of lymph vessels in the dental pulp is questioned by some and agreed upon by other investigators. Support for this system stems from investigators who use injection of fine particulate substances into the dentin or peripheral pulp, which are subsequently reported present in some of the thin-walled vessels that exit through the apical foramen. Lymph capillaries are described as endothelium-lined tubes that join thin-walled lymph venules or veins in the central pulp. The larger vessels have an irregular-shaped lumen composed of endothelial cells surrounded by an incomplete layer of pericytes or smooth muscle cells, or both. They are further characterized by absence of red blood cells and presence of lymphocytes. Absence of basal lamina adjacent to the endothelium has also been reported. Lymph vessels draining the pulp and periodontal ligament have a common outlet. Those draining the anterior teeth pass to the submental lymph nodes; those of the posterior teeth pass to the submandibular and deep cervical lymph nodes.

*Nerves.* The abundant nerve supply in the pulp follows the distribution of the blood vessels. Most nerves that enter the pulp are myelinated (Fig. 5-19). They mediate the sensation of pain caused by external stimuli. The nonmyelinated nerves are found in close association with the blood vessels of the pulp and are sympathetic in nature. They have terminals on the muscle cells of the larger vessels and function in vasoconstriction. Thick nerve bundles enter the apical foramen and proceed to the coronal area where they branch with their fibers radiating peripherally to the odontogenic zone (Fig. 5-21). The number of fibers in these bundles varies greatly from as few as 150 to more than 1200. The larger fibers range between 5 and 13 microns although the majority are smaller than 4 microns. The peripheral axons form a network of nerves located adjacent to the cell-rich zone. This is termed the "parietal layer of nerves," also known as the plexus of Raschkow (Fig. 5-22). Both myelinated axons ranging from 2 to 5 microns in diameter and minute nonmyelinated fibers of approximately 2000 to 16,000 Å in size make up this layer of nerves. The parietal layer develops gradually, becoming prominent when root formation is complete. From this layer nerve axons arise by passing through the cell-rich and cell-free zones and then either terminate among or pass between the odontoblasts where they then terminate adjacent to the odontoblast processes at the pulp-predentin border or in the dentinal tubules (Fig. 5-23). Nerve terminals consisting of round or oval enlargements of the terminal filaments contain microvesicles, small dark granular bodies, and mitochondria (Fig. 5-24). These terminals are very close to the

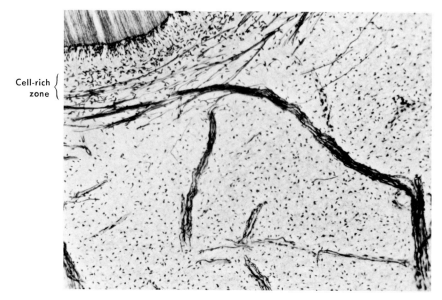

Cell-rich
zone

Fig. 5-21. Major nerve trunks branch in pulp and pass to parietal layer, which lies adjacent to cell-rich zone. Cell-rich zone curves upward to right.

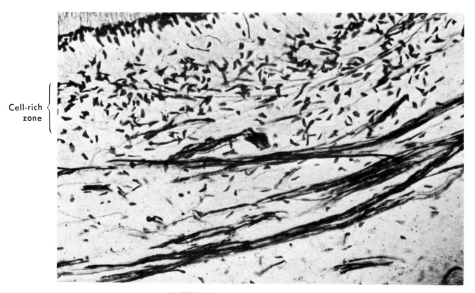

Cell-rich
zone

Fig. 5-22. Parietal layer of nerves is composed of myelinated nerve fibers. Cell-rich zone curves upward to right.

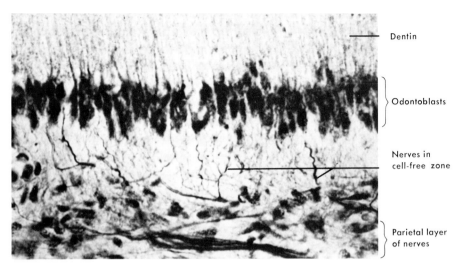

**Fig. 5-23.** Terminal nerve endings located among odontoblasts. These arise from subjacent parietal layer.

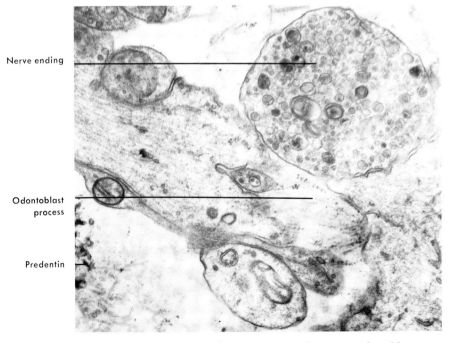

**Fig. 5-24.** Vesiculated nerve endings in predentin in zone adjacent to odontoblast process.

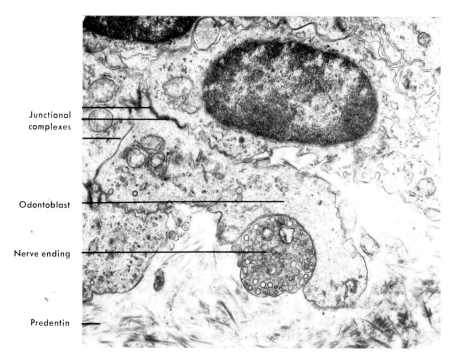

Junctional complexes

Odontoblast

Nerve ending

Predentin

**Fig. 5-25.** Vesiculated nerve ending lying in apposition to odontoblast process adjacent to predentin. Junctional complexes appear between odontoblasts.

odontoblast plasma membrane, separated only by a 200 Å cleft (Fig. 5-25). Most of the nerve endings located among the odontoblasts are believed to be sensory receptors. Some however are sympathetic. Whether they have some function relative to the odontoblast in dentinogenesis or to the capillaries in this area is not known. The nerve axons found among the odontoblasts and in the cell-free and cell-rich zone are nonmyelinated but are enclosed in a Schwann cell covering. It is presumed that these fibers lost their myelin sheath as they passed peripherally from the parietal zone.

More nerve fibers and endings are found in the pulp horns than in other peripheral areas of the coronal or radicular pulp (Fig. 5-5, *C*).

It is a feature unique to dentin receptors that environmental stimuli always elicit pain as a response. Sensory response in the pulp cannot differentiate between heat, touch, pressure, or chemicals. This is because the pulp organs lack those types of receptors that specifically distinguish these other stimuli.

## FUNCTIONS

*Inductive.* The first role of the pulp anlage is to induce oral epithelial differentiation into dental lamina and enamel organ formation and also to determine the identity of the tooth formed.

*Formative.* The pulp organ produces the dentin that surrounds it. The pulpal odontoblasts develop the organic matrix and function in its calcification. Through the development of the odontoblast processes, tubular dentin is formed.

*Nutritive.* The pulp nourishes the dentin through the odontoblasts and their processes. The nutritional elements are contained in the tissue fluid.

*Protective.* The sensory nerves in the tooth respond with pain to all stimuli such as heat, cold, pressure, operative cutting procedures, and chemical agents. The nerves also initiate reflexes that control circulation in the pulp. This sympathetic function is a reflux providing stimulation to visceral motor fibers terminating on the muscles of the blood vessels.

*Defensive or reparative.* The pulp is an organ with remarkable reparative abilities. It responds to irritation, whether mechanical, thermal, chemical, or bacterial, by producing reparative dentin and mineralizing any effected dentinal tubules. Both the reparative dentin created in the pulp or the calcification of the tubules (sclerosis) is an attempt to wall off the pulp from the source of irritation. Also, the pulp may be inflamed because of the irritation that is apparent during the formation of reparative dentin. However, the pulp has macrophages, lymphocytes, and leukocytes, all of which aid in the process of repair of the pulp. Although the rigid dentinal wall has to be considered as a protection to the pulp, it also endangers its existence under these conditions. During inflammation of the pulp, hyperemia and exudate may lead to the accumulation of excess fluid outside the capillaries. An imbalance of this type, limited by the unyielding enclosure tends to be self-perpetuating and may be followed by the total destruction of the pulp. In most cases, if the inflammation is not too severe, the pulp will heal.

## PRIMARY AND PERMANENT PULP ORGANS

*Primary pulp organs.* The primary pulp organs function for a relatively shorter period of time than do the permanent pulps. The average length of time a primary pulp functions in the oral cavity is only about 8.3 years. This amount of time may be divided into three time periods—that of *pulp organ growth* during the time the crown and roots are developing; that period of time after the root is completed until root resorption begins, which is termed "*pulp maturation*"; and finally the period of *pulp regression,* which is the time from root resorption until exfoliation. Let us consider the average time of pulp life based on figures for the entire primary dentition. These three periods (growth, maturation, and regression) are not of equal lengths. Tooth eruption to root completion is about 1 year (11.85 months), and the time of root completion to beginning root loss (based on completion of the permanent crown) is 45.3 months, or 3 years, 9 months. Finally, the time of pulp regression based on the beginning of root resorption to exfoliation is 3 years, 6 months. The amount of time the primary pulp is undergoing changes relative to growth based on both the *prenatal* crown formation to the postnatal root completion is about 4 years, 2 months, 11 months of which are involved in crown completion from the time of beginning of crown calcification to its completion. The period of time the primary radicular pulp is regressing is based on the time from when the permanent crown is completed till the time of permanent tooth eruption. In some cases, root loss commences before the root is entirely complete. The maximum life of the primary pulp including both prenatal and postnatal times of development and the period of regression is approximately 9.6 years.

*Permanent pulp organs.* During crown formation the pulps of primary and permanent teeth are morphologically nearly identical. In the permanent teeth this is a process requiring about 5 years. During this time the organs are highly cellular, exhibiting a high mitotic rate especially in the cervical region. The young differentiating odontoblasts exhibit few organelles until dentin formation begins; then they rapidly change into protein-synthesizing cells. Both the primary pulp and permanent are highly vascularized; however, the primary never attains the extent of neural development of the permanent teeth. This is caused in part by the loss of neural elements during the root-resorption period. The greater the extent of root resorption, the greater the degenerative changes seen in the primary pulps. The architecture of the primary and permanent pulps is similar in appearance to the cell-free and cell-rich zones, parietal layer, and presence of the large nerve trunks and vessels in the central pulp.

The periods of development for the pulps of the permanent teeth are, as might be expected, longer than those required for completion of the same processes in the primary teeth. As mentioned above, crown completion, based on the time during which the crown is completing formation and calcification average 5 years, 5 months. From the time of crown completion to eruption the time in both arches average 3 years, 6 months. From the time of eruption to root completion is 3 years, 11 months. Thus the pulp of the permanent teeth undergoes development for about 12 years, 4 months (based on the time from beginning prenatal crown calcification to root completion). This is in contrast to the 4 years, 2 months it takes in the primary teeth. Furthermore, the permanent roots take over twice as long to reach completion (7 years, 5 months) as do those of the primary pulps (average 3 years, 3 months).

The period of pulp aging is much accelerated in the primary teeth and occupies the time from root completion to exfoliation or about 7 years, 5 months. Aging of the pulp in the permanent teeth, on the other hand, requires much of the adult life-span.

Finally, one should note in passing that for both the primary and permanent teeth the maxillary arches require slightly longer to complete each process of development than do the mandibular arches.

## REGRESSIVE CHANGES

*Cell changes.* In addition to the appearance of fewer cells in the aging pulp, the cells are characterized by a decrease in size and number of various cytoplasmic organelles. The typical active pulpal fibrocyte or fibroblast has abundant rough-surfaced endoplasmic reticulum, noteable Golgi complex, and numerous mitochondria with well-developed cristae. The fibroblasts in the aging pulp exhibit less perinuclear cytoplasm and possess long thin cytoplasmic processes. The intracellular organelles are small and reduced in number as in the endoplasmic reticulum. Mitochondria are decreased in size with inconspicuous cristae. Intercellular fibers are in abundance among the cells.

*Fibrosis.* In the aging pulp accumulations of both diffuse fibrillar components as well as bundles of collagen fibers usually appear. Fiber bundles may appear arranged longitudinally in bundles in the radicular pulp and in a random more diffuse arrangement in the coronal area. Some older pulps show surprisingly small amounts of collagen accumulations; others have considerable amounts (Fig. 5-26). The increase in fibers in the pulp organ is gradual and is generalized throughout the organ. Any external trauma such as dental caries or deep restorations usually cause a localized fibrosis or scarring affect. Collagen increase is noted in the medial and adventitial layers of blood vessels as well. Some investigators conclude that the increase in collagen fibers is more apparent than actual, being attributable to the decrease in the size of the pulp that makes whatever fibers present occupy less space and hence become more concentrated without having increased in total overall volume.

Vascular changes occur in the aging pulp organ as they do in any organ. Plaques may appear in pulpal vessels. In other cases the diameter of vessel walls becomes greater as collagen fibers increase in the medial and adventitial layers. Also calcifications are found that surround vessels (Fig. 5-27). Calcification in

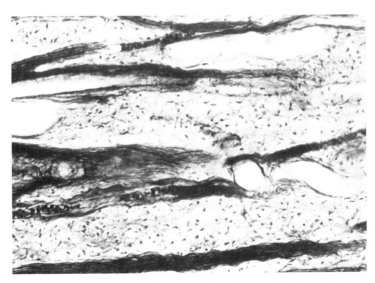

**Fig. 5-26.** Bundles of collagen fibers around and among blood vessels of pulp.

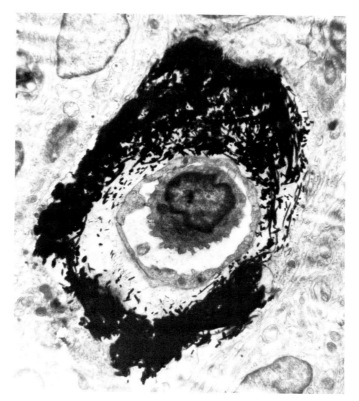

**Fig. 5-27.** Small vessel containing a lymphocyte. Its wall exhibits no basement membrane around the endothelial cells. It is probably a lymphatic capillary. Calcification appears around periphery of vessel.

the walls of blood vessels is found most often in the region near the apical foramen.

*Pulp stones or denticles.* Pulp stones, or denticles, are nodular calcified masses appearing in either or both the coronal or root portions of the pulp organ. They often develop in teeth that appear to be quite normal in other respects. They have been seen in functional as well as embedded teeth.

Pulp stones are classified, according to their structure, as true denticles, false denticles, and diffuse calcifications. The structure of true denticles is similar to dentin because they exhibit dental tubuli containing the processes of the odontoblasts that formed them and that exist on their surface (Fig. 5-28, *A*). True denticles are comparatively rare and are usually located close to the apical foramen. A theory has been advanced that the development of this type of pulp stone is caused by remnants of epithelial root sheath that have become enclosed in the pulp possibly as a result of a local disturbance at the root apex during development. These epithelial remnants then induce the cells of the pulp to differentiate into odontoblasts and form the dentin masses called true pulp stones.

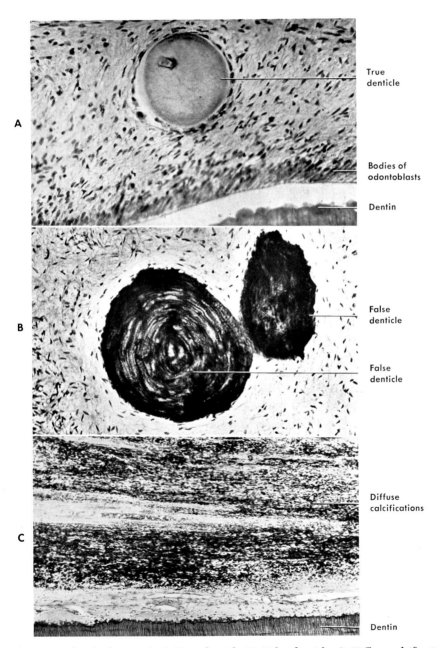

True
denticle

Bodies of
odontoblasts

Dentin

False
denticle

False
denticle

Diffuse
calcifications

Dentin

**Fig. 5-28.** Denticles (pulpstones). **A,** True denticle. **B,** False denticle. **C,** Diffuse calcifications.

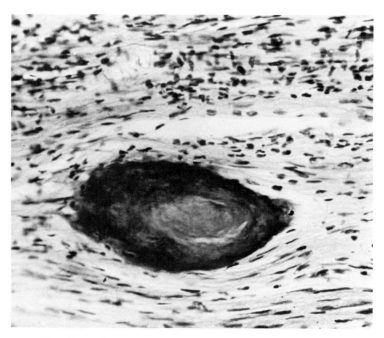

**Fig. 5-29.** Pulp stone within a collagen bundle of coronal pulp.

It is well known that the epithelial root sheath cells cause differentiation of odontoblasts along their pulpal boundary as they grow apically during root development.

False denticles do not exhibit dentinal tubules but appear instead as concentric layers of calcified tissue (Fig. 5-28, *B*). In some cases these calcification sites appear within a bundle of collagen fibers (Fig. 5-29). Other times they appear in a location in the pulp free of collagen accumulations (Fig. 5-28, *B*). Some false pulp stones undoubtedly arise around vessels as seen in Fig. 5-27. In the center of these concentric layers of calcified tissue there may be remnants of necrotic and calcified cells. Calcification of thrombi in blood vessels, called phleboliths, may also serve as niduses for false denticles. All denticles begin as small nodules but increase in size by incremental growth on their surface. The surrounding pulp tissue may appear quite normal. These pulp stones may eventually fill substantial parts of the pulp chamber.

Diffuse calcifications appear as irregular calcific deposits in the pulp tissue, usually following collagenous fiber bundles or blood vessels (Fig. 5-28, *C*). Sometimes they develop into larger masses but usually persist as fine spicules. The pulp organ may appear quite normal in its coronal portion without signs of inflammation or other pathologic changes but may exhibit these calcifications in the roots. Diffuse calcifications thus usually are found in the root canal, less often in the coronal area, whereas denticles are seen more frequently in the coronal pulp.

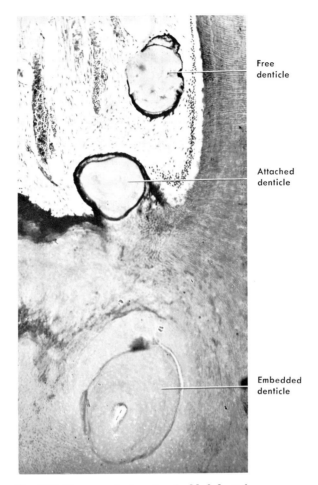

Free
denticle

Attached
denticle

Embedded
denticle

**Fig. 5-30.** Free, attached, and embedded denticles.

In addition to being classified according to their structure as true or false denticles and diffuse calcifications, pulp stones are also classified according to their location in relation to the surrounding dentinal wall. Free, attached, and embedded denticles can be distinguished (Fig. 5-30). The free denticles are entirely surrounded by pulp tissue, attached denticles are partly fused with the dentin, and embedded denticles are entirely surrounded by dentin. All are believed to be formed free in the pulp and become attached or embedded as dentin formation progresses. Pulp stones may appear close to blood vessels and nerve trunks (Fig. 5-31). This is believed to be because they are large and grow out such that they impinge on whatever structures are in their paths. The occurrence of pulp stones has been shown to be more prevalent through histologic study of human teeth than can be determined radiographically. It is believed only a relatively small number of them can be detected on roentgenograms. The incidence as well as the size of the pulp stones increases with age. According to

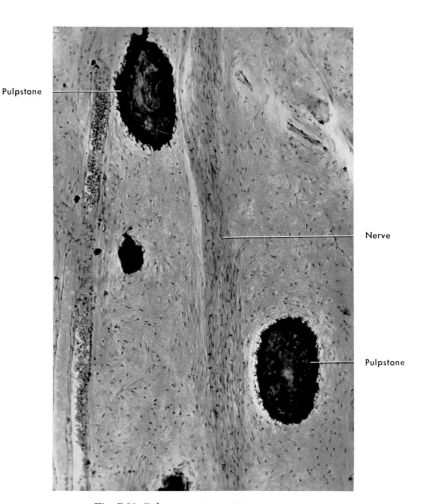

Fig. 5-31. Pulpstones in proximity to a nerve.

Fig. 5-32. These four diagrams depict the pulp organ throughout life. Observe first the decrease in size of the pulp organ. **A** to **D**, Dentin is formed circumpulpally but especially in the
bifurcation zone. Note the decrease in cells and increase in fibrous tissue. The blood vessels
*(white)* early organize into an odontoblastic plexus and later are more prominent in the subodontoblastic zone, indicating a decrease in active dentinogenesis. Observe the sparse number
of nerves in the young pulp, the organization of the parietal layer of nerves. They are less
prominent in the aging pulp. Reparative dentin and pulp stones are apparent in the oldest
pulp, at lower right, **D.**

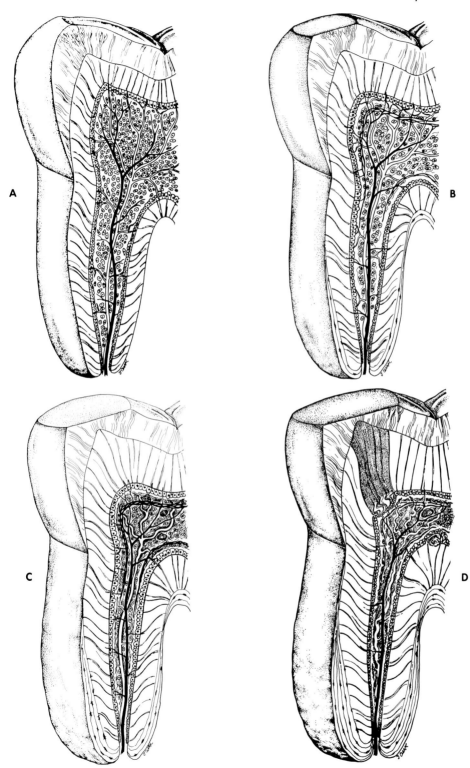

**Fig. 5-32.** For legend see opposite page.

one estimate, 66% of teeth in persons 10 to 30 years of age, 80% in those between 30 and 50 years, and 90% in those after 50 years of age contain calcifications of some type.

## CLINICAL CONSIDERATIONS

For all operative procedures the shape of the pulp chamber and its extensions into the cusps, the pulpal horns, is important to remember. The wide pulp chamber in the tooth of a young person will make a deep cavity preparation hazardous, and it should be avoided, if possible. In some instances of developmental disturbances the pulpal horns project high into the cusps, and in such cases the exposure of a pulp can occur when it is least anticipated. Sometimes a roentgenogram will help to determine the size of a pulp chamber and the extent of the pulpal horns.

If opening a pulp chamber for treatment becomes necessary, its size and variation in shape must be taken into consideration. With advancing age, the pulp chamber becomes smaller (Fig. 5-32), and because of excessive dentin formation at the roof and floor of the chamber, it is sometimes difficult to locate the root canals. In such cases it is advisable, when one opens the pulp chamber, to advance toward the distal root in the lower molar and toward the lingual root in the upper molar. In this region one is most likely to find the opening of the pulp canal without risk of perforating the floor of the pulp chamber. In the anterior teeth the coronal part of the pulp chamber may be filled with secondary dentin; thus locating the root canal is made difficult. Pulpstones lying at the opening of the root canal may cause considerable difficulty when an attempt is made to locate the canals (Fig. 5-1).

The shape of the apical foramen and its location may play an important part in the treatment of root canals. When the apical foramen is narrowed by cementum, it is more readily located because further progress of the broach will be stopped at the foramen. If the apical opening is at the side of the apex, as shown in Fig. 5-3, *B*, not even roentgenograms will reveal the true length of the root canal, and this may lead to misjudgment of the length of the canal and the root canal filling.

Since accessory canals are rarely seen in roentgenograms, they are not treated in root canal therapy. In any event it would be mechanically difficult or impossible to reach them. Fortunately, however, the majority of them do not affect the success of endodontic therapy.

When accessory canals are located near the coronal part of the root or in the bifurcation area (Fig. 5-4, *B*), a deep periodontal pocket may cause inflammation of the dental pulp. Thus periodontal disease can have a profound influence on pulp integrity. Conversely, a necrotic pulp can cause disease of the periodontium through an accessory canal. It has been recently recognized that this interrelationship between the pulpal and periodontal diseases is further exaggerated by their communicating blood supply.

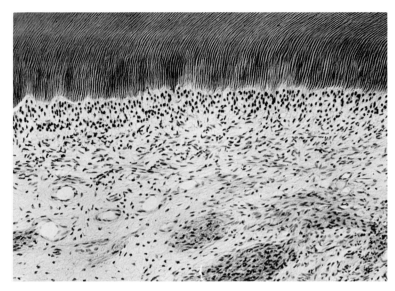

**Fig. 5-33.** Mild pulp response with loss of odontoblast identity and inflammatory cells obliterating cell-free zone.

For a long time it was believed that an exposed pulp meant a lost pulp. The fact that defense cells have been recognized in the pulp has changed this concept. Extensive experimental work has shown that exposed pulps can be preserved if proper pulp capping or pulp amputation procedures are applied. This is especially so in noninfected, accidentally exposed pulps in young individuals. In many instances dentin is formed at the site of the exposure; thus a dentin barrier or bridge is made and the pulp may remain vital. Pulp capping of primary teeth has been shown to be remarkably successful.

All operative procedures cause an initial response on the pulp, which is dependent on the severity of the insult. The pulp is highly responsive to stimuli. Even a slight stimulus will cause inflammatory cell infiltration (Fig. 5-33). A severe reaction is characterized as one with increased inflammatory cell infiltration adjacent to the cavity site, hyperemia, or localized abscesses. Hemorrhage may be present, and the odontoblast layer is either destroyed or greatly disrupted. It is of interest that most compounds such as calcium hydroxide readily induce reparative dentin underlying a cavity (Fig. 5-34). After 5 weeks most composite filling materials also induce reparative dentin formation (Fig. 5-35). Usually the closer a restoration is to the pulp organ the greater the response will be.

Since dehydration causes pulpal damage, operative procedures producing this state should be avoided. When filling materials contain harmful chemicals (e.g., acid in silicate cements and monomer in the composites), an appropriate cavity base should be used prior to the insertion of restorations.

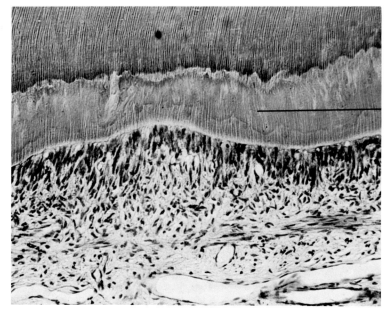

Reparative
dentin

**Fig. 5-34.** Moderate cell response with formation of reparative dentin underlying cavity. Note viable odontoblasts have functional reparative dentin deposition.

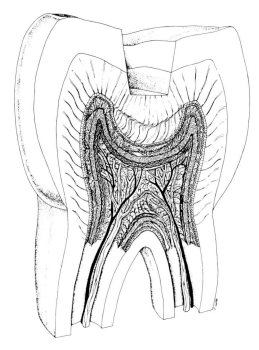

**Fig. 5-35.** Diagram of reparative function of the pulp organ to cavity preparation and subsequent restoration. Reparative dentin is limited to zone of stimulation.

A vital pulp is essential to good dentition. Although modern endodontic procedures can prolong the usefulness of a tooth, a nonvital tooth is brittle and subject to fractures. Therefore, every precaution should be taken to preserve the vitality of a pulp.

In clinical practice instruments called vitalometers or thermal stimuli (heat and cold) are often used to test the "vitality" of the pulp. These methods test the reaction of the pulp to electrical stimulus and thus provide information about the status of the nerves supplying the pulpal tissue. These devices therefore check the "sensitivity" of the pulp and not its "vitality." The vitality of the pulp depends on its blood supply, and one can have teeth with damaged nerve but normal blood supply (as in cases of traumatized teeth). Such pulps do not respond to electrical or thermal stimuli but are completely viable in every respect.

The preservation of the health of the pulp during operative procedures and its successful management in cases of disease is one of the most important challenges to the clinical dentist.

## REFERENCES

Avery, J. K.: Structural elements of the young normal human pulp. In Siskin, M., editor: The biology of the human dental pulp, St. Louis, 1973, The C. V. Mosby Co. (Available only through American Association of Endodontists, Atlanta, Ga.)

Avery, J. K., and Han, S. S.: The formation of collagen fibrils in dental pulp, J. Dent. Res. 40(6):1248-1261, Nov.-Dec. 1961.

Beveridge, E. E., and Brown, A. C.: The measurement of human dental intrapulpal pressure and its response to clinical variables, Oral Surg. 19(5):655-668, May 1965.

Bhussry, B. R.: Modification of the dental pulp organ during development and aging. In Finn, S. B., editor: Biology of the dental pulp organ: A symposium, University, Ala., 1968, University of Alabama Press.

Bradford, E. W.: Microanatomy and histochemistry of dentine. In Miles, A. E. W., editor: Structural and chemical organization of teeth. Vol. 2, New York, 1967, Academic Press Inc.

Corpron, R. E., and Avery, J. K.: The ultrastructure of intradental nerves in developing mouse molars, Anat. Rec. 175(3):585-606, March 1973.

Corpron, R. C., Avery, J. K., and Lee, S. D.: Ultrastructure of terminal pulpal blood vessels in mouse molars, Anat. Rec. 179(4):527-541, Aug. 1974.

Dahl, E., and Mjör, I. A.: The fine structure of the vessels in the human dental pulp, Acta Odontol. Scand. 31(4):223-230, Oct. 1973.

Fanibunda, K. B.: Volume of the dental pulp cavity-method of measurement. British I.A.D.R. Abstr. No. 150, J. Dent. Res. (Suppl.) 52:971, 1973.

Fanibunda, K. B.: A preliminary study of the volume of the pulp in the permanent human teeth. Unpublished. Personal communication, 1975.

Fearnhead, R. W.: The histological demonstration of nerve fibers in human dentin. In Anderson, D. J., editor: Sensory mechanisms in dentin, Oxford, 1963, Pergamon Press.

Finn, S. B.: Biology of the dental pulp organ: A symposium, University, Ala., 1968, University of Alabama Press.

Graf, W., and Björlin, G.: Diameters of nerve fibers in human tooth pulps, J. Am. Dent. Assoc. 43:186-193, 1951.

Green, D. A.: Stereoscopic study of the root apices of 400 maxillary and mandibular anterior teeth, Oral Surg. 9:1224-1232, Nov. 1956.

Griffin, C. J., and Harris, R.: Ultrastructure of collagen fibrils and fibroblasts of the developing human dental pulp, Arch. Oral Biol. 11:659-666, 1966.

Griffin, C. J., and Harris, R.: The ultrastructure of the blood vessels of the human dental pulp following injury. I to IV, Aust. Dent. J. 17:303-308, 355-362, 441, 1972; 18:88-96, 1973.

Han, S. S., and Avery, J. K.: The ultrastructure of capillaries and arterioles of the hamster dental pulp, Anat. Rec. **145**(4): 549-572, 1963.

Han, S. S., Avery, J. K., and Hale, L. E.: The fine structure of differentiating fibroblasts in the incisor pulp of the guinea pig, Anat. Rec. **153**(2):187-210, 1965.

Han, S. S., and Avery, J. K.: The fine structure of intercellular substances and rounded cells in the incisor pulp of the guinea pig, Anat. Rec. **15**(1):41-58, 1965.

Harris, R., and Griffin, C. J.: Fine structure of nerve endings in the human dental pulp, Arch. Oral Biol. **13**:773-778, 1968.

Harris, R., and Griffin, C. J.: The ultrastructure of small blood vessels of the human dental pulp, Aust. Dent. J. **16**: 220-226, 1971.

Harrop, T. J., and MacKay, B.: Electron microscopic observations of healing in dental pulp in the rat, Arch. Oral Biol. **13**(43):365-385, 1968.

Kollar, E. J., and Baird, G. R.: The influence of the dental papilla on the development of tooth shape in embryonic mouse tooth germs, J. Embryol. Exp. Morphol. **21**:131-148, 1969.

Kollar, E. J., and Baird, G. R.: Tissue interactions in embryonic mouse tooth germs. I. Reorganization of the dental epithelium during tooth-germ reconstruction, J. Embryol. Exp. Morphol. **24**:159-170, 1970.

Kollar, E. J., and Baird, G. R.: Tissue interactions in embryonic mouse tooth germs. II. The indicative role of the dental papilla, **24**:173-186, 1970.

Kovacs, I.: A systematic description of dental roots. In Dahlberg, A. A., editor: Dental morphology and evaluation, Chicago, 1971, University of Chicago Press.

Kramer, I. R. H.: The vascular architecture of the human dental pulp, Arch. Oral Biol. **2**:177-189, 1960.

Langeland, K.: Tissue changes in the dental pulp, Odont. Tidskr. **65**(4):239-386, 1957.

Mjör, I. A., and Pindborg, J. J.: Histology of the human tooth, Copenhagen, 1973, Munksgaard, International Booksellers & Publishers, Ltd.

Nishijima, S., Imanishi, I., and Aka, M.: An experimental study on the lymph circulation in dental pulp, J. Osaka Dent. School **5**:45-49, 1965.

Nygaard-Ostby, B., and Hjortdal, O.: Tissue formation in the root canal following pulp removal, Scand. J. Dent. Res. **79**:333-349, 1971.

Ogilvie, A. L., and Ingle, J. E.: An atlas of pulpal and periapical biology, Philadelphia, 1965, Lea & Febiger.

Organ, B. J.: Contribution to the histology of the dental pulp and periodontal membrane, with special reference to the cells of "defense" of these tissues, J. Am. Dent. Assoc. **16**(6):965-981, 1929.

Provenza, V. D.: Fundamentals of oral histology and embryology, Philadelphia, 1972, J. B. Lippincott Co.

Rapp, R., Avery, J. K., and Rector, R. A.: A study of the distribution of nerves in human teeth, J. Can. Dent. Assoc. **23**:447-453, 1957.

Rapp, R., Avery, J. K., and Strachan, D. S.: The distribution of nerves in human primary teeth, Anat. Rec. **159**(1):89-104, 1967.

Ruben, M. P., Prieto-Hernandez, J. R., Gott, F. K., Kramer, G. M., and Bloom, A. A.: Visualization of lymphatic microcirculation of oral tissues. II. Vital retrograde lymphography, J. Periodontol. **42**:774-784, Dec. 1971.

Saunders, R. L. de C. H., and Röckert, H. O. E.: Vascular supply of dental tissues, including lymphatics. In Miles, A. E. W., editor: Structural and chemical organization of teeth, vol. 1, New York, 1967, Academic Press Inc.

Schroff, F. R.: Physiologic path of changes in the dental pulp, Oral Surg. **6**:1455-1460, 1953.

Seltzer, S., and Bender, I. B.: The dental pulp, Philadelphia, 1965, J. B. Lippincott Co.

Shumaker, D. B., and El Hadray, M. S.: Roentgenographic study of eruption, J. Am. Dent. Assoc. **61**:19, 535-541, 1960.

Sicher, H.: Oral anatomy, ed. 4, St. Louis, 1965, The C. V. Mosby Co.

Stanley, H. R., and Rainey, R. R.: Age changes in the human dental pulp, Oral Surg. **15**:1396-1404, 1962.

Torneck, C. D.: Changes in the fine structure of the dental pulp in human caries pulpitis. I. Nerves and blood vessels, J. Oral Pathol. **3**:71-82, 1974.

Torneck, C. D.: Changes in the fine structure of the dental pulp in human caries pulpitis. II. Inflammatory infiltration, J. Oral Pathol. **3**:83-99, 1974.

Weinstock, M., and Leblond, C. P.: Formation of collagen, Fed. Proc. 33(5):1205-1218, 1974.

Weinstock, M., and Leblond, C. P.: Synthesis migration and release of precursor collagen by odontoblasts as visualized by radioautography after [³H] proline administration, J. Cell Biol. 60:92-127, 1974.

Yankowitz, D.: An investigation of the existence and magnitude of intrapulpal pressure in dog teeth. Master's thesis, University of Washington, Seattle, 1963.

Zachrisson, B. V.: Mast cells in human dental pulp, Arch. Oral Biol. 16:555-556, 1971.

Zerlotti, E.: Histochemical study of the connective tissue of the dental pulp, Arch. Oral Biol. 9:149-160, 1964.

# 6 Cementum

Cementum is the mineralized dental tissue covering the anatomic roots of human teeth. It was first demonstrated microscopically in 1835 by two pupils of Purkinje. It begins at the cervical portion of the tooth at the cementoenamel junction and continues to the apex. Cementum furnishes a medium for the attachment of collagen fibers that bind the tooth to surrounding structures. It is a specialized connective tissue that shares some physical, chemical, and structural characteristics with compact bone. Unlike bone, however, human cementum is avascular.

## PHYSICAL CHARACTERISTICS

The hardness of fully mineralized cementum is less than that of dentin. Cementum is light yellow in color and can be distinguished from enamel by its lack of luster and its darker hue. Cementum is somewhat lighter in color than dentin. The difference in color, however, is slight, and under clinical conditions it is not possible to distinguish cementum from dentin based on color alone. Under some experimental conditions cementum has been shown to be permeable to a variety of materials.

## CHEMICAL COMPOSITION

On a dry weight basis, cementum from fully formed permanent teeth contains about 45% to 50% inorganic substances and 50% to 55% organic material and water. The inorganic portion consists mainly of calcium and phosphate in the form of hydroxyapatite. Numerous trace elements are found in cementum in varying amounts. It is of interest that cementum has the highest fluoride content of all the mineralized tissues.

The organic portion of cementum consists primarily of collagen and protein polysaccharides. Amino acid analyses of collagen obtained from the cementum of human teeth indicate close similarities to the collagens of dentin and alveolar bone. The chemical nature of the protein polysaccharides or ground substance of cementum is virtually unknown.

## CEMENTOGENESIS

Cementum formation in the developing tooth is preceded by the deposition of dentin along the inner aspect of Hertwig's epithelial root sheath. Once dentin formation is underway, breaks occur in the epithelial root sheath allowing the newly formed dentin to come in direct contact with connective tissue of the dental follicle (Fig. 6-1). Cells derived from this connective tissue are responsible for cementum formation.

At the ultrastructural level, breakdown of Hertwig's epithelial root sheath involves degeneration or loss of its basal lamina on the cemental side. Loss of

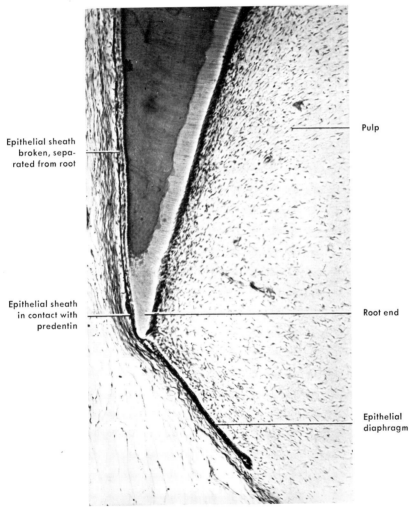

Epithelial sheath broken, separated from root

Epithelial sheath in contact with predentin

Pulp

Root end

Epithelial diaphragm

**Fig. 6-1.** Hertwig's epithelial root sheath at end of forming root. At side of root the sheath is broken up, and cementum formation begins. (From Gottlieb, B.: J. Periodont. **13**:13, 1942.)

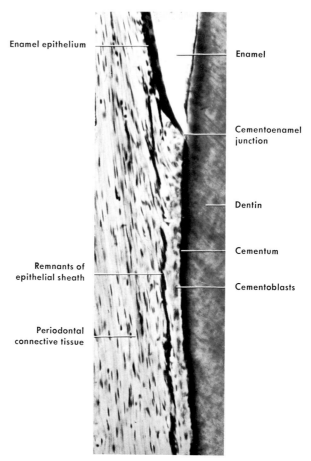

Enamel epithelium

Enamel

Cementoenamel junction

Dentin

Cementum

Remnants of epithelial sheath

Cementoblasts

Periodontal connective tissue

**Fig. 6-2.** Epithelial sheath is broken and separated from root surface by connective tissue.

continuity of the basal lamina is soon followed by the appearance of collagen fibrils and cementoblasts between epithelial cells of the root sheath. Some sheath cells migrate away from the dentin toward the dental sac, whereas others remain near the developing tooth and ultimately are incorporated into the cementum. Sheath cells that migrate toward the dental sac become the epithelial rests of Malassez found in the periodontal ligament of fully developed teeth.

**Cementoblasts.** Soon after Hertwig's sheath breaks up, undifferentiated mesenchymal cells from adjacent connective tissue differentiate into cementoblasts (Fig. 6-2). Cementoblasts synthesize collagen and protein polysaccharides, which make up the organic matrix of cementum. These cells have numerous mitochondria, a well-formed Golgi apparatus, and large amounts of granular endoplasmic reticulum (Fig. 6-3). These ultrastructural features are not unique to cementoblasts and can be observed in other cells actively producing proteins and polysaccharides.

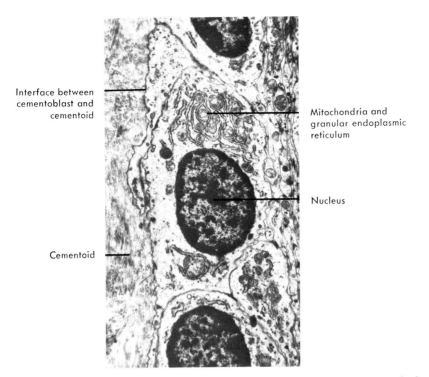

Interface between
cementoblast and
cementoid

Mitochondria and
granular endoplasmic
reticulum

Nucleus

Cementoid

**Fig. 6-3.** Cementoblasts on surface of cementoid. Mitochondria and granular endoplasmic reticulum are visible. (Electron micrograph; ×8000.) (Courtesy S. D. Lee, Ann Arbor, Mich.)

After some cementum matrix has been laid down, its mineralization begins. Calcium and phosphate ions present in tissue fluids are deposited into the matrix and are arranged as unit cells of hydroxyapatite. Mineralization of cementoid is a highly ordered event and not the random precipitation of ions into an organic matrix.

*Cementoid tissue.* Under normal conditions growth of cementum is a rhythmic process, and as a new layer of cementoid is formed, the old one calcifies. A thin layer of cementoid can usually be observed on the cemental surface (Fig. 6-4). This cementoid tissue is lined by cementoblasts. Connective tissue fibers from the periodontal ligament pass between the cementoblasts into the cementum. These fibers are embedded in the cementum and serve to attach the tooth to surrounding bone. Their embedded portions are known as Sharpey's fibers (Fig. 6-5). Each Sharpey's fiber is composed of numerous collagen fibrils that pass well into the cementum (Fig. 6-6).

## STRUCTURE

With the light microscope two kinds of cementum can be differentiated: acellular and cellular. The term "acellular cementum" is unfortunate. As a living tissue, cells are an integral part of cementum at all times. However, some layers of cementum do not *incorporate* cells, the spiderlike cementocytes, whereas other layers do contain such cells in their lacunae. It is probably best to view cementum as a unit consisting of cementoblasts, cementoid, and fully mineralized tissue.

Acellular cementum may cover the root dentin from the cementoenamel junction to the apex, but it is often missing on the apical third of the root. Here the cementum may be entirely of the cellular type. Cementum is thinnest at the cementoenamel junction (20 to 50 microns) and thickest toward the apex (150 to 200 microns). The apical foramen is surrounded by cementum. Sometimes cementum extends to the inner wall of the dentin for a short distance, and so a lining of the root canal is formed.

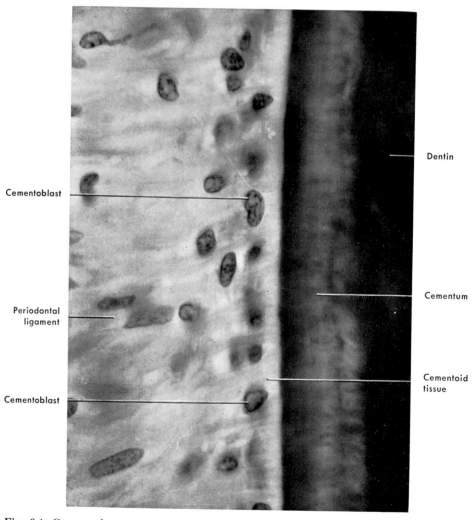

**Fig. 6-4.** Cementoid tissue on surface of calcified cementum. Cementoblasts between fibers.

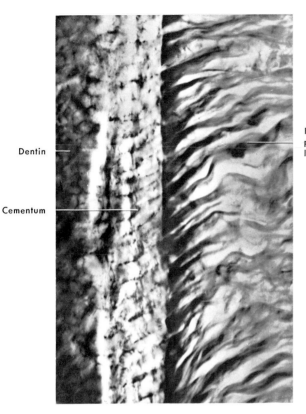

Dentin

Cementum

Fibers of
periodontal
ligament

**Fig. 6-5.** Fibers of periodontal ligament continue into surface layer of
cementum as Sharpey's fibers.

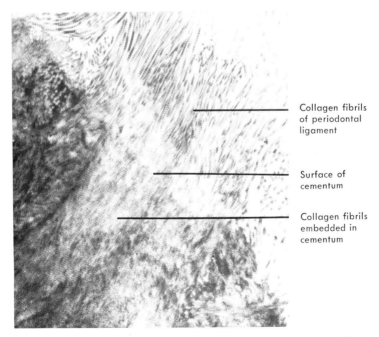

Collagen fibrils
of periodontal
ligament

Surface of
cementum

Collagen fibrils
embedded in
cementum

**Fig. 6-6.** Collagen fibrils from periodontal ligament continue into cementum. The numerous
collagen fibrils embedded in cementum are collectively referred to as Sharpey's fibers. (Decalcified human molar; electron micrograph; ×17,000.)

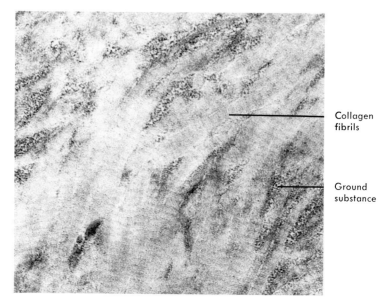

Collagen
fibrils

Ground
substance

**Fig. 6-7.** Electron micrograph of human cementum showing ground substance interspersed between collagen fibrils. (Decalcified specimen; ×42,000.)

In decalcified specimens of cementum, collagen fibrils make up the bulk of the organic portion of the tissue. Interspersed between some collagen fibrils are electron-dense reticular areas, which probably represent protein polysaccharide materials of the ground substance (Fig. 6-7). Collagen fibrils of both acellular and cellular cementum are arranged in a very complex fashion with little discernible pattern. In some areas, however, relatively discrete bundles of collagen fibrils can be seen, particularly in tangential sections (Fig. 6-8). These bundles are Sharpey's fibers, which make up a substantial portion of cementum.

In mineralized specimens it has been observed that cemental collagen is not totally mineralized. This is particularly true in a zone 10 to 50 microns wide near the cementodentinal junction. The unmineralized areas in cementum are about 1 to 5 microns in diameter. They appear to be poorly mineralized cores of Sharpey's fibers.

The cells incorporated into cellular cementum, cementocytes, are similar to osteocytes. They lie in spaces designated as lacunae. A typical cementocyte has numerous cell processes or canaliculi radiating from its cell body. These processes may branch, and they frequently anastomose with those of a neighboring cell. Most of the processes are directed toward the periodontal surface of the cementum. The full extent of these processes does not show up in routinely prepared histologic sections. They are best viewed in mineralized ground sections (Fig. 6-9). The cytoplasm of cementocytes in deeper layers of cementum contains few organelles, the endoplasmic reticulum appears dilated, and mitochon-

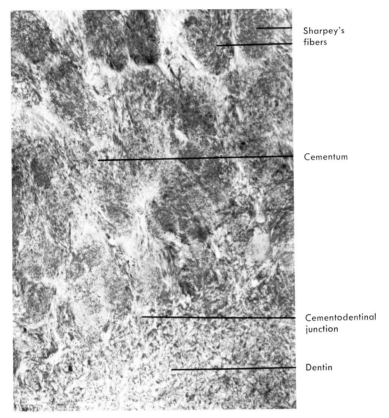

Sharpey's
fibers

Cementum

Cementodentinal
junction

Dentin

**Fig. 6-8.** Ultrastructural view of cementodentinal junction of human incisor. In this tangential section, Sharpey's fibers are visible as discrete bundles of collagen fibrils. (Decalcified specimen; electron micrograph; ×5000.)

dria are sparse. These characteristics indicate that cementocytes are either degenerating or are marginally active cells. At a depth of 60 microns or more cementocytes show definite signs of degeneration, such as cytoplasmic clumping and vesiculation. At the light microscopic level, lacunae in the deeper layers of cementum appear to be empty, suggesting complete degeneration of cementocytes located in these areas (Fig. 6-10).

Both acellular and cellular cementum are separated by incremental lines into layers, which indicate periodic formation (Figs. 6-10 and 6-11). Incremental lines can be seen best in decalcified specimens prepared for light microscopic observation. They are difficult to identify at the ultrastructural level. Histochemical studies indicate that incremental lines are highly mineralized areas with less collagen and more ground substance than other portions of the cementum.

When cementum remains relatively thin, Sharpey's fibers cross the entire thickness of the cementum. With further apposition of cementum, a larger part of the fibers is incorporated in the cementum. The attachment proper is confined

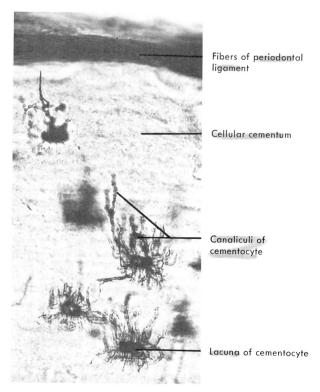

Fibers of periodontal ligament

Cellular cementum

Canaliculi of cementocyte

Lacuna of cementocyte

Fig. 6-9. Cellular cementum from human premolar. Note lacunae of spiderlike cementocytes with numerous canaliculi or cell processes. (Ground section; ×480.)

to the most superficial or recently formed layer of cementum (Fig. 6-5). This would seem to indicate that the thickness of cementum does not enhance functional efficiency by increasing the strength of attachment of the individual fibers.

The location of acellular and cellular cementum is not definite. As a general rule, however, acellular cementum usually predominates on the coronal half of the root, whereas cellular cementum is more frequent on the apical half. Layers of acellular and cellular cementum may alternate in almost any pattern. Acellular cementum can occasionally be found on the surface of cellular cementum (Fig. 6-10). Cellular cementum is frequently formed on the surface of acellular cementum (Fig. 6-10), but it may comprise the entire thickness of apical cementum (Fig. 6-12). It is always thickest around the apex and, by its growth, contributes to the length of the root (Fig. 6-13).

Extensive variations in the surface topography of cementum can be observed with the scanning electron microscope. Resting cemental surfaces, where mineralization is more or less complete, exhibit low rounded projections corresponding to the centers of Sharpey's fibers (Fig. 6-14). Cemental surfaces with actively mineralizing fronts have numerous small openings that correspond to sites where

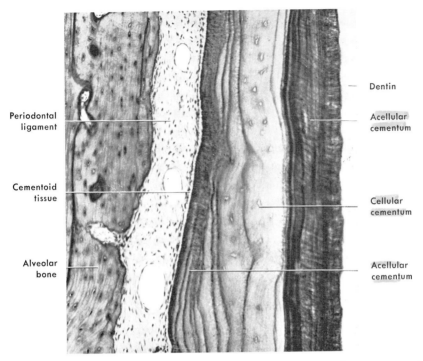

Periodontal ligament

Cementoid tissue

Alveolar bone

Dentin

Acellular cementum

Cellular cementum

Acellular cementum

**Fig. 6-10.** Cellular cementum on surface of acellular cementum and again covered by acellular cementum (incremental lines). Lacunae of cellular cementum appear empty, indicating degeneration of cementocytes.

individual Sharpey's fibers enter the tooth (Fig. 6-15). These openings represent unmineralized cores of the fibers. Numerous resorption bays and irregular ridges of cellular cementum are also frequently observed on root surfaces (Fig. 6-16).

## CEMENTODENTINAL JUNCTION

The dentin surface upon which cementum is deposited is relatively smooth in permanent teeth. The cementodentinal junction in deciduous teeth, however, is sometimes scalloped. The attachment of cementum to dentin in either case is quite firm although the nature of this attachment is not fully understood.

The interface between cementum and dentin is clearly visible in decalcified and stained histologic sections using the light microscope (Figs. 6-10 and 6-11). In such preparations cementum usually stains more intensely than does dentin. When observed with the electron microscope, the cementodentinal junction is not as distinct as when observed with the light microscope. A narrow interface zone between the two tissues, however, can be detected with the electron microscope. In decalcified preparations, cementum is more electron dense than dentin and some of its collagen fibrils are arranged in relatively distinct bundles while those of dentin are arranged somewhat haphazardly (Fig. 6-8). Since collagen

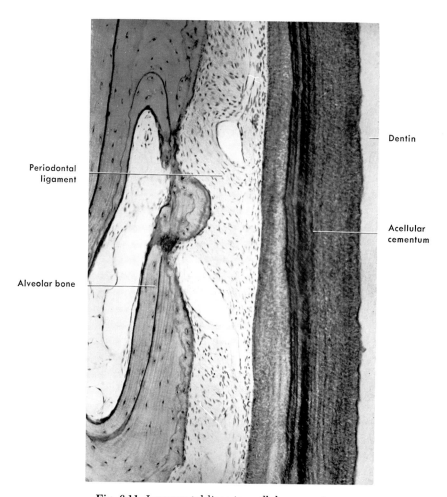

Fig. 6-11. Incremental lines in acellular cementum.

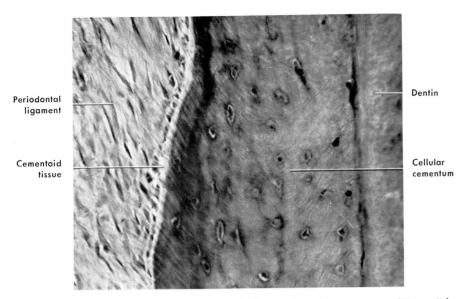

Periodontal ligament

Cementoid tissue

Dentin

Cellular cementum

Fig. 6-12. Cellular cementum forming entire thickness of apical cementum. (From Orban, B.: Dental histology and embryology, Philadelphia, 1929, P. Blakiston's Son & Co.)

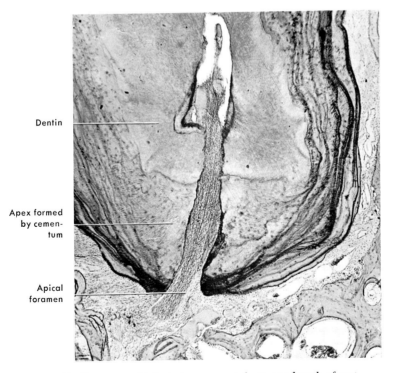

Dentin

Apex formed by cementum

Apical foramen

Fig. 6-13. Cementum thickest at apex, contributing to length of root.

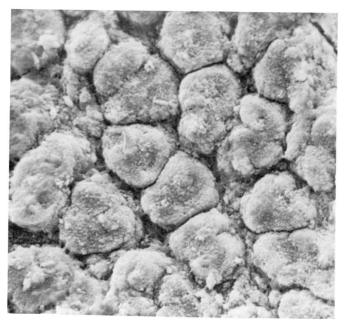

**Fig. 6-14.** Scanning electron micrograph of resting cemental surface of human premolar. Rounded projections correspond to insertion sites of Sharpey's fibers. (Anorganic preparation; ×3400.) (Courtesy A. Boyde, London, England.)

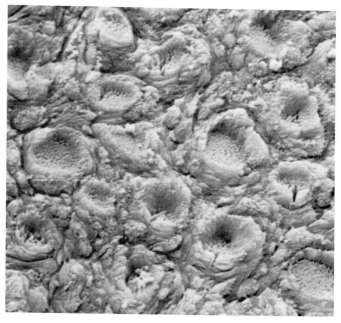

**Fig. 6-15.** Scanning electron micrograph of cemental surface of human molar with actively mineralizing front. Peripheral portions of Sharpey's fibers are more mineralized than their centers. (Anorganic preparation; approximately ×1500.) (From Jones, S. J., and Boyde, A.: Z. Zellforsch. **130:**318, 1972.)

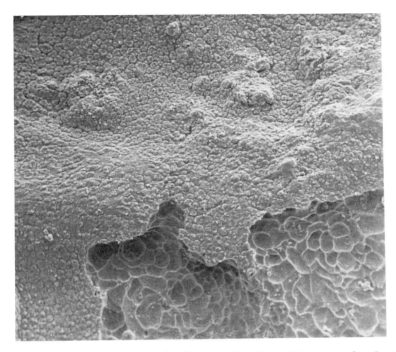

**Fig. 6-16.** Scanning electron micrograph of cemental surface of human molar showing numerous projections of Sharpey's fibers. Note large multiloculate resorption bay at bottom of field. (Anorganic preparation; ×250.) (From Jones, S. J., and Boyde, A.: Z. Zellforsch. **130**:318, 1972.)

fibrils of cementum and dentin intertwine at their interface in a very complex fashion, it is not possible to precisely determine which fibrils are of dentinal origin and which are of cemental origin.

Sometimes dentin is separated from cementum by a zone known as the "intermediate cementum layer," which does not exhibit characteristic features of either dentin or cementum (Fig. 6-17). This layer is predominately seen in the apical two thirds of roots of molars and premolars and is only rarely observed in incisors or deciduous teeth. It is believed that this layer represents areas where cells of Hertwig's epithelial sheath become trapped in a rapidly deposited dentin or cementum matrix. Sometimes it is a continuous layer. Sometimes it is found only in isolated areas.

## CEMENTOENAMEL JUNCTION

The relation between cementum and enamel at the cervical region of teeth is variable. In approximately 30% of all teeth, cementum meets the cervical end of enamel in a relatively sharp line (Fig. 6-18, A). In about 10% of the teeth, enamel and cementum do not meet. Presumably this occurs when enamel epithelium in the cervical portion of the root is delayed in its separation from dentin. In such cases there is no cementonenamel junction. Instead, a zone of the root is devoid of cementum and is, for a time, covered by reduced enamel epithelium.

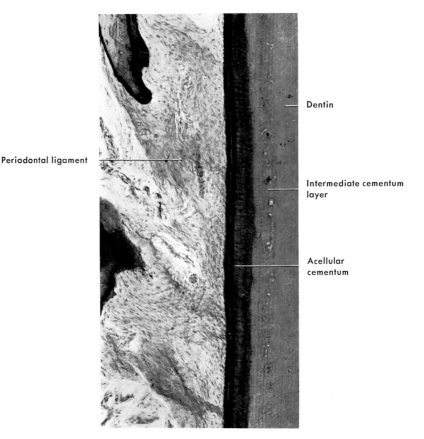

Periodontal ligament

Dentin

Intermediate cementum layer

Acellular cementum

Fig. 6-17. Intermediate layer of cementum.

In approximately 60% of the teeth, cementum overlaps the cervical end of enamel for a short distance (Fig. 6-18, *B*). This occurs when the enamel epithelium degenerates at its cervical termination, permitting connective tissue to come in direct contact with the enamel surface. Electron microscopic evidence indicates that when connective tissue cells, probably cementoblasts, come in contact with enamel they produce a laminated, electron-dense, reticular material termed "afibrillar cementum." Afibrillar cementum is so named because it does not possess collagen fibrils with a 640 Å periodicity. If such afibrillar cementum remains in contact with connective tissue cells for a long enough time, fibrillar cementum with characteristic collagen fibrils may subsequently be deposited on its surface; thus the thickness of cementum that overlies enamel increases.

## FUNCTION

The primary function of cementum is to furnish a medium for the attachment of collagen fibers that bind the tooth to alveolar bone. Since collagen fibers of the periodontal ligament cannot be incorporated into dentin, a connective tissue

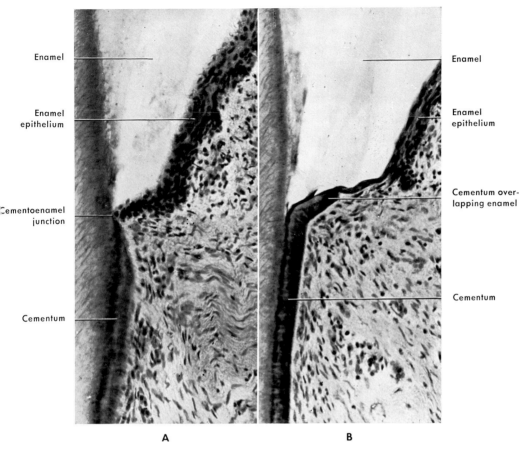

Fig. 6-18. Variations at cementoenamel junction. **A,** Cementum and enamel meet in a sharp line. **B,** Cementum overlaps enamel.

attachment to the tooth is impossible without cementum. This is dramatically demonstrated in some cases of hypophosphatasia, a rare hereditary disease, where loosening and premature loss of anterior deciduous teeth occurs. The exfoliated teeth are characterized by an almost total absence of cementum.

The continuous deposition of cementum is of considerable functional importance. In contrast to the alternating resorption and new formation of bone, cementum is not resorbed under normal conditions. As the most superficial layer of cementum ages, a new layer of cementum must be deposited to keep the attachment apparatus intact. The repeated apposition of cemental layers represents the aging of the tooth as an organ. In other words, a tooth is, functionally speaking, only as old as the last layer of cementum laid down on its root. The "functional age" of a tooth may be considerably less than its chronologic age.

Cementum serves as the major reparative tissue for root surfaces. Damage to roots such as fractures and resorptions can be repaired by the deposition of new cementum. Cementum can also be viewed as the tissue that makes functional adaptation of teeth possible. For example, deposition of cementum in an apical area can compensate for loss of tooth substance from occlusal wear.

## HYPERCEMENTOSIS

Hypercementosis is an abnormal thickening of cementum. It may be diffuse or circumscribed, it may affect all teeth of the dentition, it may be confined to a single tooth, or it may even affect only parts of one tooth. If the overgrowth improves the functional qualities of the cementum, it is termed a "cementum hypertrophy." If the overgrowth occurs in nonfunctional teeth or if it is not cor-related with increased function, it is termed "hyperplasia."

In localized hypertrophy a spur or pronglike extension of cementum may be formed (Fig. 6-19). This condition frequently is found in teeth that are exposed to great stress. The pronglike extensions of cementum provide a larger surface

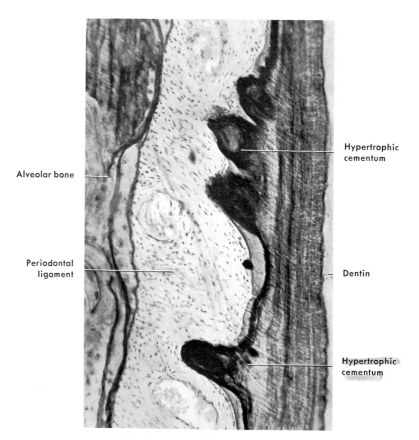

Fig. 6-19. Pronglike excementoses.

area for the attaching fibers; thus a firmer anchorage of the tooth to the surrounding alveolar bone is assured.

Localized hypercementosis may sometimes be observed in areas in which enamel drops have developed on the dentin. The hyperplastic cementum covering the enamel drops (Fig. 6-20) occasionally is irregular and sometimes contains round bodies that may be calcified epithelial rests. The same type of embedded calcified round bodies frequently are found in localized areas of hyperplastic cementum (Fig. 6-21). Such knoblike projections are designated as excementoses. They, too, develop around degenerated epithelial rests.

Extensive hyperplasia of cementum is occasionally found in connection with chronic periapical inflammation. Here the hyperplasia is circumscribed and surrounds the root like a cuff.

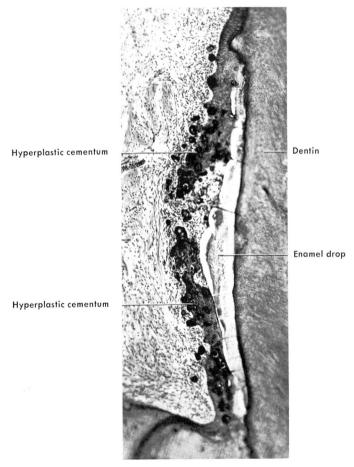

Fig. 6-20. Irregular hyperplasia of cementum on surface of enamel drop.

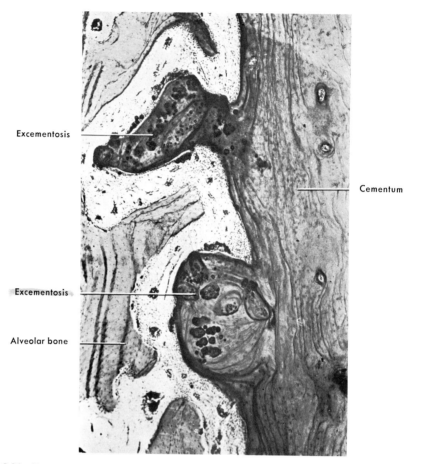

Fig. 6-21. Excementoses in bifurcation of molar. (From Gottlieb, B.: Oesterr. Z. Stomatol. 19:515, 1921.)

A thickening of cementum is often observed on teeth that are not in function. The hyperplasia may extend around the entire root of the nonfunctioning teeth or may be localized in small areas. Hyperplasia of cementum in nonfunctioning teeth is characterized by a reduction in the number of Sharpey's fibers embedded in the root.

The cementum is thicker around the apex of all teeth and in the furcation of multirooted teeth than it is on other areas of the root. This thickening can be observed in embedded as well as in newly erupted teeth.

In some cases an irregular overgrowth of cementum can be found, with spike-like extensions and calcification of Sharpey's fibers and accompanied by numerous cementicles. This type of cemental hyperplasia can occasionally be observed on many teeth of the same dentition and is, at least in some cases, the sequela of injuries to the cementum (Fig. 6-22).

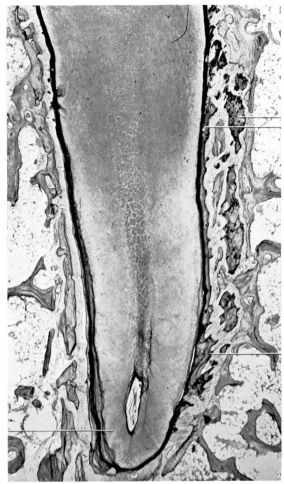

Remnants of
fractured cementum
Hyperplastic cementum

Hyperplastic cementum

Apex

**Fig. 6-22.** Extensive spikelike hyperplasia of cementum formed during the healing of cemental tear.

## CLINICAL CONSIDERATIONS

Cementum is more resistant to resorption than is bone, and it is for this reason that orthodontic tooth movement is made possible. When a tooth is moved by means of an orthodontic appliance, bone is resorbed on the side of the pressure, and new bone is formed on the side of tension. On the side toward which the tooth is moved, pressure is equal on the surfaces of bone and cementum. Resorption of bone as well as of cementum may be anticipated. However, in careful orthodontic treatment, cementum resorption, is minimal or absent but bone resorption leads to tooth migration.

The difference in the resistance of bone and cementum to "pressure" may be caused by the fact that bone is richly vascularized, whereas cementum is avas-

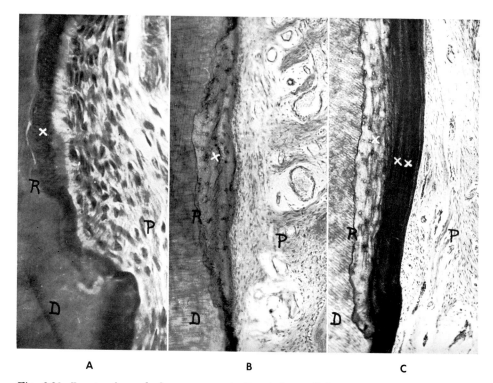

**Fig. 6-23.** Repair of resorbed cementum. **A,** Repair by acellular cementum, *x.* **B,** Repair by cellular cementum, *x.* **C,** Repair first by cellular, *x,* and later by acellular, *xx,* cementum. *D,* Dentin. *R,* Line of resorption. *P,* Periodontal ligament.

cular. Thus degenerative processes are much more easily affected by interference with circulation in bone, whereas cementum with its slow metabolism (as in other avascular tissues) is not damaged by a pressure equal to that exerted on bone.

Cementum resorption can occur after trauma or excessive occlusal forces. In severe cases cementum resorption may continue into the dentin. After resorption has ceased, the damage usually is repaired, either by formation of acellular (Fig. 6-23, *A*) or cellular (Fig. 6-23, *B*) cementum or by alternate formation of both (Fig. 6-23, *C*). In most cases of repair there is a tendency to reestablish the former outline of the root surface. This is called *anatomic repair.* However, if only a thin layer of cementum is deposited on the surface of a deep resorption, the root outline is not reconstructed, and a baylike recess remains. In such areas sometimes the periodontal space is restored to its normal width by formation of a bony projection, so that a proper functional relationship will result. The outline of the alveolar bone in these cases follows that of the root surface (Fig. 6-24). In contrast to anatomic repair, this change is called *functional repair.*

If teeth are subjected to a severe blow, smaller or larger fragments of ce-

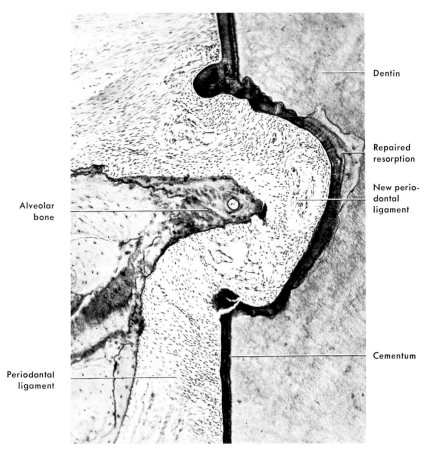

Dentin

Repaired resorption

New perio-dontal ligament

Alveolar bone

Cementum

Periodontal ligament

**Fig. 6-24.** Functional repair of cementum resorption by bone apposition. Normal width of periodontal ligament reestablished.

mentum may be severed from the dentin. The tear occurs frequently at the cementodentinal junction, but it may also be in the cementum or dentin.

Transverse fractures of the root may occur after trauma, and these may heal by formation of new cementum.

Frequently, hyperplasia of cementum is secondary to periapical inflammation or extensive occlusal stress. The fact is of practical significance because the extraction of such teeth may necessitate the removal of bone. This also applies to extensive excementoses, as shown in Fig. 6-21. These can anchor the tooth so tightly to the socket that the jaw or parts of it may be fractured in an attempt to extract the tooth. This possibility indicates the necessity for taking roentgenograms before any extraction. Small fragments of roots left in the jaw after extraction of teeth may be surrounded by cementum and remain in the jaw without causing any disturbance.

Gingival recession or periodontal surgery lead to exposure of cervical cementum. Whereas this may not cause any symptoms, in some cases it produces cervical sensitivity. The sensitivity is caused by the fact that the thin layer of cementum at the cervical area cannot protect the underlying dentin from the oral environment. Such cases are corrected by coagulation of the odontoblastic processes in the dentinal tubules with chemical coagulants (calcium hydroxide).

In periodontal pockets the plaque and its by-products can penetrate the cementum and through the dentinal tubules reach the pulp. In such cases, a periodontal pocket may produce a pulpal lesion (pulpitis). In differential diagnosis of tooth (pulpal) pain therefore, a periodontal origin must be considered, and if so established, the periodontal pocket should either be surgically eliminated or patients instructed to keep it meticulously clean and free of plaque.

## REFERENCES

Beumer, J., Trowbridge, H. O., Silverman, S., Jr., and Eisenberg, E.: Childhood hypophosphatasia and the premature loss of teeth. A clinical and laboratory study of seven cases, Oral Surg. **35**:631, 1973.

Blackwood, H. J. J.: Intermediate cementum, Br. Dent. J. **102**:345, 1957.

Bruckner, R. J., Rickles, N. H., and Porter, D. R.: Hypophosphatasia with premature shedding of teeth and aplasia of cementum, Oral Surg. **15**:1351, 1962.

Denton, G. B.: The discovery of cementum, J. Dent. Res. **18**:239, 1939.

Eastoe, J. E.: Composition of the organic matrix of cementum, J. Dent. Res. **54** (special issue, abstr. L547):L137, 1975.

El Mostehy, M. R., and Stallard, R. E.: Intermediate cementum, J. Periodont. Res. **3**:24, 1968.

Furseth, R.: A microradiographic and electron microscopic study of the cementum of human deciduous teeth, Acta Odontol. Scand. **25**:613, 1967.

Furseth, R.: The fine structure of the cellular cementum of young human teeth, Arch. Oral Biol. **14**:1147, 1969.

Gedalia, I., Nathan, H., Schapira, J., Hass, N., and Feldmann, J.: Fluoride concentration of surface enamel, cementum, lamina dura and subperiosteal bone from the mandibular angle of Hebrews, J. Dent. Res. **44**:452, 1965.

Gottlieb, B.: Zementexostosen, Schmelztropfen und Epithelnester [Exostosis of cementum, enamel drops, and epithelial rests], Osterr. Z. Stomatol. **19**:515, 1921.

Gottlieb, B.: Biology of the cementum, J. Periodont. **13**:13, 1942.

Jones, S. J., and Boyde, A.: A study of human root cementum surfaces as prepared for and examined in the scanning electron microscope, Z. Zellforsch. **130**:318, 1972.

Kronfeld, R.: The biology of cementum, J. Am. Dent. Assoc. **25**:1451, 1938.

Kronfeld, R.: Coronal cementum and coronal resorption, J. Dent. Res. **17**:151, 1938.

Lester, K. S.: The incorporation of epithelial cells by cementum, J. Ultrastruct. Res. **27**:63, 1969.

Lindén, L.-Å.: Microscopic observations of fluid flow through cementum and dentine. An *in vitro* study on human teeth, Odontol. Revy **19**:367, 1968.

Listgarten, M. A.: Phase-contrast and electron microscopic study of the junction between reduced enamel epithelium and enamel in unerupted human teeth, Arch. Oral Biol. **11**:999, 1966.

Nihei, I.: A study on the hardness of human teeth, J. Osaka Univ. Dent. Soc. **4**:1, 1959.

Olsen, T., and Johansen, E.: Inorganic composition of sound and carious human cementum. Preprinted abstracts, Fiftieth General Meeting of the International Association for Dental Research, Abstr. no. 174, p. 91, 1972.

Orban, B.: Dental histology and embryology, ed. 2, Philadelphia, 1929, P. Blakiston's Son & Co.

Paynter, K. J., and Pudy, G.: A study of the structure, chemical nature, and development of cementum in the rat, Anat. Rec. **131**:233, 1958.

Rautiola, C. A., and Craig, R. G.: The microhardness of cementum and underlying dentin of normal teeth and teeth exposed to periodontal disease, J. Periodont. **32**:113, 1961.

Rodriguez, M. S., and Wilderman, M. N.:

Amino acid composition of the cementum matrix from human molar teeth, J. Periodont. **43**:438, 1972.

Schroeder, H. E., and Listgarten, M. A.: Fine structure of the developing epithelial attachment of human teeth. In Wolsky, A., editor: Monographs in developmental biology, vol. 2, Basel, 1971, S. Karger, AG.

Selvig, K. A.: Electron microscopy of Hertwig's epithelial root sheath and of early dentin and cementum formation in the mouse incisor, Acta Odontol. Scand. **21**: 175, 1963.

Selvig, K. A.: An ultrastructural study of cementum formation, Acta Odontol. Scand. **22**:105, 1964.

Selvig, K. A.: The fine structure of human cementum, Acta Odontol. Scand. **23**:423, 1965.

Sherman, D. B., Ruben, M. P., Goldman, H. M., Breck, F., and Healy, M.: Laser spectrochemical microanalysis of cementum. Preprinted abstracts, Forty-fourth General Meeting of the International Association for Dental Research, Abstr. no. 85, p. 59, 1966.

Van Kirk, L. E.: Variations in structure of human enamel and dentin, J. Am. Dent. Assoc. **15**:1270, 1928.

Zander, H A., and Hürzeler, B.: Continuous cementum apposition, J. Dent. Res. **37**: 1035, 1958.

Zipkin, I.: The inorganic composition of bones and teeth, In Schraer, H., editor: Biological calcification, New York, 1970, Appleton-Century-Crofts.

# 7 Periodontal ligament

EVOLUTION

DEVELOPMENT

CELLS

Synthetic cells
Osteoblasts
Fibroblasts
Cementoblasts

Resorptive cells
Osteoclasts
"Fibroclasts"
Cementoclasts

Progenitor cells

Relationship between cells

Epithelial rests of Malassez

Mast cells

Macrophages

EXTRACELLULAR SUBSTANCE
Fibers
Collagen
Oxytalan

Ground substance
Interstitial tissue

STRUCTURES PRESENT IN CONNECTIVE TISSUE
Blood vessels
Lymphatics
Nerves
Cementicles

FUNCTIONS
Supportive
Sensory
Nutritive
Homeostatic

CLINICAL CONSIDERATIONS

The periodontium is a connective tissue organ, covered by epithelium, that attaches the teeth to the bones of the jaws and provides a continually adapting apparatus for support of the teeth during function. The periodontium comprises four connective tissues, two mineralized and two fibrous. The two mineralized connective tissues comprise cementum and alveolar bone (Chapters 6 and 8) and the two fibrous connective tissues, periodontal ligament and lamina propria of the gingiva (Chapter 9). The periodontium is attached to the dentin of the root of the tooth by cementum and to the bone of the jaws by alveolar bone. The periodontal ligament occupies the periodontal space, which is located between the cementum and the periodontal surface of the alveolar bone, and extends coronally to the most apical part of the lamina propria of the gingiva. By definition, therefore, the coronal part of the periodontal ligament is marked by the most superficial fibers appearing to extend from cementum to alveolar bone. Collagen fibers of the periodontal ligament are embedded in cementum and alveolar bone, so that the ligament provides soft-tissue continuity between the mineralized connective tissues of the periodontium.

The periodontal ligament is a fibrous connective tissue that is noticeably cellular (Fig. 7-1) and vascular. All connective tissues, the periodontal ligament included, comprise cells and extracellular substance consisting of fibers and ground substance. The majority of the fibers of the periodontal ligament are collagen, and the ground substance comprises a variety of macromolecules, the basic constituents of which are proteins and polysaccharides. It is important to remember that the extracellular substance is produced and can be removed by the cells of the connective tissue.

The periodontal ligament has a number of functions, which include attachment and support, nutrition, synthesis and resorption, and proprioception. Over

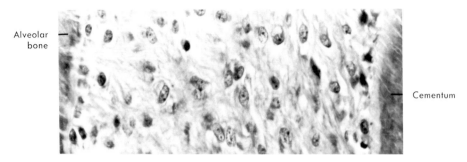

Alveolar bone

Cementum

Fig. 7-1. Oblique section of periodontal ligament from pig molar showing its cellularity. (Hematoxylin and eosin; ×600.)

the years it has been described by a number of terms. Among these are desmodont, gomphosis, pericementum, dental periosteum, alveolodental ligament, and periodontal membrane. Periodontal membrane and periodontal ligament are the terms that are now most commonly used. Neither term describes the structure and its functions adequately. It is neither a typical membrane nor a typical ligament. However, as it is a quite complex soft connective tissue providing continuity between two mineralized connective tissues, the term "periodontal ligament" appears to be the most appropriate.

## EVOLUTION

There is a fundamental difference in the attachment of reptilian and mammalian teeth. In the ancestral reptiles the teeth are ankylosed to the bone. In mammals they are suspended in their sockets by ligaments. The evolutionary step from reptile to mammal included a series of coordinated changes in the jaws. The central point of these changes is the radical "reconstruction" of the mandible. In the reptiles the mandible consists of a series of bones united by sutures. Only the uppermost bone, the dentary, carries the ankylosed teeth. The mandibular articulation is formed by a separate bone of the mandible, the articulare, and a separate bone of the cranium, the quadratum. During the period of transition from advanced types of reptiles to the first mammals, the dentary attains larger proportions, whereas the other mandibular bones are reduced in size. Finally, only the dentary forms the mammalian mandible. The other bony components of the reptilian mandible are either lost or changed into two of the ossicles of the middle ear: the articulare survives as the malleus and the quadratum as the incus. Before this change could take place, the dentary, growing a condylar process, formed a "new" temporomandibular articulation that, for a time, functioned together with the old articulare-quadratum joint. Such "double-jointed" forms are now known.

The change from the many-boned reptilian to the single-boned mammalian mandible brings with it a radical change in the mode of growth. In the reptile the growth of the mandible is "sutural," in the same manner as the growth of the cranium. In the mammal the newly acquired cartilage of the condyle takes over as the most important growth site of the mandible. In the reptile, growth of the mandibular body in height occurs in the mandibular sutures, whereas in the mammal it occurs by growth at the free margins of the alveolar process. In the reptile the mandibular (and maxillary) teeth "move" with the bones to which they are fused. In the mammal the teeth have to "move" as units independent of the bones, and this movement is made possible by the remodeling of the ligament. The evolutionary change from the reptiles to mammals replaces the ankylosis of tooth and bone to a ligamentous suspension of the tooth.

## DEVELOPMENT

The dental organ (enamel organ) and, later in tooth development, Hertwig's epithelial root sheath are surrounded by the dental sac (see p. 23). It consists of a thin layer of cells that are continuous with the cells of the dental papilla. It has been suggested that the term *dental follicle* be reserved for those cells, and the term *perifollicular mesenchyme* for the cells that surround the dental follicle (Fig. 7-2). The cells of the dental follicle give origin to the cementoblasts that deposit cementum on the developing root, to the fibroblasts of the developing periodontal ligament, and possibly to the osteoblasts of the developing alveolar bone. The formation of the periodontal ligament occurs after the cells of Hertwig's epithelial root sheath (see p. 37) have separated, forming the strands known as the *epithelial rests of Malassez* (see p. 37). This separation permits the cells of the dental follicle to migrate to the external surface of the newly formed root dentin. These migrant follicle cells then differentiate into cementoblasts and deposit the first-formed cementum on the surface of the dentin. Other cells of the dental follicle differentiate into fibroblasts, which synthesize the fibers and ground substance of the periodontal ligament. The fibers become embedded in newly developed cementum and alveolar bone and, as the tooth erupts, are orientated in characteristic fashion (Chapter 11).

## CELLS

The principle cells of the healthy, functioning periodontal ligament are the differentiated cells and their progenitors. The differentiated cells are concerned with the synthesis and resorption of alveolar bone, the synthesis and resorption of the fibrous connective tissue of the ligament, and the synthesis and, on occasions, resorption of cementum. Consequently, the cells of the periodontal ligament may be divided into three main categories:

Synthetic cells
    Osteoblasts
    Fibroblasts
    Cementoblasts
Resorptive cells
    Osteoclasts
    "Fibroclasts"
    Cementoclasts
Progenitor cells

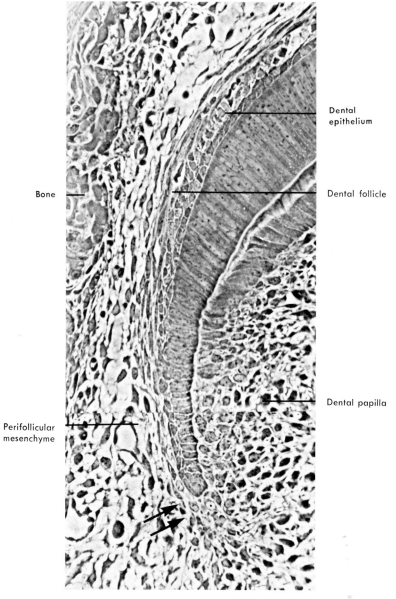

**Fig. 7-2.** Montage phase-contrast photomicrograph of first molar tooth germ of a 1-day-old mouse showing dental follicle, which is continuous with dental papilla around cervical loop (*arrows*). (×450.) (From Freeman, E., and Ten Cate, A. R.: J. Periodontol. **42:**387, 1971.)

There are, in addition, epithelial cells present in the ligament:

Epithelial rests of Malassez

And there are other types of connective tissue cells:

Mast cells
Macrophages

### Synthetic cells

There are certain general cytologic criteria that distinguish all cells that are synthesizing proteins for secretion (e.g., extracellular substance of connective tissue), and these criteria can be applied equally to osteoblasts, cementoblasts, and fibroblasts. For a cell to produce protein, it must, among other activities, transcribe ribonucleic acid (RNA), synthesize ribosomes in the nucleolus and transport them to the cytoplasm, and increase its complement of rough endoplasmic reticulum (RER) and Golgi membranes for translation and transport of the protein. It must also have the means to produce an adequate supply of energy. Each of these functional activities is reflected morphologically when synthetically active tissues are viewed by the electron and light microscopes. Increased transcription of RNA and production of ribosomes is reflected by a large open-faced or vesicular nucleus containing prominent nucleoli. The development of large quantities of rough endoplasmic reticulum covered by ribosomes is readily recognized in the electron microscope and is reflected by hematoxyphilia of the cytoplasm when the cell is seen in the light microscope after staining by hematoxylin and eosin. The hematoxyphilia is the result of interaction of the RNA with the acid hematein in the stain. The Golgi saccules and vesicles are also readily seen in the electron microscope but are not stained by acid hematein and so, in the light microscope, they are seen in appropriate sections as a clear, unstained area in the otherwise hematoxyphilic cytoplasm. The increased requirement for energy is reflected in the electron microscope by the presence of relatively large numbers of mitochondria. Accommodation of all these organelles in the cell requires a large amount of cytoplasm. Thus, a cell that is actively secreting extracellular substance will be seen in the light microscope to exhibit a large, open-faced or vesicular nucleus with prominent nucleoli and to have abundant cytoplasm that tends to be hematoxyphilic, with, if the plane of section is favorable, a clear area representing the Golgi membranes.

Cells with the morphology described above, if applied to the periodontal surface of the alveolar bone, are active osteoblasts; if lying in the body of the soft connective tissue, they are active fibroblasts; and, if applied to cementum, they are active cementoblasts. These cells all have, in addition to the features described above, the particular characteristics of osteoblasts, fibroblasts, and cementoblasts. Descriptions of the first two types of cells can be found in appropriate textbooks and of the third, in the chapter on cementum (Chapter 6).

Synthetic cells in all stages of activity are present in the periodontal ligament, and this is reflected directly by the degree to which the characteristics described above are developed in each cell. Cells having a paucity of cytoplasm (that is, cytoplasm that virtually cannot be distinguished in the light microscope) and having very few organelles and a close-faced nucleus, are also found in the ligament. Some cells that are not actively synthesizing extracellular substance are progenitor cells and will be discussed below.

**Osteoblasts.** The osteoblasts covering the periodontal surface of the alveolar bone constitute a modified endosteum and not a periosteum. A periosteum can be recognized by the fact that it comprises at least two distinct layers, an inner cellular or cambium layer and an outer fibrous layer. A cellular layer, but not an outer fibrous layer, is present on the periodontal surface of the alveolar bone. The surface of the bone lining the dental socket must therefore be regarded as an interior surface of bone, akin to that lining medullary cavities, and not an external surface, which would be covered by periosteum. The surface of the bone is covered largely by osteoblasts in various stages of differentiation, by progenitor cells, as well as by occasional osteoclasts. Collagen fibers of the ligament that penetrate the alveolar bone intervene between the cells.

**Fibroblasts.** Fibroblasts in various stages of differentiation, and their pro-

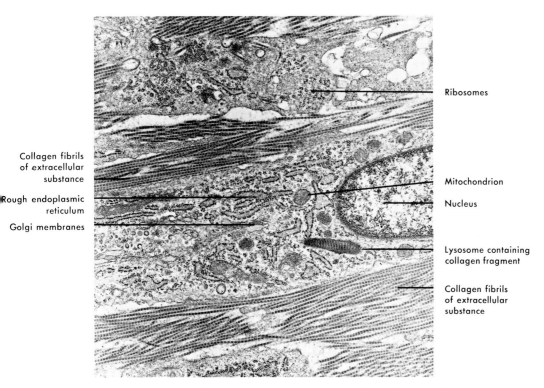

Collagen fibrils of extracellular substance

Rough endoplasmic reticulum

Golgi membranes

Ribosomes

Mitochondrion

Nucleus

Lysosome containing collagen fragment

Collagen fibrils of extracellular substance

**Fig. 7-3.** Fibroblasts of mouse molar periodontal ligament. (×9250.) (Courtesy Dr. A. R. Ten Cate, Toronto.)

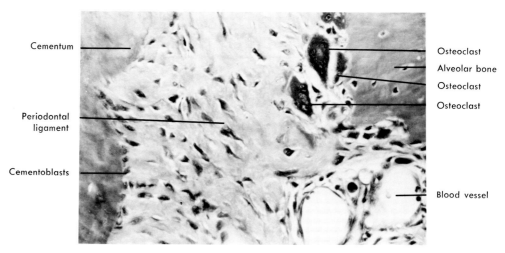

Cementum

Periodontal
ligament

Cementoblasts

Osteoclast
Alveolar bone
Osteoclast
Osteoclast

Blood vessel

**Fig. 7-4.** Osteoclasts on periodontal surface of alveolar bone in monkey periodontal ligament. (Hematoxylin and eosin; ×400.)

genitors, are found in the periodontal ligament where they are surrounded by fibers and ground substance (Fig. 7-3). In longitudinal sections viewed by light microscopy, the cells of the ligament appear to be orientated parallel to the orientated bundles of collagen fibers.

*Cementoblasts.* The distribution on the tooth surface of variously differentiated cementoblasts (Fig. 7-4) and their progenitors is similar to the distribution of osteoblasts on the bone surface.

### Resorptive cells

*Osteoclasts.* These cells resorb bone, tend to be large and multinucleated, but can be small and mononuclear. Multinucleated osteoclasts are formed by fusion of precursor cells. The characteristic multinucleated giant cells usually exhibit an eosinophilic cytoplasm and are easily recognizable. The cells may sometimes occupy bays in bone, Howship's lacunae, or surround the end of the bone spicules when viewed in the light microscope. In the electron microscope their cytoplasm is seen to exhibit numerous mitochondria and lysosomes, abundant Golgi saccules and free ribosomes, but little RER. The part of the plasma membrane lying adjacent to bone that is being resorbed is raised in characteristic folds and is termed the ruffled or striated border. The ruffled border is separated from the rest of the plasma membrane by a zone of specialized membrane that is closely applied to the bone. The bone related to the ruffled border can be seen to be undergoing resorption. Resorption occurs in two stages: the mineral is first removed from a narrow zone at the bone margin, and this is followed by disintegration of the recognizable exposed organic matrix. The osteoclast appears to accomplish both demineralization and disaggregation of the organic matrix, the latter apparently being achieved by the secretion of appropriate enzymes. The ruffled border disappears in inactive osteoclasts. Light and electron microscopic histochemical tests can be used to show that osteoclasts are rich in acid phosphatase, which is contained in lysosomes.

The presence of osteoclasts on the periodontal surface of the alveolar bone (Fig. 7-4) indicates that resorption was active, or had recently ceased, in that area at the time the tissue was removed. Osteoclasts are seen regularly in normal functioning periodontal ligament, in which the cells play a part in the removal and deposition of bone that constitutes its remodeling, a process that allows functional changes in the position of teeth to be accommodated by the supporting tissues (Chapter 11).

"**Fibroclasts.**" It has recently become evident that the collagen fibrils of mammalian periodontal ligament can be resorbed under physiologic conditions by mononuclear cells resembling fibroblasts. These cells exhibit lysosomes that contain fragments of collagen that appear to be undergoing digestion (Fig. 7-3). The activity of these fibroclastic cells does not necessarily appear to be restricted to destruction of collagen, as large portions of their cytoplasm may be filled with the organelles normally associated with protein synthesis. Thus the term "fibroclast" is used here purely to describe cells apparently engaged in resorption of collagen. It must be made clear that there does not appear to be a unique cell that resorbs the extracellular substance of soft connective tissue, but that the cell commonly termed a "fibroblast" may be capable of both synthesis and resorption. Collagen-resorbing fibroblasts are inhabitants of normal functioning periodontal ligament and their presence, like that of osteoclasts in relation to bone, indicates resorption of fibers occurring during physiologic turnover or remodeling of periodontal ligament.

**Cementoclasts.** These cells resemble osteoclasts and are only occasionally found in normal functioning periodontal ligament. This observation is consistent with the knowledge that cementum is not remodeled in the fashion of alveolar bone and periodontal ligament, but that it undergoes continual deposition during life. However, resorption of cementum can occur under certain circumstances, and in these instances mononuclear cementoclasts or multinucleated giant cells, often located in Howship's lacunae, are found on the surface of the cementum.

### Progenitor cells

All connective tissues, including periodontal ligament, contain undifferentiated progenitor cells that have the capacity to undergo mitotic division. If they were not present, there would be no cells available to replace differentiated cells dying at the end of their life-span or as a result of trauma. It is believed that generally, after division, one of the daughter cells differentiates into a functional type of connective tissue cell (i.e., any one of the cell types described above) while the other remains an undifferentiated progenitor cell retaining the capacity to divide when stimulated appropriately. Progenitor cells have a small, close-

faced nucleus and very little cytoplasm and are intermingled with the other cells
of the periodontal ligament.

Almost nothing is known about the progenitor cells of the ligament. It is not
known, e.g., whether they are located perivascularly as in some other soft connective tissues. It is also not known whether a single population of progenitor
cells gives rise to all of the specialized cells in the ligament or if there are a
number of populations, each of which gives rise to a different specialized cell.
That progenitor cells are present is evident from the burst of mitoses that occur
after application of pressure to a tooth as in orthodontic therapy, or after wound-
ing, maneuvers that stimulate differentiation of cells of periodontal ligament.

### Relationship between cells

The cells of the periodontal ligament form a three-dimensional network and,
in appropriately orientated sections, their processes can be seen to surround the
collagen fibers of the extracellular substance. Cells of periodontal ligament associated with bone, fibrous connective tissue, and cementum are not separated
from one another, but adjacent cells generally are in contact with their neighbors,
usually through their processes (Fig. 7-5). The site of some of the contacts between adjacent cells may be marked by modification of the structure of the
contiguous plasma membranes. The nature of these junctions has not yet been
elucidated satisfactorily. Although many appear to be zonulae occludentes, it is

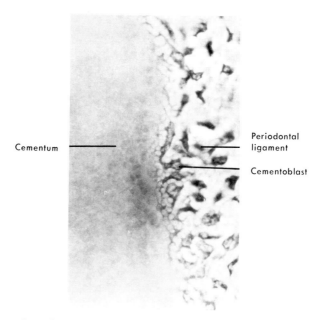

Cementum — Periodontal ligament

Cementoblast

**Fig. 7-5.** Surface of monkey cementum illustrating cementoblast processes. (Hematoxylin and eosin; ×600.)

conceivable that they are in fact gap junctions. Gap junctions in other tissues occur between cells that have been found to be in direct communication with one another. It is evident that some form of communication must exist between the cells of the periodontal ligament, otherwise it is difficult to see how the homeostatic mechanisms that are known to operate in the periodontal ligament could function.

### Epithelial rests of Malassez

The periodontal ligament contains epithelial cells that are found close to the cementum but not in contact with it (Fig. 7-6). These cells were first described by Malassez in 1884 and are the remnants of the epithelium of Hertwig's

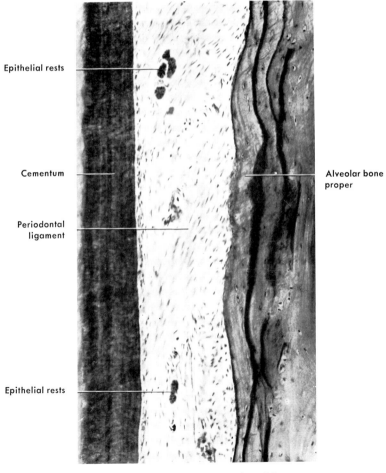

**Fig. 7-6.** Epithelial rests in periodontal ligament.

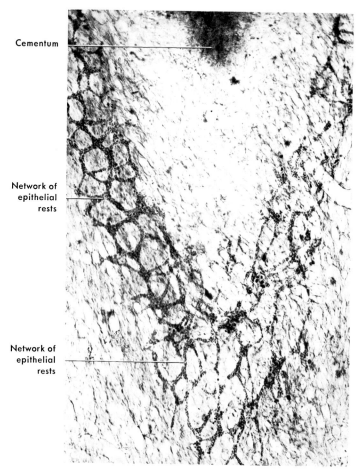

Cementum

Network of epithelial rests

Network of epithelial rests

**Fig. 7-7.** Network of epithelial rests in periodontal ligament. (Tangential section almost parallel to root surface.)

epithelial root sheath (Chapter 2). At the time of cementum formation the continuous layer of epithelium that covers the surface of the newly formed dentin breaks into lace-like strands (Fig. 7-7). These persist as a network, strands, or tubules near and parallel to the surface of the root (Figs. 7-6 to 7-8).

Only in sections almost parallel to the root can the true arrangement of these epithelial strands be seen. When the tooth is sectioned longitudinally or transversely, the strands of the network are cut in cross section or obliquely and, as a result, appear as isolated islands when viewed in the light microscope. The cause of disintegration of the epithelium and any inductive influence that it may have on the cells of the dental follicle have not been elucidated.

In rat and mouse molars, most but not all of the epithelium of the developing root is incorporated into the cementum, and consequently the epithelial rests of Malassez are sparse.

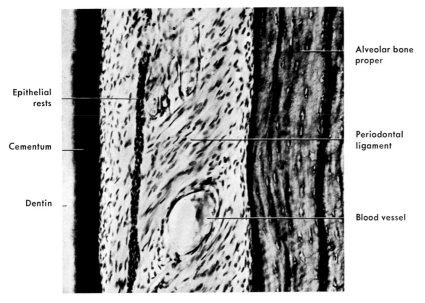

**Fig. 7-8.** Long strand of epithelium in periodontal ligament.

Electron microscopic observations show the epithelial rests to be isolated from the connective tissue cells by a basal lamina, similar to that occurring at the junction of epithelium and connective tissue elsewhere in the body. It is evident from their ultrastructure, response to histochemical tests, and behavior in cell, tissue, and organ culture that, although the epithelial cells appear in some mammals to decrease with age, they are not effete. However, their physiologic role, if any, in the functioning periodontal ligament is unknown. Under certain pathologic conditions they can undergo rapid proliferation and produce a variety of cysts and tumors that are unique to the jaws.

### Mast cells

Mast cells may be found in the periodontal ligament, and their characteristic morphology is described in most textbooks of general histology.

### Macrophages

Macrophages may also be present in the ligament. However, it is important to understand that the only criterion by which macrophages can be recognized in the light microscope is the presence of phagocytosed material in their cytoplasm and, further, that differentiated cells in the periodontal ligament are capable of phagocytosis. The wandering type of macrophage, probably derived from blood monocytes, has a characteristic ultrastructure that is also well described in general textbooks of histology.

## EXTRACELLULAR SUBSTANCE

The extracellular substance of the periodontal ligament comprises the following:

Fibers
    Collagen
    Oxytalan
Ground substance
    Proteoglycans
    Glycoproteins

### Fibers

The fibers in human periodontal ligament comprise collagen and oxytalan. Elastic fibers are restricted almost entirely to the walls of the blood vessels. The majority of fibers in the periodontal ligament are collagen.

*Collagen.* Collagen is a specific, high-molecular-weight protein to which is attached a small number of sugars. There are at least four different types of collagen, all of identical basic physical and chemical structure, but each exhibiting certain specific and unique chemical characteristics. Periodontal ligament appears to comprise predominantly type I collagen. Collagen *macromolecules* are rodlike, being very long in relation to their diameter, and are arranged to form *fibrils*. These fibrils show a highly ordered periodic banding pattern that is definitive for collagen when viewed in the electron microscope (Fig. 7-3), but because of their small diameter, they cannot be resolved by light microscopy. However, the fibrils are packed side by side to form bundles or *fibers*, which, when of diameter greater than 0.2 microns, can be seen at the highest magnifica-

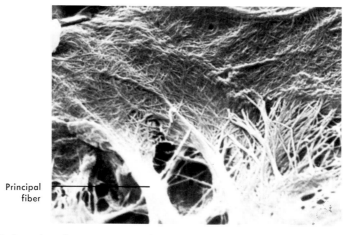

Principal
fiber

**Fig. 7-9.** Scanning electron micrograph of cross section of human periodontal ligament close to cementum (not shown). Principal fibers lose their identity as they blend with fibrils orientated in apparently random fashion *(upper half of picture).* (×4000.) (From Shackleford, J. M.: Am. J. Anat. **131:**427, 1971.)

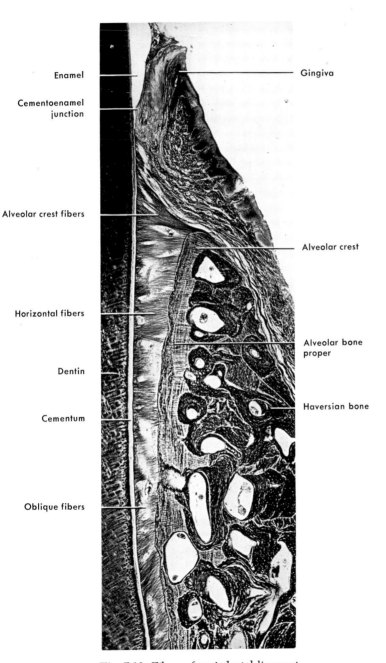

Enamel

Cementoenamel
junction

Alveolar crest fibers

Horizontal fibers

Dentin

Cementum

Oblique fibers

Gingiva

Alveolar crest

Alveolar bone
proper

Haversian bone

**Fig. 7-10.** Fibers of periodontal ligament.

tion of the light microscope. Fibers are the smallest order of collagen that can be resolved by light microscopy. Collagen fibers are further gathered together to form bundles, and these are readily resolved by light microscopy.

The collagen fibrils of periodontal ligament, when examined by transmission electron microscopy, are seen to be gathered together to form fibers. When examined in the light microscope, many of the collagen fibers are found to be gathered into bundles having clear orientation relative to the periodontal space, and these are termed *principal fibers*. When viewed by scanning electron microscopy, however, many of the fibrils are seen not to be gathered into fibers, but rather to be distributed in apparently random fashion (Fig. 7-9), ramifying with and between the fibers. These observations suggest that the collagen fibrils of the periodontal ligament are gathered together either in fibers, bundles of which constitute the highly orientated and readily identifiable principal fibers, or else are arranged in apparently unorientated fashion, forming a meshwork between the principal fibers.

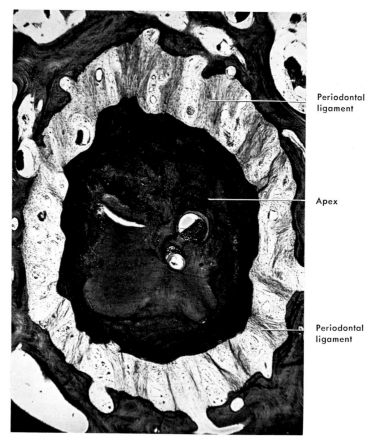

Periodontal ligament

Apex

Periodontal ligament

**Fig. 7-11.** Apical fibers of periodontal ligament. (From Orban, B.: Dental histology and embryology, Philadelphia, 1929, P. Blakiston's Son & Co.)

The principal fibers of the periodontal ligament (Figs. 7-10 to 7-12) are arranged in five particular groups, each group having a name, as follows:

1. *Alveolar crest group.* The fibers bundles of this group radiate from the crest of the alveolar process and attach themselves to the cervical part of the cementum.

2. *Horizontal group.* The bundles run at right angles to the long axis of the tooth, from the cementum to the bone.

3. *Oblique group.* The bundles run obliquely. They are attached in the cementum somewhat apically from their attachment to the bone. These fiber bundles are most numerous and constitute the main attachment of the tooth.

4. *Apical group.* The bundles are irregularly arranged and radiate from the apical region of the root to the surrounding bone.

5. *Interradicular group.* From the crest of the interradicular septum, bundles extend to the furcation of multirooted teeth.

There are also fiber bundles in the lamina propria of the gingiva that have specific orientation, and some of them lie immediately coronal to the periodontal ligament (Chapter 9). The most superficial fibers of the alveolar crest group of principal fibers mark the coronal extremity of the periodontal ligament.

Collagen fibers are embedded into cementum on one side of the periodontal space and into alveolar bone on the other. The embedded fibers are termed *Sharpey's fibers.* There is some evidence from small rodents and monkeys that Sharpey's fibers can traverse the bone of the alveolar process, to continue interdentally as principal fibers in the adjacent periodontal ligament or to mingle

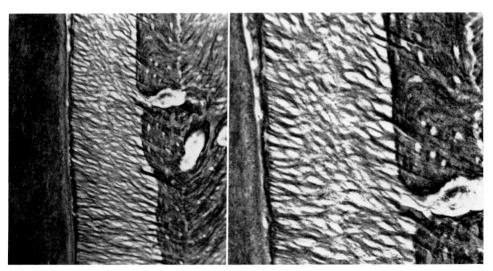

**A**

**B**

Fig. 7-12. **A,** Periodontal ligament of monkey premolar demonstrating principal fibers. **B,** Higher magnification of an area of **A.** Zone described as intermediate plexus is evident. (**A,** silver impregnation, ×400; **B,** ×800.) (Courtesy Dr. Ino Sciaky, Jerusalem.)

buccally and lingually with the fibers of the periosteum covering the alveolar process.

The principal fibers run a wavy course from cementum to bone. It may appear in some sections examined in the light microscope as though fibers arising from cementum and bone are joined in the midregion of the periodontal space giving rise to a zone of distinct appearance, the so-called *intermediate plexus* (Fig. 7-12, *B*) (see also Chapter 11). It used to be believed that the intermediate plexus provides a site where rapid remodeling of fibers occurs, allowing adjustments in the ligament to be made to accommodate small movements of the tooth. However, evidence derived from radioautography and surgical experiments provide no support for this belief. The so-called intermediate plexus is evidently an artifact arising out of the plane of section and may be attributable to the fact that the collagen fibers do not course only in one bundle but may move from one bundle to the other. This is most readily seen in horizontal sections of the liga-

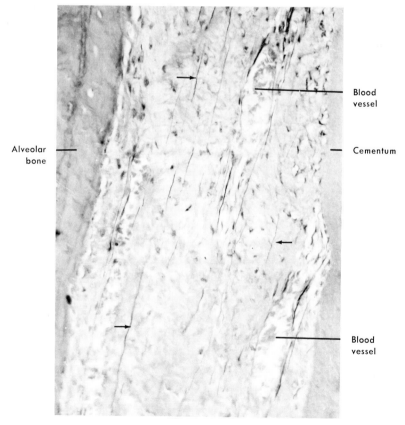

Fig. 7-13. Oxytalan fibers (*arrows*) in monkey periodontal ligament. (×245.)

ment, where the fibers are found to be arranged in many small bundles on the tooth side but in a few large bundles on the bone side.

It no longer seems important to question whether fibers run continuously from tooth to bone. First, the length of a single fibril is not known; second, the fibers evidently run from one bundle to the other, probably to be spliced with, and incorporated into, their new neighbors; and, third, the protein of the periodontal ligament is continually being remodeled, and so parts of fibrils must continually be removed and new pieces added, an alteration that does not necessarily reestablish continuity in the old orientation.

**Oxytalan.** Although elastic fibers are found in the periodontal ligaments of some animals, they are restricted to the walls of the blood vessels in humans. A fiber, termed oxytalan, which appears to be an immature elastic fiber, is found in human periodontal ligaments. They can be demonstrated in the light microscope in tissue stained by certain methods used to color elastic fibers, provided that the tissues are oxidized prior to staining. In the electron microscope, fibers believed to be oxytalan, resemble developing elastic fibers.

The orientation of the oxytalan fibers is quite different from the collagen fibers. Instead of running from bone to tooth, they tend to run in an axial direction (Fig. 7-13), one end being embedded in bone or possibly cementum and the other often in the wall of a blood vessel. In the vicinity of the apex they form a complex network. The function of the oxytalan fibers is unknown, but it has been suggested that they may play a part in supporting the blood vessels of the periodontal ligament.

### Ground substance

The space between cells, fibers, blood vessels, and nerves in the periodontal space is occupied by ground substance. Indeed, the ground substance is present in every nook and cranny, including the interstices between fibers and between fibrils. It is important to understand that all anabolites reaching the cells from the microcirculation in the ligament and all catabolites passing in the opposite direction must pass through the ground substance. It is therefore evident that its integrity is essential if the cells of the ligament are to function properly. The importance of the ground substance is frequently overlooked, and this is possibly because it is a difficult substance to investigate and perhaps because it is not demonstrated and therefore not recognizable in tissue prepared by routine methods for light and electron microscopy.

In essence, the ground substance comprises two major groups of substances, *proteoglycans* (or acid mucopolysaccharides) and *glycoproteins*. Both groups comprise proteins and polysaccharides, but of different type and arrangement, and proteoglycans carry a much stronger negative charge than do glycoproteins. The interested reader will find detailed descriptions of protein polysaccharides and glycoproteins in texts concerned with connective tissue biochemistry.

It was mentioned above that neither of these substances is demonstrated by routine histologic or electron-microscopic methods; they are demonstrated only by histochemical methods. A histochemical method is in essence a technique that attaches a material that can be recognized microscopically to specific chemical groups in the substance to be demonstrated (Chapter 15). For light microscopy, the specific substance is a dye that can be recognized by its color, and for electron microscopy an electron-dense material. In the case of the proteoglycans, a number of methods that utilize their strong negative charges have been developed to demonstrate the location of these substances in both the light and electron microscopes. Examples of the chemicals used are alcian blue 8GX and toluidine blue for light microscopy and ruthenium red for electron microscopy.

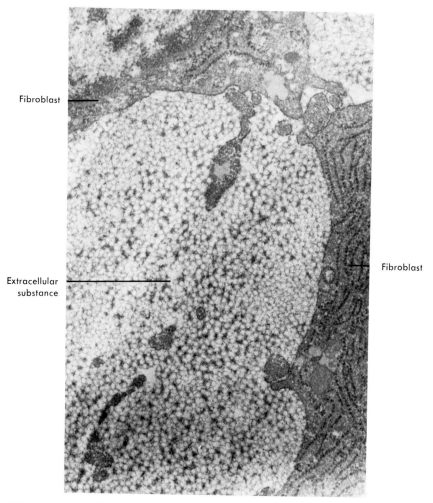

**Fig. 7-14.** Mouse periodontal ligament "stained" with ruthenium red to demonstrate proteoglycan of ground substance. Collagen fibrils are electron lucent, and ground substance is electron dense. (×33,000.)

Glycoproteins possess comparatively unique chemical groups (1, 2, glycols) that can be demonstrated in light microscopy by the periodic acid–Schiff method and in electron microscopy by the periodic acid–silver methenamine technique. These methods show quite clearly that ground substance is a significant constituent of the periodontal ligament (Fig. 7-14).

### Interstitial tissue

Some of the blood vessels, lymphatics, and nerves of the periodontal ligament are surrounded by loose connective tissue, and these areas can readily be recognized in the light microscope (Fig. 7-15). These areas have been termed *interstitial tissue*, but it is not known whether they have any particular biologic significance.

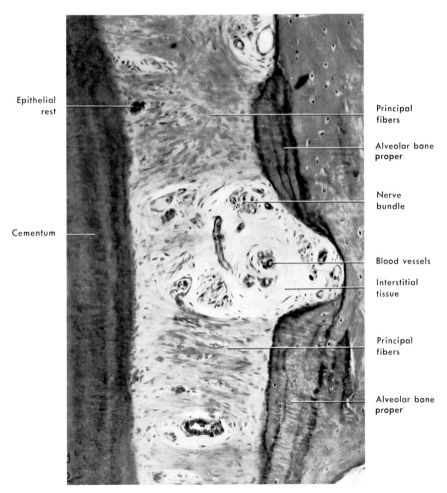

Epithelial rest

Cementum

Principal fibers

Alveolar bone proper

Nerve bundle

Blood vessels

Interstitial tissue

Principal fibers

Alveolar bone proper

**Fig. 7-15.** Interstitial spaces in periodontal ligament contain loose connective tissue, vessels, and nerves. (From Orban, B.: J. Am. Dent. Assoc. **16:**405, 1929.)

## STRUCTURES PRESENT IN CONNECTIVE TISSUE

The following discrete structures are present in the connective tissue of the periodontal ligament:

Blood vessels
Lymphatics
Nerves
Cementicles

*Blood vessels.* The arterial vessels of the periodontal ligament are derived from three sources:

Branches in the periodontal ligament from apical vessels that supply the dental pulp.
Branches from intra-alveolar vessels. These branches run horizontally, penetrating the alveolar bone to enter the periodontal ligament (Fig. 7-16) (Chapter 8).
Branches from gingival vessels. These enter the periodontal ligament from the coronal direction.

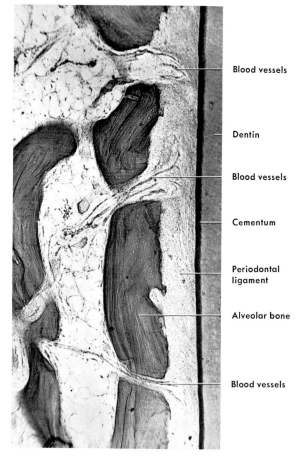

Blood vessels

Dentin

Blood vessels

Cementum

Periodontal
ligament

Alveolar bone

Blood vessels

**Fig. 7-16.** Blood vessels enter periodontal ligament through openings in alveolar bone. (From Orban, B.: Dental histology and embryology, Philadelphia, 1929, P. Blakiston's Son & Co.)

The arterial vessels of the microcirculation ramify in the periodontal ligament, forming a rich network of arcades that is more evident in the half of the periodontal space adjacent to bone than that adjacent to cementum. There is a particularly rich vascular plexus at the apex and in the cervical part of the ligament. The venous vessels tend to run axially and to drain to the apex. There are numerous arteriovenous anastamoses between the two sides of the microcirculation, as well as glomerulus-like structures, and these are possibly involved in the role that the circulation plays in supporting the teeth during function.

**Lymphatics.** A network of lymphatic vessels, following the path of the blood vessels, provides the lymph drainage of the periodontal ligament. The flow is from the ligament toward and into the adjacent alveolar bone.

**Nerves.** Nerves, which usually are associated with blood vessels, pass

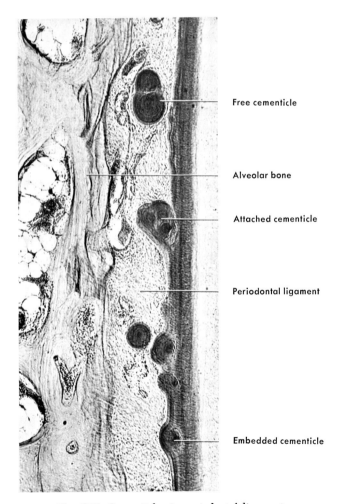

Free cementicle

Alveolar bone

Attached cementicle

Periodontal ligament

Embedded cementicle

Fig. 7-17. Cementicles in periodontal ligament.

through foramina in the alveolar bone to enter the periodontal ligament. In the region of the apex, they run toward the cervix, whereas along the length of the root they branch and run both coronally and apically. The nerve fibers are either of large diameter and myelinated or of small diameter, in which case they may or may not be myelinated. The small fibers appear to end in fine branches throughout the ligament, and the large fibers in a variety of endings, e.g., knob-like, spindle-like, and Meissner-like, but these seem to vary among the species. The large-diameter fibers appear to be concerned with discernment of touch and the small-diameter ones, with pain. Some of the unmyelinated small-diameter fibers evidently are associated with blood vessels and presumably are autonomic.

*Cementicles.* Calcified bodies called cementicles are sometimes found in the periodontal ligament. These bodies are seen in older individuals, and they may remain free in the connective tissue, they may fuse into large calcified masses, or they may be joined with the cementum (Fig. 7-17). As the cementum thickens with advancing age, it may envelop these bodies. When they are adherent to the cementum, they form excementoses. The origin of these calcified bodies is not established. It is possible that degenerated epithelial cells form the nidus for their calcification.

## FUNCTIONS

The periodontal ligament has the following functions:

Supportive
Sensory
Nutritive
Homeostatic

*Supportive.* When a tooth is moved in its socket as a result of forces acting on it during mastication or through application of an orthodontic force, part of the periodontal space will be narrowed and the periodontal ligament contained in these areas will be compressed. Other parts of the periodontal space will be widened. The compressed periodontal ligament provides support for the loaded tooth. The collagen fibers in the compressed ligament act as a cushion for the displaced tooth. The ground substance, which, as a result of its chemical constitution, binds large quantities of water, does the same. The pressure of blood in the numerous vessels also provides a hydraulic mechanism for the support of the teeth. It has often been suggested that the collagen fibers in the widened parts of the periodontal space are extended to their limit when a force is applied to a tooth and, being nonelastic, prevent the tooth from being moved too far. How-ever, evidence to support this contention appears to be lacking, and the role of the collagen fibers seems to be restricted to attaching the cementum that is fused to the dentin of the root to alveolar bone and to acting as a cushion.

*Sensory.* The periodontal ligament, through its nerve supply, provides a most efficient proprioceptive mechanism, allowing the organism to detect the application of the most delicate forces to the teeth and very slight displacement of the teeth. Anyone who has bitten into soft food containing a small hard object such as stone or shot knows the importance of this mechanism in protecting both the supporting structures of the tooth and the substance of the crown from the effects of excessively vigorous masticatory movements.

*Nutritive.* The ligament transmits blood vessels, which provide anabolites and other substances required by the cells of the ligament, by the cementocytes, and presumably by the more superficial osteocytes of the alveolar bone. The blood vessels are also concerned with removal of catabolites. Occlusion of blood vessels leads to necrosis of cells in the affected part of the ligament; this occurs when too heavy a force is applied to a tooth in orthodontic therapy.

*Homeostatic.* It is evident that the cells of the periodontal ligament have the capacity to resorb and synthesize the extracellular substance of the connective tissue of the ligament, alveolar bone, and cementum. It is also evident that these processes are not activated sporadically or haphazardly but function continuously, with varying intensity, throughout the life of the tooth. Alveolar bone appears to be resorbed and replaced (i.e., remodeled) at a rate higher than other bone tissue in the jaws. Furthermore, the periodontal ligament is also continually remodeled and the cells in the bone half of the ligament are more active than those on the cementum side. On the other hand, deposition of cementum by cementoblasts appears to be a slow, continuous process, and resorption is not a regular occurrence.

The mechanisms whereby the cells responsible for these processes of synthesis and resorption are controlled is unfortunately unknown. It is evident that the processes are exquisitely controlled as, under normal conditions of function, the various tissues of the periodontium maintain their integrity and relationship to one another. However, when these homeostatic mechanisms are upset, derangement of the periodontium occurs. If periodontal ligament, either in part or whole, is irreparably destroyed, bone will be deposited in the periodontal space, obliterating it, and this will result in ankylosis between bone and tooth. If the balance between synthesis and resorption is disturbed, the quality of the tissues will be changed. For example, if an experimental animal is deprived of substances essential for collagen synthesis, such as vitamin C or protein, resorption of collagen will continue unabated, but its synthesis and replacement will stop. This will result in progressive destruction and loss of extracellular substance of periodontal ligament, more advanced on the bone side of the ligament than on the cementum side. This eventually will lead to loss of attachment between bone and tooth and finally to loss of the tooth, such as occurs in scurvy when vitamin C is absent from the diet.

Another aspect of homeostasis relates to function. A periodontal ligament supporting a fully functional tooth exhibits all the structural features described above. However, with loss of function, much of the extracellular substance of the ligament is lost, possibly because of diminished synthesis of substances required to replace structural molecules resorbed during normal turnover, and the width of the periodontal space is subsequently decreased. These changes are accompanied by increased deposition of cementum but by a decrease in the mass of alveolar bone tissue per unit volume. The process is reversible if the tooth is returned to function, but the precise nature of the stimuli that control the changed activity of the cells is unknown.

## CLINICAL CONSIDERATIONS

The primary role of the periodontal ligament is to support the tooth in the bony socket. Its thickness varies in different individuals, different teeth in the same person, and different locations on the same tooth, as is illustrated in Tables 3 and 4.

The measurements shown in the tables indicate that it is not feasible to refer to an average figure of normal width of the periodontal ligament. Measurements of a large number of ligaments range from 0.15 to 0.38 mm. The fact that the periodontal ligament is thinnest in the middle region of the root seems to indicate that the fulcrum of physiologic movement is in this region. The thickness of the periodontal ligament seems to be maintained by the functional movements of the tooth. It is thin in functionless and embedded teeth and wide in teeth that are under excessive occlusal stresses (Fig. 7-18).

**Table 3.** Thickness of periodontal ligament of 154 teeth from 14 human jaws*†

|  | Average at alveolar crest (mm.) | Average at midroot (mm.) | Average at apex (mm.) | Average for entire tooth (mm.) |
|---|---|---|---|---|
| Ages 11-16 (83 teeth from 4 jaws) | 0.23 | 0.17 | 0.24 | 0.21 |
| Ages 32-50 (36 teeth from 5 jaws) | 0.20 | 0.14 | 0.19 | 0.18 |
| Ages 51-67 (35 teeth from 5 jaws) | 0.17 | 0.12 | 0.16 | 0.15 |

*From Coolidge, E. D.: J. Am. Dent. Assoc. **24:**1260, 1937.
†The table shows that the width of the periodontal ligament decreases with age and that it is wider at the crest and at the apex than at the midroot.

**Table 4.** Comparison of periodontal ligament in different locations around the same tooth (subject 11 years of age)*†

|  | Mesial (mm.) | Distal (mm.) | Labial (mm.) | Lingual (mm.) |
|---|---|---|---|---|
| Upper right central incisor, mesial and labial drift | 0.12 | 0.24 | 0.12 | 0.22 |
| Upper left central incisor, no drift | 0.21 | 0.19 | 0.24 | 0.24 |
| Upper right lateral incisor, distal and labial drift | 0.27 | 0.17 | 0.11 | 0.15 |

*From Coolidge, E. D.: J. Am. Dent. Assoc. **24:**1260, 1937.
†The table shows the variation in width of the mesial, distal, labial, and lingual sides of the same tooth.

For the practice of restorative dentistry the importance of these changes in structure is obvious. The supporting tissues of a tooth long out of function are unable to carry the load suddenly placed upon the tooth by a restoration. This applies to bridge abutments, teeth opposing bridges or dentures, and teeth used as anchorage for removable bridges. This may account for the inability of a patient to use a restoration immediately after its placement. Some time must elapse before the supporting tissues become adapted again to the new functional demands. An adjustment period, likewise, must be permitted after orthodontic treatment.

Acute trauma of the periodontal ligament, accidental blows, condensing of foil, or rapid mechanical separation may produce pathologic changes such as fractures or resorption of the cementum, tears of fiber bundles, hemorrhage, and

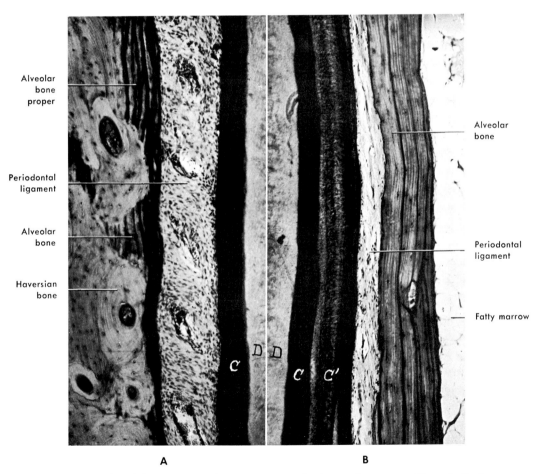

**Fig. 7-18.** Periodontal ligament of a functioning, **A,** and of a nonfunctioning, **B,** tooth. In the functioning tooth the periodontal ligament is wide, and principal fibers are present. Cementum, *C,* is thin. In the nonfunctioning tooth the periodontal space is narrow, and no principal fiber bundles are seen. Cementum is thick, *C* and *C'.* Alveolar bone is lamellated. *D,* Dentin.

necrosis. The adjacent alveolar bone is resorbed, the periodontal ligament is widened, and the tooth becomes loose. When trauma is eliminated, repair usually takes place. Occlusal trauma is always restricted to the intra-alveolar tissues and does not cause changes of the gingiva such as recession or pocket formation or gingivitis.

Orthodontic tooth movement depends on bone resorption and bone formation stimulated by properly regulated pressure and tension. These stimuli are transmitted through the medium of the periodontal ligament. If the movement of teeth is within physiologic limits (which may vary with the individual), the initial compression of the periodontal ligament on the pressure side is compensated for by bone resorption, whereas on the tension side bone apposition is seen.

The periodontal ligament in the periapical area of the tooth is often the site of a pathologic lesion. Inflammatory diseases of the pulp progress to the apical periodontal ligament and replace its fiber bundles with granulation tissue. This lesion, called a dental granuloma, contains epithelial cells that may undergo proliferation and produce a cyst. The dental granuloma and the apical cyst are the two most common pathologic lesions of the jaws.

Safeguarding the integrity of the periodontal ligament (and the alveolar bone) is one of the most important challenges for the clinician. Gingivitis, or the inflammation of the gingiva, is the most common disease of man. If not controlled or treated, it invariably extends to the periodontal ligament and bone and produces their slow but progressive destruction. Once destroyed by this slow inflammatory process, the periodontal ligament and the alveolar bone are very difficult to regenerate. Therefore, the diseases of the periodontal ligament are often irreversible. Their control is the primary aim of good clinical practice and much of what is called preventive dentistry is directed toward these goals.

## REFERENCES

Anderson, D. J., Hannam, A. G., and Mathews, B.: Sensory mechanisms in mammalian teeth and their supporting structures, Physiol. Rev. **50**:171, 1970.

Arnim, S. S., and Hagerman, D. A.: The connective tissue fibers of the marginal gingiva, J. Am. Dent. Assoc. **47**:271, 1953.

Bernick, S.: Innervation of teeth and periodontium after enzymatic removal of collagenous elements, Oral Surg. **10**:323, 1957.

Box, K. F.: Evidence of lymphatics in the periodontium, J. Can. Dent. Assoc. **15**:8, 1949.

Bruszt, P.: Ueber die netzartige Anordnung des paradentalen Epithels [The network arrangement of the epithelium in the periodontal membrane], Z. Stomatol. **30**:679, 1932.

Carmichael, G. G., and Fullmer, H. M.: The fine structure of the oxytalan fiber, J. Cell Biol. **28**:33, 1966.

Cohn, S. A.: Disuse atrophy of the periodontium in mice, Arch. Oral Biol. **10**:909, 1965.

Cohn, S. A.: A re-examination of Sharpey's fibres in alveolar bone of the mouse, Arch. Oral Biol. **17**:255, 1972.

Cohn, S. A.: A re-examination of Sharpey's fibres in alveolar bone of the marmoset (*Saguinus fuscicollis*), Arch. Oral Biol. **17**:261, 1972.

Coolidge, E. D.: The thickness of the human periodontal membrane, J. Am. Dent. Assoc. **24**:1260, 1937.

Deporter, D. A., and Ten Cate, A. R.: Fine structural localization of acid and alkaline phosphatase in collagen-containing vesicles of fibroblasts, J. Anat. **114**:457, 1973.

Folke, L. E. A., and Stallard, R. E.: Periodontal microcirculation as revealed by plastic microspheres, J. Periodont. Res. **2:** 53, 1967.

Freeman, E., and Ten Cate, A. R.: Development of the periodontium: An electron microscopic study, J. Periodontol. **42:**387, 1971.

Fullmer, H. M.: Connective tissue components of the periodontium. In Miles, A. E. W., editor: Structural and chemical organization of the teeth, vol. 2, New York, 1967, Academic Press Inc.

Garfunkel, A., and Sciaky, I.: Vascularization of the periodontal tissues in the adult laboratory rat, J. Dent. Res. **50:**880, 1971.

Goldman, H. M.: The effects of dietary deprivation and of age on periodontal tissues of the rat and spider monkey, J. Periodontol. **25:**87, 1954.

Goldman, H. M., and Gianelly, A. A.: Histology of tooth movement, Dent. Clin. N. Am. **16:**439, 1972.

Griffin, C. J.: Unmyelinated nerve endings in the periodontal membrane of human teeth, Arch. Oral Biol. **13:**1207, 1968.

Holtrop, M. E., Raisz, L. G., and Simmons, H. A.: The effects of parathormone, colchicine and calcitonin on the ultrastructure and the activity of osteoclasts in organ culture, J. Cell Biol. **60:**346, 1974.

Ishimitsu, K.: Beitrag zur Kenntnis der Morphologie und Entwicklungsgeschichte der Glomeruli periodontii [Contribution to the knowledge of morphology and development of the periodontal glomeruli], Yokohama Med. Bull. **11:**415, 1960.

Kindlova, M., and Matena, V.: Blood vessels of the rat molar, J Dent. Res. **41:**650, 1962.

Malassez, M. L.: Sur l'existence de masses épithéliales dans le ligament alvéolodentaire [On the existence of epithelial masses in the periodontal membrane], Comp. Rend. Soc. Biol. **36:**241, 1884.

Malkani, K., Luxembourger, M.-M., and Rebel, A.: Cytoplasmic modifications at the contact zone of osteoclasts and calcified tissue in the diaphyseal growing plate of foetal guinea-pig tibia, Calcif. Tissue Res. **11:**258, 1973.

Melcher, A. H.: Repair of wounds in the periodontium of the rat. Influence of periodontal ligament on osteogenesis, Arch. Oral Biol. **15:**1183, 1970.

Melcher, A. H., and Correia, M. A.: Remodelling of periodontal ligament in erupting molars of mature rats, J. Periodont. Res. **6:**118, 1971.

Picton, D. C. A.: The effects of external forces in the periodontium. In Melcher, A. H., and Bowen, W. H., editors: Biology of the periodontium, New York, 1969, Academic Press Inc.

Revel, J. P., and Karnovsky, M. J.: Hexagonal array of subunits in intercellular junctions of the mouse heart and liver, J. Cell Biol. **33:**C7, 1967.

Roberts, W. E., Chase, D. C., and Jee, W. S. S.: Counts of labelled mitoses in the orthodontically-stimulated periodontal ligament in the rat, Arch. Oral Biol. **19:**665, 1974.

Rygh, P.: Ultrastructural cellular reactions in pressure zones of rat molar periodontium incident to orthodontic tooth movement, Acta Odontol. Scand. **30:**575, 1972.

Sakamoto, S., Goldhaber, P., and Glimcher, M. J.: The further purification and characterization of mouse bone collagenase, Calcif. Tissue Res. **10:**142, 1972.

Shackleford, J. M.: The indifferent fiber plexus and its relationship to principal fibers of the periodontium, Am. J. Anat. **131:**427, 1971.

Shackleford, J. M.: Scanning electron microscopy of the dog periodontium, J. Periodont. Res. **6:**45, 1971.

Sicher, H.: The principal fibers of the periodontal membrane, Bur **55:**2, 1954.

Stallard, R. E.: The utilization of ³H-proline by the connective tissue elements of the periodontium, Periodontics **1:**185, 1963.

Ten Cate, A. R., Mills, C., and Solomon, G.: The development of the periodontium. A transplantation and autoradiographic study, Anat. Rec. **170:**365, 1971.

Ten Cate, A. R., and Mills, C.: The development of the periodontium: The origin of alveolar bone, Anat. Rec. **173:**69, 1972.

Vaes, G.: Excretion of acid and of lysosomal hydrolytic enzymes during bone resorption induced in tissue culture by parathyroid extract, Exp. Cell Res. **39:**470, 1965.

Valderhaug, J. P., and Nylen, M. U.: Function of epithelial rests as suggested by their ultrastructure, J. Periodont. Res. **1:**69, 1966.

Waerhaug, J.: Effect of C-avitaminosis on the supporting structures of the teeth, J. Periodontol. **29:**87, 1958.

Zwarych, P. D., and Quigley, M. B.: The intermediate plexus of the periodontal ligament: History and further observations, J. Dent. Res. **44:**383, 1965.

# 8 Maxilla and mandible (alveolar process)

## DEVELOPMENT OF MAXILLA AND MANDIBLE

In the beginning of the second month of fetal life the skull consists of three parts:

1. The chondrocranium, which is cartilaginous, comprises the base of the skull with the otic and nasal capsules.
2. The desmocranium, which is membranous, forms the lateral walls and roof of the braincase.
3. The appendicular or visceral part of the skull consists of the cartilaginous skeletal rods of the branchial arches.

The bones of the skull develop either by endochondral ossification, replacing the cartilage, or by intramembranous ossification in the mesenchyme. Intramembranous bone may develop in proximity to cartilaginous parts of the skull or directly in the desmocranium, which is the membranous capsule of the brain. (See Plate 2.)

The endochondral bones are the bones of the base of the skull: ethmoid bone; inferior concha (turbinate bone); body, lesser wings, basal part of the greater wings, and the lateral plate of the pterygoid process of the sphenoid bone; petrosal part of the temporal bone; and basilar, lateral, and lower part of the squamous portion of the occipital bone. The following bones develop in the desmocranium: frontal bones; parietal bones; squamous and tympanic parts of the temporal bone; parts of the greater wings and the medial plate of the pterygoid process of the sphenoid bone; and the upper part of the squamous portion of the occipital bone. All the bones of the upper face develop by intramembranous ossification, most of them close to the cartilage of the nasal capsule. The mandible develops as intramembranous bone, lateral to the cartilage of the mandibular arch. This cartilage, Meckel's cartilage, is in its proximal parts the primordium for two of the auditory ossicles: the incus (anvil) and the malleus (hammer). The third auditory ossicle, the stapes (stirrup), develops from the proximal part of the skeleton in the second branchial arch, which also gives rise to the styloid process, the stylohyoid ligament, and part of the hyoid bone. The latter is completed by the derivatives of the third arch. The fourth and fifth arches form the skeleton of the larynx.

**234**

**A**

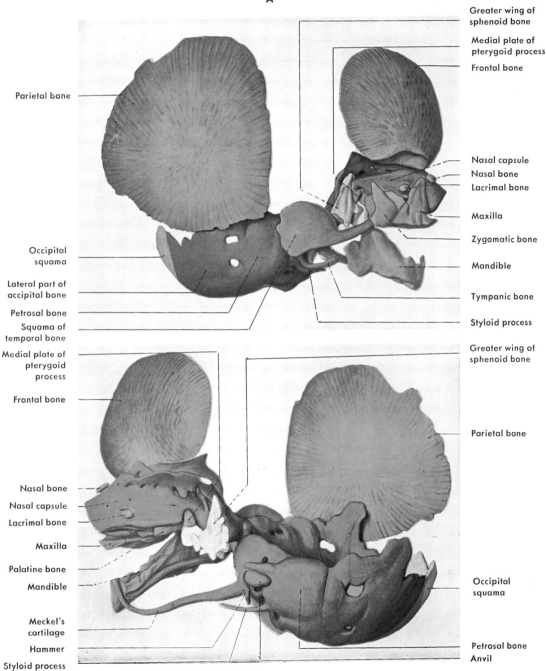

Greater wing of
sphenoid bone

Medial plate of
pterygoid process

Frontal bone

Parietal bone

Nasal capsule
Nasal bone
Lacrimal bone

Maxilla

Zygomatic bone

Occipital
squama

Mandible

Lateral part of
occipital bone

Tympanic bone

Petrosal bone

Squama of
temporal bone

Styloid process

Medial plate of
pterygoid
process

Greater wing of
sphenoid bone

Frontal bone

Parietal bone

Nasal bone
Nasal capsule
Lacrimal bone

Maxilla

Palatine bone
Mandible

Occipital
squama

Meckel's
cartilage

Hammer

Petrosal bone

Styloid process

Anvil

**B**

**Plate 2.** Reconstruction of skull of human embryo 80 mm. in length. Cartilage, *green*. Intramembranous bones, *pink*. Endochondral bones, *white*. **A,** Right lateral view. **B,** Left lateral view after removal of left intramembranous bones. (From Sicher, H., and Tandler, J.: Anatomie für Zahnärzte [Anatomy for dentists], Vienna, 1928, Julius Springer Verlag.)

*Maxilla.* The human maxilla is homologous to two bones, the maxilla proper and the premaxilla. The latter, in most animals a separate bone, carries the incisors and forms the anterior part of the hard palate and the rim of the piriform aperture. The ossification centers of the premaxilla and maxilla may be separate for a very short time, or only one center of ossification, common to both the premaxilla and maxilla, appears. That man therefore may not have an independent premaxilla, even in the first developmental stages, does not change the fact that man possesses the homolog of a premaxilla. The composition of the human maxilla from premaxilla and maxilla is indicated by the incisive fissure, which is clearly visible in young skulls. It is seen on the palate, where it extends from the incisive foramen to the alveolus of the canine.

*Mandible.* The mandible makes its appearance as a bilateral structure in the

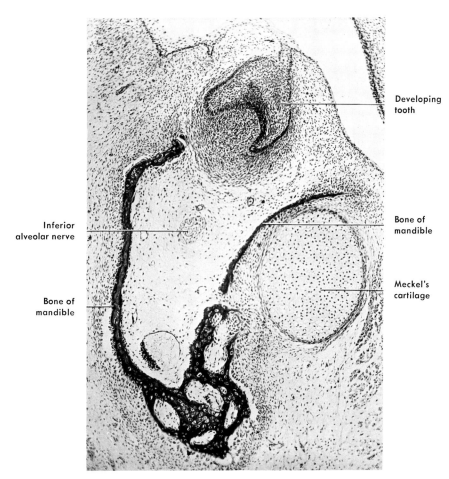

Developing tooth

Inferior alveolar nerve

Bone of mandible

Bone of mandible

Meckel's cartilage

Fig. 8-1. Development of mandible as intramembranous bone lateral to Meckel's cartilage (human embryo 45 mm. in length).

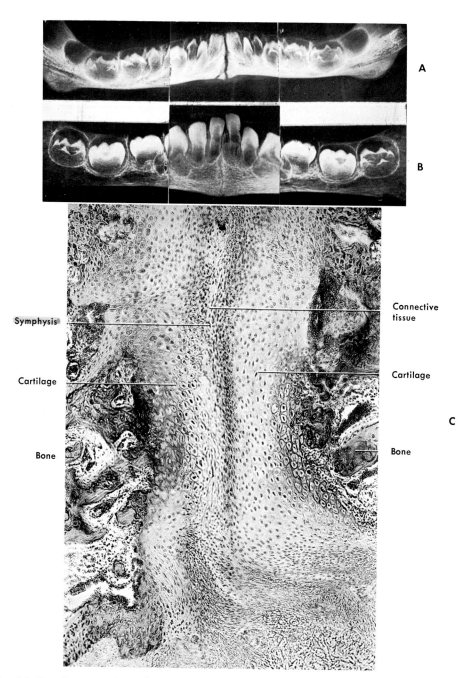

**Fig. 8-2.** Development of mandibular symphysis. **A,** Newborn infant. Symphysis wide open. Mental ossicle (roentgenogram). **B,** Child 9 months of age. Symphysis partly closed. Mental ossicles fused to the mandible (roentgenogram). **C,** Frontal section through mandibular symphysis of newborn infant. Connective tissue in midline connects plates of cartilage on either side. Cartilage is later replaced by bone.

sixth week of fetal life as a thin plate of bone lateral to, and at some distance from, Meckel's cartilage (Fig. 8-1). The latter is a cylindric rod of cartilage. Its proximal end (close to the base of the skull) is continuous with the hammer and is in contact with the anvil. Its distal end at the midline is bent upward and is in contact with the cartilage of the other side. (See Plate 2.) The greater part of Meckel's cartilage disappears without contributing to the formation of the bone of the mandible. Only a small part of the cartilage, some distance from the midline, is the site of endochondral ossification. Here the cartilage calcifies and is destroyed by chondroclasts, being replaced by connective tissue and then by bone. Throughout fetal life the mandible is a paired bone. Right and left mandibles are joined in the midline by fibrocartilage in the mandibular symphysis. The cartilage at the symphysis is not derived from Meckel's cartilage but differentiates from the connective tissue in the midline. In it, small irregular bones known as the mental ossicles develop and at the end of the first year fuse with the mandibular body. At the same time the two halves of the mandible unite by ossification of the symphyseal fibrocartilage (Fig. 8-2).

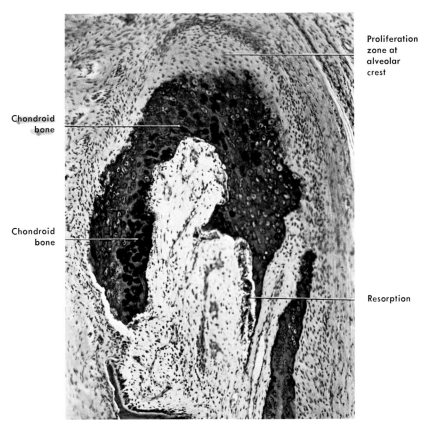

**Fig. 8-3.** Vertical growth of mandible at alveolar crest. Formation of chondroid bone that later is replaced by typical bone.

## DEVELOPMENT OF ALVEOLAR PROCESS

Near the end of the second month of fetal life the maxilla as well as the mandible forms a groove that is open toward the surface of the oral cavity (Fig. 8-1). The tooth germs are contained in this groove, which also includes the alveolar nerves and vessels. Gradually bony septa develop between the adjacent tooth germs, and much later the primitive mandibular canal is separated from the dental crypts by a horizontal plate of bone.

An alveolar process in the strict sense of the word develops only during the eruption of the teeth. It is important to realize that during growth part of the alveolar process is gradually incorporated into the maxillary or mandibular body, while it grows at a fairly rapid rate at its free borders. During the period of rapid growth a tissue may develop at the alveolar crest that combines characteristics of cartilage and bone. It is called chondroid bone (Fig. 8-3).

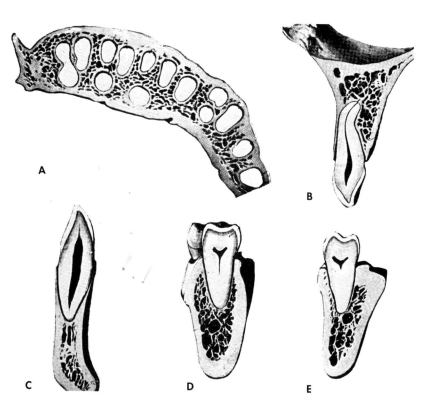

**Fig. 8-4.** Gross relations of alveolar processes. **A,** Horizontal section through upper alveolar process. **B,** Labiolingual section through upper lateral incisor. **C,** Labiolingual section through lower canine. **D,** Labiolingual section through lower second molar. **E,** Labiolingual section through lower third molar. (From Sicher, H., and Tandler, J.: Anatomie für Zahnärzte [Anatomy for dentists], Vienna, 1928, Julius Springer Verlag.)

## STRUCTURE OF ALVEOLAR PROCESS

The alveolar process may be defined as that part of the maxilla and the mandible that forms and supports the sockets of the teeth (Fig. 8-4). Anatomically, no distinct boundary exists between the body of the maxilla or the mandible and their respective alveolar processes. In some places the alveolar process is fused with, and partly masked by, bone that is not functionally related to the teeth. In the anterior part of the maxilla the palatine process fuses with the oral plate of the alveolar process. In the posterior part of the mandible the oblique line is superimposed laterally upon the bone of the alveolar process (Fig. 8-4, *D* and *E*).

As a result of its adaptation to function, two parts of the alveolar process can be distinguished. The first consists of a thin lamella of bone that surrounds the root of the tooth and gives attachment to principal fibers of the periodontal

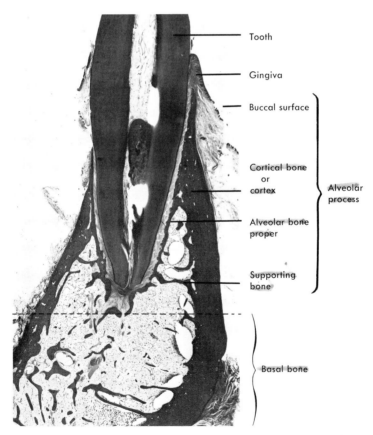

Tooth

Gingiva

Buccal surface

Cortical bone or cortex

Alveolar bone proper

Supporting bone

Alveolar process

Basal bone

Fig. 8-5. Section through mandible showing relationship of tooth to alveolar process and basal bone. (From Bhaskar, S. N.: Synopsis of oral histology, St. Louis, 1962, The C. V. Mosby Co.)

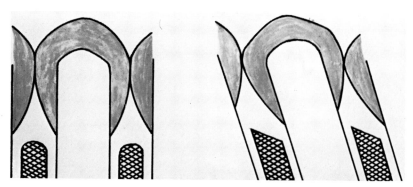

**Fig. 8-6.** Diagram of relation between cementoenamel junction of adjacent teeth and shape of crests of alveolar septa. (From Ritchey, B., and Orban, B.: J. Periodont. **24:**75, 1953.)

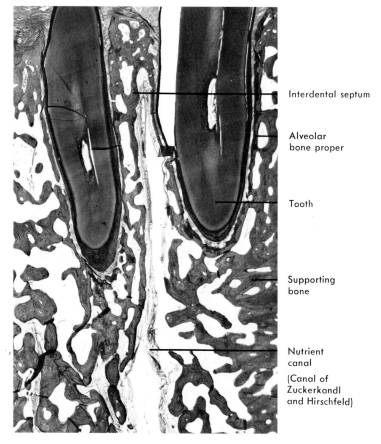

Interdental septum

Alveolar
bone proper

Tooth

Supporting
bone

Nutrient
canal

(Canal of
Zuckerkandl
and Hirschfeld)

**Fig. 8-7.** Section through jaw showing nutrient canal of Zuckerkandl and Hirschfeld in the interdental bony septum. (From Bhaskar, S. N.: Synopsis of oral histology, St. Louis, 1962, The C. V. Mosby Co.)

ligament. This is the *alveolar bone proper*. The second part is the bone that surrounds the alveolar bone and gives support to the socket. This has been called *supporting alveolar bone*. The latter, in turn, consists of two parts: (1) cortical plates, which consist of compact bone and form the outer and inner plates of the alveolar processes, and (2) the spongy bone, which fills the area between these plates and the alveolar bone proper (Figs. 8-4 and 8-5).

The cortical plates, continuous with the compact layers of the maxillary and mandibular body, are generally much thinner in the maxilla than in the mandible. They are thickest in the premolar and molar regions of the lower jaw, especially on the buccal side. In the maxilla the outer cortical plate is perforated by many small openings through which blood and lymph vessels pass. In the lower jaw the cortical bone of the alveolar process is dense. In the region of the anterior teeth of both jaws the supporting bone usually is very thin. No spongy bone is found here, and the cortical plate is fused with the alveolar bone proper (Fig. 8-4, *B* and *C*). In such areas, notably in the premolar and molar regions of the maxilla, defects of the outer alveolar wall are fairly common. Such defects, where periodontal tissues and covering mucosa fuse, do not impair the firm attachment and function of the tooth.

The shape of the outlines of the crest of the alveolar septa in the roentgenogram is dependent on the position of the adjacent teeth. In a healthy mouth the distance between the cementoenamel junction and the free border of the alveolar bone proper is fairly constant. If the neighboring teeth are inclined, therefore, the alveolar crest is oblique. In the majority of individuals the inclination is most pronounced in the premolar and molar regions, with the teeth being tipped mesially. Then the cementoenamel junction of the mesial tooth is situated in a more occlusal plane than that of the distal tooth, and the alveolar crest therefore slopes distally (Fig. 8-6).

The interdental and interradicular septa contain the perforating canals of Zuckerkandl and Hirschfeld (nutrient canals), which house the interdental and interradicular arteries, veins, lymph vessels, and nerves (Fig. 8-7).

Histologically, the cortical plates consists of longitudinal lamellae and haversian systems (Fig. 8-8). In the lower jaw, circumferential or basic lamellae reach from the body of the mandible into the cortical plates.

The study of roentgenograms permits the classification of the spongiosa of the alveolar process into two main types. In type I the interdental and interradicular trabeculae are regular and horizontal in a ladderlike arrangement (Fig. 8-9, *A* to *C*). Type II shows irregularly arranged, numerous, delicate interdental and interradicular trabeculae (Fig. 8-9, *D*). Both types show a variation in thickness of trabeculae and size of marrow spaces. The architecture of type I is seen most often in the mandible and fits well into the general idea of a trajectory pattern of spongy bone. Type II, although evidently functionally satisfactory, lacks a distinct trajectory pattern, which seems to be compensated for by the greater number of trabeculae in any given area. This arrangement is more com-

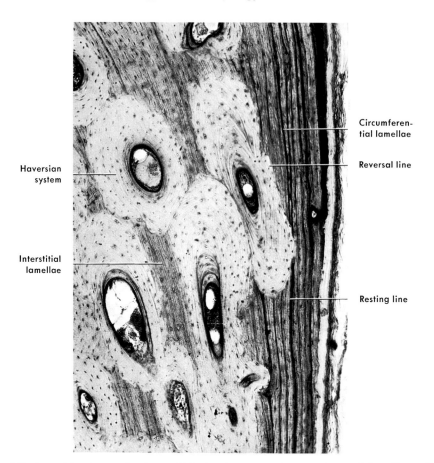

Haversian system

Interstitial lamellae

Circumferential lamellae

Reversal line

Resting line

Fig. 8-8. Appositional growth of mandible by formation of circumferential lamellae. These are replaced by haversian bone; remnants of circumferential lamellae in the depth persisting as interstitial lamellae.

mon in the maxilla. From the apical part of the socket of lower molars, trabeculae are sometimes seen radiating in a slightly distal direction. These trabeculae are less prominent in the upper jaw because of the proximity of the nasal cavity and the maxillary sinus. The marrow spaces in the alveolar process may contain hematopoietic marrow, but usually they contain fatty marrow. In the condylar process, in the angle of the mandible, in the maxillary tuberosity, and in other isolated foci, hematopoietic cellular marrow is found.

The alveolar bone proper, which forms the inner wall of the socket (Fig. 8-10), is perforated by many openings that carry branches of the interalveolar nerves and blood vessels into the periodontal ligament (Chapter 7), and it is therefore called the *cribriform plate*. The alveolar bone proper consists partly of *lamellated* and partly of *bundle bone*. Some lamellae of the lamellated bone are arranged roughly parallel to the surface of the adjacent marrow spaces, whereas others form haversian systems. Bundle bone is that bone in which the

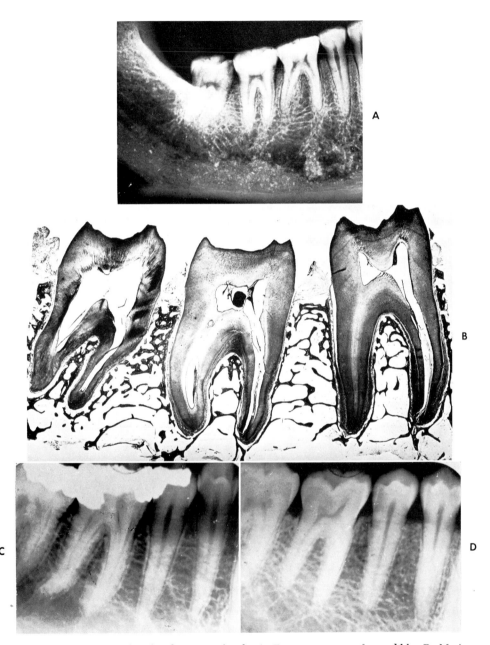

**Fig. 8-9.** Supporting trabeculae between alveoli. **A,** Roentgenogram of mandible. **B,** Mesiodistal section through mandibular molars showing alveolar bone proper and supporting bone. **C,** Type I of alveolar spongiosa. Note regular horizontal trabeculae. **D,** Type II of alveolar spongiosa. Note irregularly arranged trabeculae. (Courtesy Dr. N. Brescia, Chicago, Ill.)

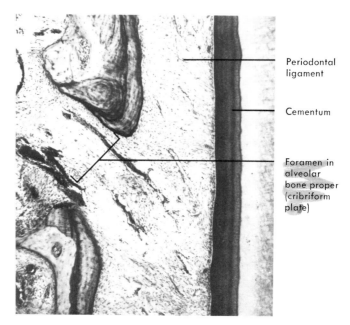

Periodontal
ligament

Cementum

Foramen in
alveolar
bone proper
(cribriform
plate)

Fig. 8-10. Histologic section showing foramen in alveolar bone proper (cribriform plate). (From Bhaskar, S. N.: Synopsis of oral histology, St. Louis, 1962, The C. V. Mosby Co.)

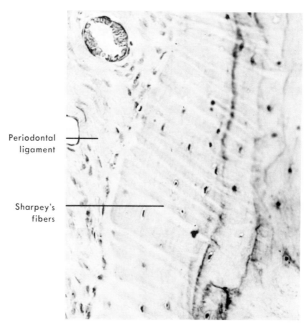

Periodontal
ligament

Sharpey's
fibers

Fig. 8-11. Histologic section showing Sharpey's fibers in alveolar bone proper. (From Bhaskar, S. N.: Synopsis of oral histology, St. Louis, 1962, The C. V. Mosby Co.)

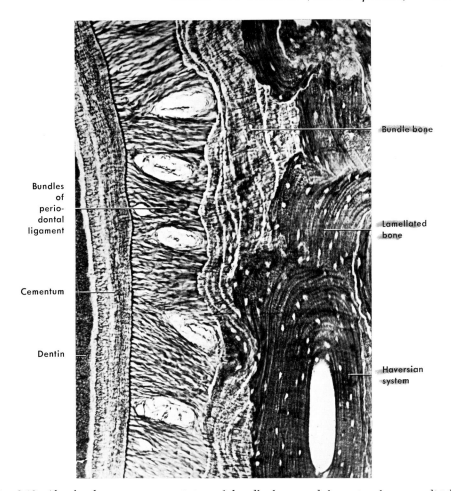

**Fig. 8-12.** Alveolar bone proper consisting of bundle bone and haversian bone on distal alveolar wall. A reversal line separates the two (silver impregnation).

principal fibers of the periodontal ligament are anchored. The term "bundle bone" was chosen because the bundles of the principal fibers continue into the bone as Sharpey's fibers (Fig. 8-11). The bundle bone is characterized by the scarcity of the fibrils in the intercellular substance. These fibrils, moreover, are all arranged at right angles to Sharpey's fibers. The bundle bone contains less fibrils than does lamellated bone and therefore it appears dark in routine sections and much lighter in preparations stained with silver than does lamellated bone (Fig. 8-12). In some areas the alveolar bone proper consists mainly of bundle bone. Such areas are visible in a roentgenogram by their greater radiopacity.

## PHYSIOLOGIC CHANGES IN ALVEOLAR PROCESS

The internal structure of bone is adapted to mechanical stresses. It changes continuously during growth and alteration of functional stresses. In the jaws, structural changes are correlated to the growth, eruption, movements, wear, and loss of teeth. All these processes are made possible only by a coordination of destructive and formative activities. Specialized cells, the osteoclasts, have the function of eliminating overaged bony tissue or bone that is no longer adapted to mechanical forces, whereas osteoblasts produce new bone.

Osteoclasts are, as a rule, multinucleated giant cells (Fig. 8-13, *A*). The number of nuclei in one cell may rise to a dozen or more. However, occasionally uninucleate osteoclasts are found. The nuclei are vesicular, showing a prominent nucleolus and little chromatin. The cell body is irregularly oval or club shaped and may show many branching processes. In general, osteoclasts are found in baylike depressions in the bone that are called *Howship's lacunae.* They are formed by the activity of the osteoclasts. The cytoplasm that is in contact with the bone is striated. The osteoclasts seem to be able to produce demineralization of bone as well as to produce proteolytic enzymes that destroy or dissolve the organic constituents of the bone matrix.

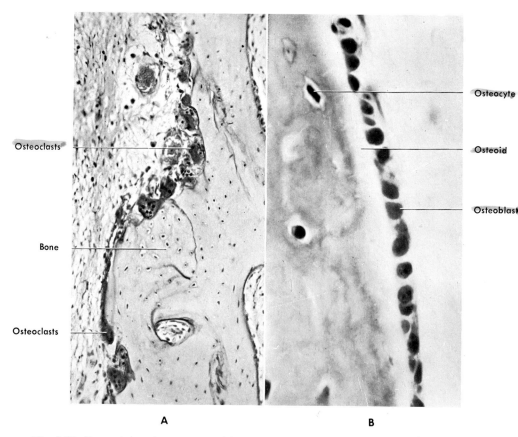

Fig. 8-13. Resorption and apposition of bone. **A,** Osteoclasts in Howship's lacunae. **B,** Osteoblasts along a bone trabecula. Layer of osteoid tissue is a sign of bone formation.

Osteoclasts differentiate from undifferentiated mesenchymal reserve cells, most probably by fusion of several cells. The stimulus that leads to the differentiation of mesenchymal cells into osteoclasts is not known. Osteoclastic resorption of bone is partly genetically patterned and partly functionally determined. Overaged bone seems to stimulate the differentiation of osteoclasts, possibly by chemical changes that are the consequence of degeneration and final necrosis of the osteocytes.

New bone is produced by the activity of osteoblasts (Fig. 8-13, *B*). These cells also differentiate from undifferentiated mesenchymal reserve cells of the loose connective tissue. Functioning osteoblasts are arranged along the surface of the growing bone in a continuous layer.

The osteoblasts produce the intercellular substance of bone consisting of collagenous fibrils bound together by mucopolysaccharides. It is at first devoid of mineral salts and at this stage is termed *osteoid tissue*. While the intercellular substance is being produced, some of the osteoblasts become embedded in it as osteocytes. Normally the organic matrix calcifies immediately after formation.

## INTERNAL RECONSTRUCTION OF BONE

The bone in the alveolar process is identical to bone elsewhere in the body and is in a constant state of flux. During the growth of the maxilla and the man-

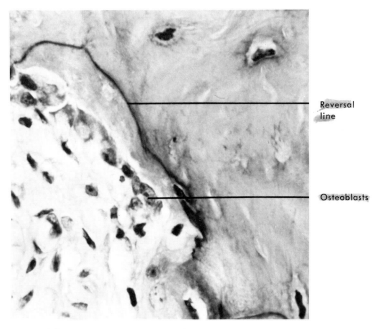

Reversal line

Osteoblasts

**Fig. 8-14.** Reversal line in bone. (From Bhaskar, S. N.: Synopsis of oral histology, St. Louis, 1962, The C. V. Mosby Co.)

dible, bone is deposited on the outer surfaces of the cortical plates. In the mandible, with its thick, compact cortical plates, bone is deposited in the shape of basic or circumferential lamellae (Fig. 8-8). When the lamellae reach a certain thickness, they are replaced from the inside by haversian bone. This reconstruction is correlated to the functional and nutritional demands of the bone. In the haversian canals, closest to the surface, osteoclasts differentiate and resorb the haversian lamellae and part of the circumferential lamellae. The resorbed bone is replaced by proliferating loose connective tissue. After a time the resorption ceases and new bone is apposed onto the old. The scalloped outline of Howship's lacunae that turn their convexity toward the old bone remains visible as a darkly stained cementing line, a *reversal line* (Fig. 8-14). This is in contrast to those cementing lines that correspond to a rest period in an otherwise continuous process of bone apposition. They are called *resting lines* (Fig. 8-8). Resting and reversal lines are found between layers of bone of varying age.

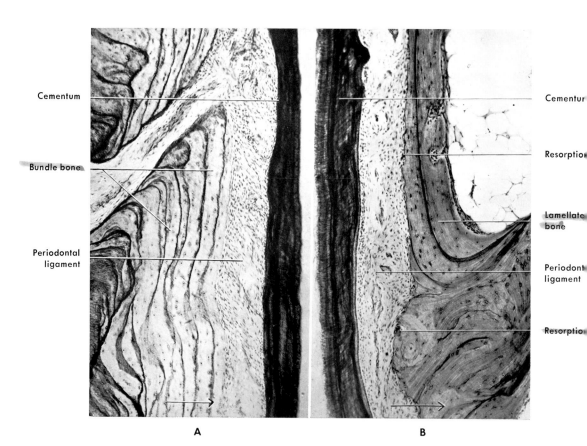

Cementum

Bundle bone

Periodontal ligament

Cementum

Resorption

Lamellate bone

Periodontal ligament

Resorption

A                                                   B

Fig. 8-15. Mesial drift indicated by *arrow.* **A,** Apposition of bundle bone on distal alveolar wall. **B,** Resorption of bone on mesial alveolar wall. (From Weinmann, J. P.: Angle Orthodont. **11:**83, 1941.)

Wherever a muscle, tendon, or ligament is attached to the surface of bone, Sharpey's fibers can be seen penetrating the basic lamellae. During replacement of the latter by haversian systems, fragments of bone containing Sharpey's fibers remain in the deeper layers. Thus the presence of these lamellae containing Sharpey's fibers indicates the former level of the surface.

Alterations in the structure of the alveolar bone are of great importance in connection with the physiologic eruptive movements of the teeth. These movements are directed mesiocclusally. At the alveolar fundus the continual apposition of bone can be recognized by resting lines separating parallel layers of bundle bone. When the bundle bone has reached a certain thickness, it is resorbed partly from the marrow spaces and then replaced by lamellated bone or spongy trabeculae. The presence of bundle bone indicates the level at which the alveolar fundus was situated previously. During the mesial drift of a tooth, bone is apposed on the distal and resorbed on the mesial alveolar wall (Fig. 8-15).

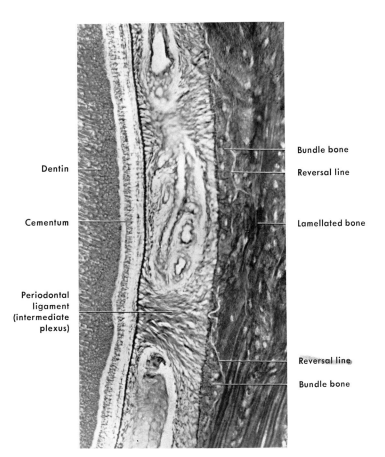

Dentin

Cementum

Periodontal ligament (intermediate plexus)

Bundle bone

Reversal line

Lamellated bone

Reversal line

Bundle bone

**Fig. 8-16.** Mesial alveolar wall where the alveolar bone proper consists mostly of lamellated bone and islands of bundle bone, which anchor principal fibers of periodontal ligament.

The distal wall is made up almost entirely of bundle bone. However, the osteoclasts in the adjacent marrow spaces remove part of the bundle bone when it reaches a certain thickness. In its place, lamellated bone is laid down (Fig. 8-12).

On the mesial alveolar wall of a drifting tooth, signs of active resorption are the presence of Howship's lacunae containing osteoclasts (Fig. 8-15). Bundle bone, however, on this side is always present in some areas but forms merely a thin layer (Fig. 8-16). This is due to the fact that the mesial drift of a tooth does not occur simply as a bodily movement. Thus resorption does not involve the entire mesial surface of the alveolus at one and the same time. Moreover, periods of resorption alternate with periods of rest and repair. It is during these periods of repair that bundle bone is formed, and detached periodontal fibers are again secured. Islands of bundle bone are separated from the lamellated bone by reversal lines that turn their convexities toward the lamellated bone (Fig. 8-16).

During these changes, compact bone may be replaced by spongy bone or spongy bone may change into compact bone. This type of internal reconstruc-

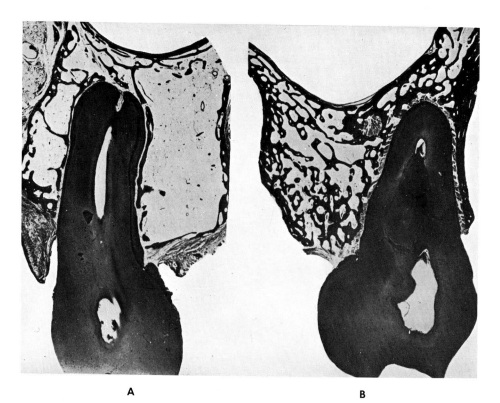

**A**                                                                                    **B**

**Fig. 8-17.** Osteoporosis of alveolar process caused by inactivity of tooth that has no antagonist. Labiolingual sections through upper molars of the same individual. **A,** Disappearance of bony trabeculae after loss of function. Plane of mesiobuccal root. Alveolar bone proper remains intact. **B,** Normal spongy bone in plane of mesiobuccal root of functioning tooth. (From Kellner, E.: Z. Stomatol. **18:**59, 1920.)

tion of bone can be observed in physiologic mesial drift or in orthodontic mesial or distal movement of teeth. In these movements an interdental septum shows apposition on one surface and resorption on the other. If the alveolar bone proper is thickened by apposition of bundle bone, the interdental marrow spaces widen and advance in the direction of apposition. Conversely, if the plate of the alveolar bone proper is thinned by resorption, apposition of bone occurs on those surfaces that face the marrow spaces. The result is a reconstructive shift of the interdental septum.

## CLINICAL CONSIDERATIONS

Bone, although one of the hardest tissues of the human body, is biologically a highly plastic tissue. Where bone is covered by a vascularized connective tissue, it is exceedingly sensitive to pressure, whereas tension acts generally as a stimulus to the production of new bone. It is this biologic plasticity that enables the orthodontist to move teeth without disrupting their relations to the alveolar bone. Bone is resorbed on the side of pressure and apposed on the side of tension; thus the entire alveolus is allowed to shift with the tooth.

The adaptation of bone to function is quantitative as well as qualitative. Whereas increase in functional forces leads to formation of new bone, decreased function leads to a decrease in the volume of bone. This can be observed in the supporting bone of teeth that have lost their antagonists. Here the spongy bone around the alveolus shows pronounced rarefaction: the bone trabeculae are less numerous and very thin (Fig. 8-17). The alveolar bone proper, however, is gen-

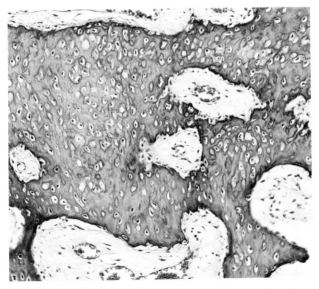

**Fig. 8-18.** Immature bone. Note many osteocytes and absence of lamellae or resting lines. (From Bhaskar, S. N.: Synopsis of oral histology, St. Louis, 1962, The C. V. Mosby Co.)

erally well preserved because it continues to receive some stimuli from the tension of the periodontal tissues.

During healing of fractures or extraction wounds an embryonic type of bone is formed, which only later is replaced by mature bone. The embryonic bone, also called immature or coarse fibrillar bone, is characterized, among other aspects, by the greater number, size, and irregular arrangement of the osteocytes than mature bone (Fig. 8-18). The greater number of cells and the reduced volume of calcified intercellular substance render this immature bone more radiolucent than mature bone. This explains why bony callus cannot be seen in roentgenograms at a time when histologic examination of a fracture reveals a well-developed union between the fragments and why a socket after an extraction wound appears to be empty at a time when it is almost filled with immature bone. The visibility in radiographs lags 2 or 3 weeks behind actual formation of new bone.

### REFERENCES

Bhaskar, S. N.: Radiographic interpretation for the dentist, ed. 2, St. Louis, 1975, The C. V. Mosby Co.

Bhaskar, S. N., Mohammed, C., and Weinmann, J.: A morphological and histochemical study of osteoclasts, J. Bone Joint Surg. 38-A:1335, 1956.

Brodie, A. G.: Some recent observations on the growth of the mandible, Angle Orthodont. 10:63, 1940.

Brodie, A. G.: On the growth pattern of the human head from the third month to the eighth year of life, Am. J. Anat. 68:209, 1941.

Ham, A., and Leeson, T.: Histology, ed. 4, Philadelphia, 1961, J. B. Lippincott Co.

Orban, B.: A contribution to the knowledge of the physiologic changes in the periodontal membrane, J. Am. Dent. Assoc. 16:405, 1929.

Ritchey, B., and Orban, B.: The crests of the interdental alveolar septa, J. Periodontol. 24:75, 1953.

Schaffer, J.: Die Verknöcherung des Unterkiefers [Ossification of the mandible], Arch. Mikrosk. Anat. 32:266, 1888.

Sicher, H., and DuBrul, E. L.: Oral anatomy, ed. 6, St. Louis, 1975, The C. V. Mosby Co.

Weinmann, J. P.: Das Knochenbild bei Störungen der physiologischen Wanderung der Zähne [Bone in disturbances of the physiologic mesial drift], Z. Stomatol. 24:397, 1926.

Weinmann, J. P.: Bone changes related to eruption of the teeth, Angle Orthodont. 11:83, 1941.

Weinmann, J. P., and Sicher, H.: Bone and bones; fundamentals of bone biology, ed. 2, St. Louis, 1955, The C. V. Mosby Co.

# 9 Oral mucous membrane

The oral cavity is unique in structure. It contains the teeth. The salivary glands discharge their secretions into it. It contains the taste buds and can be used to perceive and sense in other ways. Thus it serves a variety of functions.

Food first enters the digestive tract through the oral cavity. Here the food is tasted, masticated, and mixed with saliva. Hard inedible particles are sensed and expectorated. Saliva secreted into the oral cavity lubricates the food and facilitates swallowing. Enzymes in the saliva initiate digestion.

Body cavities that communicate with the external surface are lined by mucous membranes, which are coated by serous and mucous secretions. The surface of the oral cavity is a mucous membrane. Its structure varies in an apparent adaptation to function in different regions of the oral cavity. Areas involved in the mastication of food, such as the gingiva and the hard palate, have a much different structure than does the floor of the mouth or the mucosa of the cheek.

Based upon these functional criteria, the oral mucosa may be divided into three major types:

1. Masticatory mucosa (gingiva and hard palate)
2. Lining or reflecting mucosa (lip, cheek, vestibular fornix, alveolar mucosa, floor of mouth and soft palate)
3. Specialized mucosa (dorsum of the tongue and taste buds)

The masticatory mucosa tends to be bound to bone and does not stretch. It bears forces generated when food is chewed. The lining mucosa is not equally

**253**

exposed to such forces. However, it covers the musculature and is distensible, adapting itself to the contraction and relaxation of cheeks, lips, and tongue and to movements to the mandible produced by the muscles of mastication. It makes up all the surfaces of the mouth except for the dorsum of the tongue and the masticatory mucosa. The specialized (sensory) mucosa is so-called because it bears the taste buds, which have a sensory function. These will be discussed below as will two areas with a slightly different structure—the dentogingival junction (the attachment of the gingiva to the tooth) and the red zone or vermilion border of the lips.

## DEFINITIONS AND GENERAL CONSIDERATIONS

The structure of the oral mucous membrane resembles the skin in many ways. It is composed of two layers, epithelium and connective tissue (Fig. 9-1). The connective tissue component of oral mucosa is termed the *lamina propria*. The comparable part of skin is known as dermis or corium.

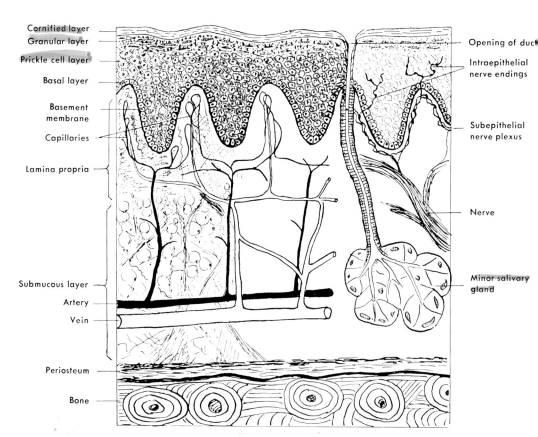

**Fig. 9-1.** Diagram of oral mucous membrane (epithelium, lamina propria, and submucosa).

The two layers form an interface that is folded into corrugations. Papillae of connective tissue protrude toward the epithelium (Fig. 9-2). The papillae carry blood vessels and nerves. Although some of the nerves actually pass into it, the epithelium does not contain blood vessels. The epithelium in turn is formed into ridges that protrude toward the lamina propria. These ridges interdigitate with the papillae and are called epithelial ridges. When the tissue is sectioned for microscopy, these ridges look like pegs as they alternate with the papillae, forming a serpentine interface. At one time, the epithelial ridges were mistakenly called epithelial pegs.

Although the two tissues are intimately connected, they are separate. At their junction, there are two different structures with very similar names, the basal lamina and the basement membrane. The basal lamina is evident at the electron microscopic level and is epithelial in origin (Fig. 9-3). The basement membrane is evident at the light microscopic level. It is found within the connective tissue,

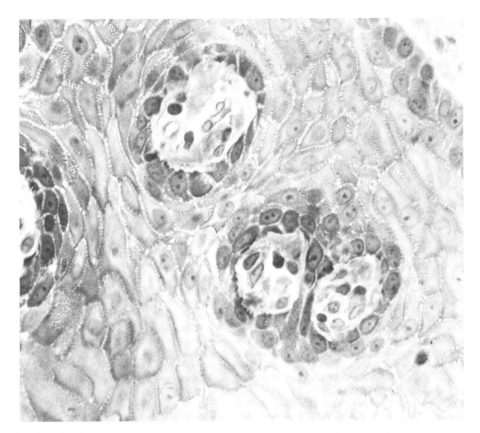

**Fig. 9-2.** Papillae of connective tissue protrude into epithelium. Blood vessels, fibroblasts, and collagen fibers are seen within them. Cells surrounding papillae are basal cells. The other cells are mainly spinous cells.

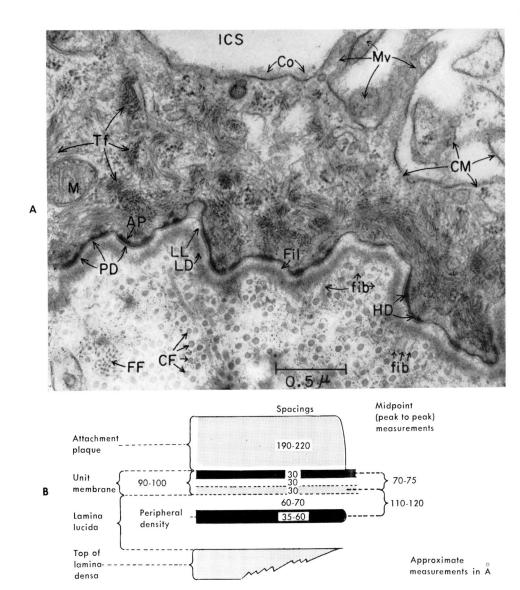

**Fig. 9-3.** Electron micrograph of human gingiva. **A,** This is a portion of a basal cell showing basal plasma membrane and also hemidesmosomes, *HD.* Lamina lucida, *LL,* and lamina densa, *LD.* Collagen fibrils, *CF,* may be seen cut in cross section in the connective tissue. There are also fine fibrils, *FF,* present as a grouping. Other special or anchoring fibrils, *fib,* may be seen inserting into connective tissue side of lamina densa. Area of intercellular space, *ICS,* is evident above epithelial cell. Microvilli, *Mv,* and coating, *Co,* on plasma membrane, *CM,* are present there. **B,** Approximate dimensions of a hemidesmosome. (From Stern, I. B.: Periodontics 3:224, 1965.)

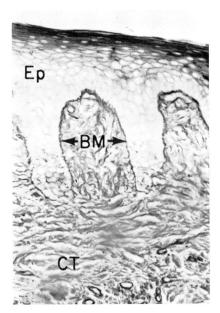

**Fig. 9-4.** Photomicrograph of human gingiva. (PAS stain.) The PAS-positive basement membrane appears as a dense line at the epithelium–connective tissue junction. Note that blood vessels in lamina propria also have a PAS-positive basement membrane. *BM,* Basement membrane; *CT,* connective tissue; *Ep,* epithelial cells. (×160.) (From Stern, I. B.: Periodontics **3:** 224, 1965.)

subjacent to the basal cells. It is a zone that is 1 to 4 microns wide and is relatively cell-free. This zone stains positively with the periodic acid–Schiff method, indicating that it contains neutral mucopolysaccharides (glycosaminoglycans) (Fig. 9-4). It also contains fine argyrophilic reticulin fibers (Fig. 9-5), as well as special anchoring fibrils (Fig. 9-6).

*Lamina propria.* The lamina propria may be described as a connective tissue of variable thickness that supports the epithelium. It is divided for descriptive reasons into two parts—papillary and reticular. The papillary portion is named for the papillae. The reticular portion is named for the reticular fibers. Since there is considerable variation in length and width of the papillae in different areas, the papillary portion is also of variable depth. A portion of the lamina propria subjacent to the basement membrane can be distinguished from the connective tissue because it has the property of taking up silver stain more strongly (argyrophilia) (Fig. 9-5). Fine immature collagen fibers that are argyrophilic and have a trellis or lattice-like arrangement are termed reticulin. This portion as well as the papillary portion contains reticular fibers. The two portions are not separate. They are a continuum but are used to describe this region in different ways. The reticular zone is always present. The papillary zone may be absent in some areas such as in the case in the alveolar mucosa when the papillae are short or lacking.

The interlocking arrangement of the connective tissue papillae and the epithe-

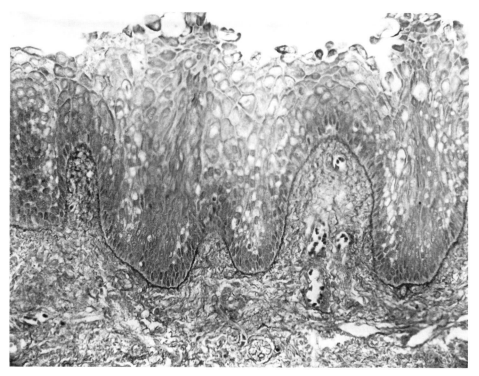

**Fig. 9-5.** Silver-stained section of human fetal tongue showing basement membrane as a dense line separating epithelium above from connective tissue below. Extending for a variable distance into connective tissue are dark-stained reticular fibers, which are found in greatest number immediately below basement membrane. This zone, known as the reticular zone, is found whether or not papillae are present. The papillae delineate extent of papillary zone.

lial ridges and the even finer undulations and projections found at the base of each epithelial cell increases the area of contact between the lamina propria and epithelium (Fig. 9-7). This additional area facilitates exchange of material between the epithelium and the blood vessels in the connective tissue.

The lamina propria may attach to the periosteum of the alveolar bone, or it may overlay the submucosa, which varies in different regions of the mouth such as the soft palate and floor of the mouth.

*Submucosa.* The submucosa consists of connective tissue of varying thickness and density. It attaches the mucous membrane to the underlying structures. Whether this attachment is loose or firm depends on the character of the submucosa. Glands, blood vessels, nerves, and also adipose tissue are present in this layer. It is in the submucosa that the larger arteries divide into smaller branches, which then enter the lamina propria. Here they again divide to form a subepithelial capillary network in the papillae. The veins originating from the capillary network course back along the path taken by the arteries. The blood vessels are accompanied by a rich network of lymph vessels. The sensory nerves

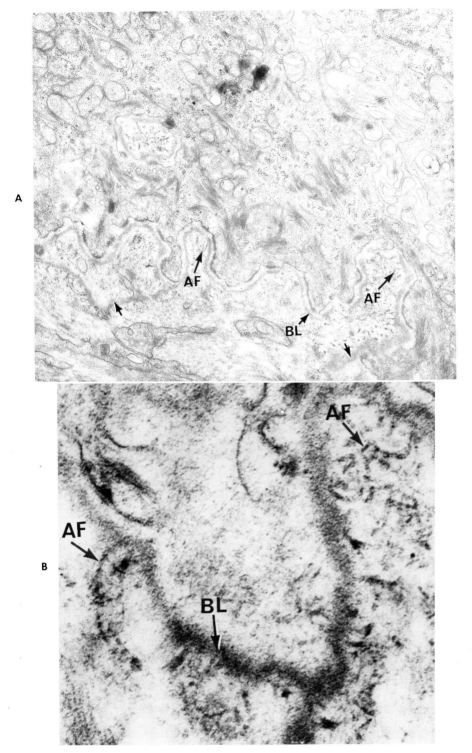

**Fig. 9-6. A,** Anchoring fibrils, *AF,* and basal lamina, *BL,* which are cut tangentially at places *(arrows).* **B,** These fibrils branch, loop, and exhibit banding.

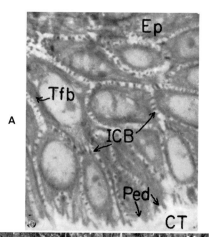

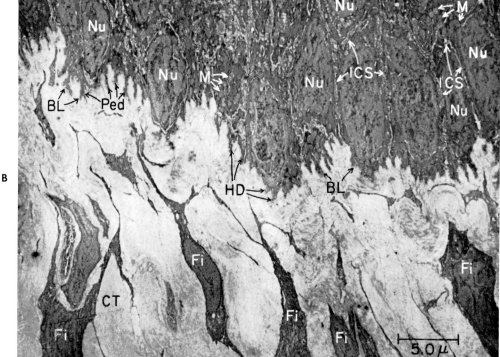

Fig. 9-7. **A,** Photomicrograph of human gingival epithelial cells, *Ep.* Pedicles, *Ped,* are present at base of basal cells and extend toward connective tissue, *CT.* Tonofibrils, *Tfb,* are evident both in the cells and apparently coursing across intercellular bridges, *ICB.* **B,** Electron micrograph of rat gingiva. Several basal cells with apparent pedicles, *Ped,* extending toward the connective tissue, *CT,* but separated from it by basement lamina, *BL,* which is barely visible. Fibroblasts, *Fi,* may be noted within the connective tissue. Epithelial cells contain a prominent nucleus, *Nu,* and are demarcated from adjacent cells by the lighter appearance of the intercellular spaces, *ICS.* Small, round, light areas in epithelial cells are mitochondria, *M.* Pedicles, *Ped,* in this electron micrograph are of a much smaller dimension than the larger undulations of basal cell surface outlined by *arrows* at *HD.* These, in turn, are smaller than the ridges shown in Fig. 9-7, *A.* (**A,** ×1400.) (From Stern, I. B.: Periodontics 3:224, 1965.)

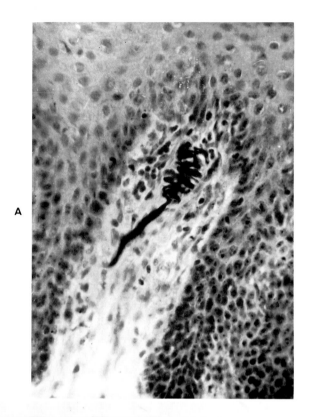

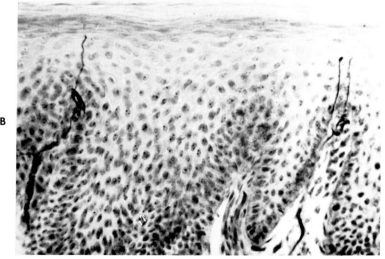

Fig. 9-8. **A,** Meissner tactile corpuscle in human gingiva. (Silver impregnation after Biel-schowsky-Gros.) **B,** Intraepithelial "ultraterminal" extensions and nerve endings in the human gingiva. (Silver impregnation after Bielschowsky-Gros.) (From Gairns, F. W., and Aitchison, J. A.: Dent. Rec. **70:**180, 1950.)

of the mucous membrane tend to be more concentrated toward the anterior part of the mouth (rugae, tip of tongue, etc.). The nerve fibers are myelinated as they traverse the submucosa but lose their myelin sheath before splitting into their end arborizations. Sensory nerve endings of various types are found in the papillae (Fig. 9-8, *A*). Some of the fibers enter the epithelium, where they terminate between the epithelial cells as free nerve endings (Fig. 9-8, *B*). The blood vessels are accompanied by nonmyelinated visceral nerve fibers that supply their smooth muscles. Other visceral fibers supply the glands.

In studying any mucous membrane, the following features should be considered: (1) type of covering epithelium, (2) structure of the lamina propria, its density, thickness, and presence or lack of elasticity, (3) the type of junction between the epithelium and lamina propria, and (4) its fixation to the underlying structures, in other words, the submucous layer. Considered as a separate and well-defined layer, submucosa may be present or absent. Looseness or density of its texture determines whether the mucous membrane is moveably or immovably attached to the deeper layers. Presence or absence and location of adipose tissue or glands should also be noted.

*Epithelium.* The epithelium of the oral mucous membrane is of the stratified squamous variety. It may be keratinized, parakeratinized, or nonkeratinized, depending on location. In man the epithelium of the gingiva and the hard palate is keratinized (Fig. 9-9, *A*), although in many individuals the gingival epithelium is parakeratinized (Fig. 9-9, *C*). The cheek, faucal, and sublingual tissues are normally nonkeratinized (Fig. 9-9, *B*).

Keratinizing oral epithelium has four cell layers: basal, spinous, granular, and cornified. These are also referred to in Latin as *stratum basale, stratum spinosum, stratum granulosum,* and *stratum corneum.* These layers take their names from their morphologic appearance.

A single cell is, at different times, a part of each layer. After mitosis, it may remain in the basal layer and divide again or as it may migrate or be pushed upward. During its migration, it becomes a specialized cell and undergoes biochemical and morphologic changes. In other words it differentiates to form a keratinocyte. A keratinocyte ultimately forms a keratinized squama when it reaches the surface and desquamates. In order for the tissue to remain in a steady state, one cell must form in the basal layer for each cell that desquamates.

The basal layer is made up of cells that synthesize DNA and undergo mitosis, thus providing new cells (Fig. 9-10). The bulk of new cells are generated in the basal layer. However, some mitotic figures may be seen in spinous cells just beyond the basal layer. Therefore, the basal cells and the parabasal spinous cells are referred to as the *stratum germinativum.*

The basal cells are a single layer of cuboid or high cuboid cells that have protoplasmic processes (pedicles) projecting from their basal surfaces toward the connective tissue (Fig. 9-7). They contain specialized structures called *hemidesmosomes,* which abut on the basal lamina (Fig. 9-3). These consist of

*Text continued on p. 267.*

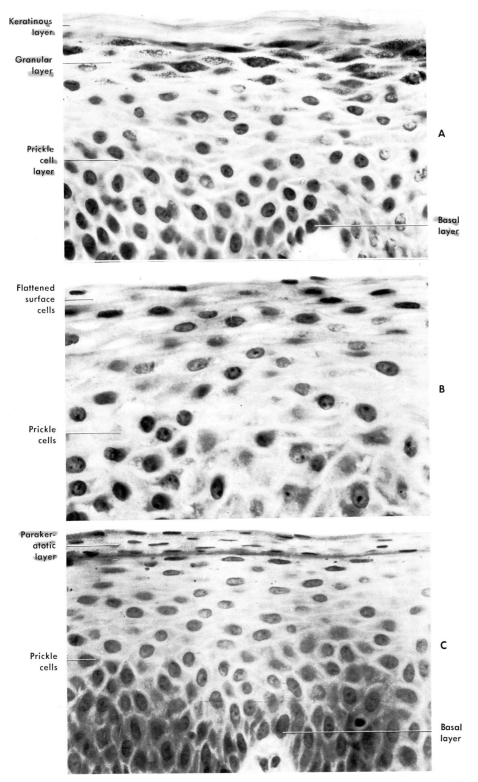

Keratinous layer

Granular layer

Prickle cell layer

Basal layer

Flattened surface cells

Prickle cells

Parakeratotic layer

Prickle cells

Basal layer

Fig. 9-9. Variations of gingival epithelium. **A,** Keratinized. **B,** Nonkeratinized. **C,** Parakeratinized.

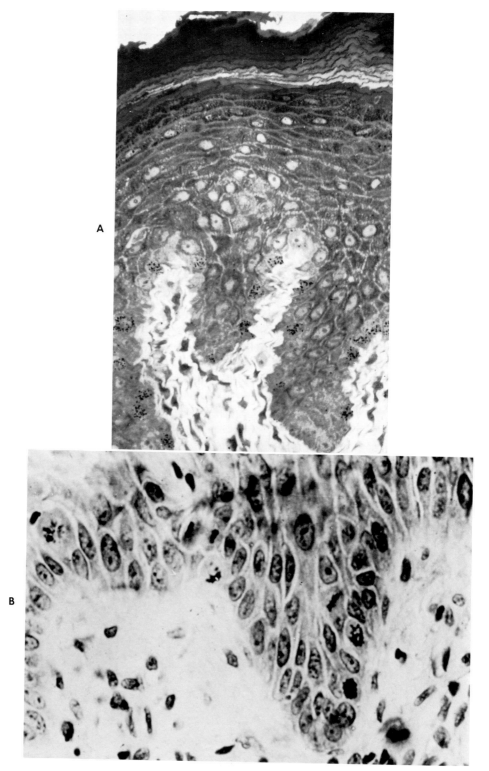

Fig. 9-10. **A,** Arrangement of labeling in oral epithelium 30 minutes after administration of tritiated thymidine. Grains are localized over nuclei in stratum basale. **B,** Oral epithelium showing many mitotic figures. (**A** from Anderson, G. S., and Stern, I. B.: Periodontics 4:115, 1966.)

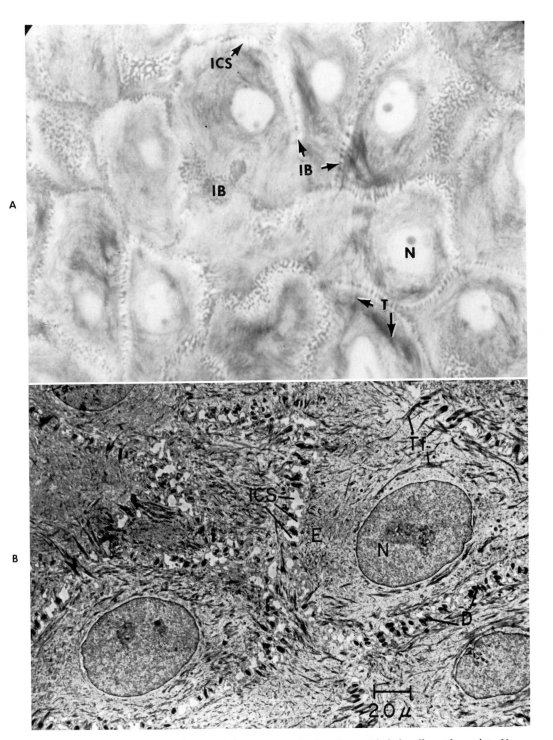

Fig. 9-11. **A,** High magnification light micrograph showing epithelial cells with nuclei, *N;* intercellular spaces, *ICS;* tonofibrils, *T;* and intercellular bridges, *IB.* Speckled areas are inter-cellular bridges (desmosomes) cut tangentially or "en face." **B,** Electron micrograph of prickle cells on human gingiva. Portions of epithelial cells, *E,* are evident, separated by intercellular space, *ICS.* Several nuclei, *N,* are evident. Tonofilaments, *Tf,* are present in the cytoplasm and extend toward desmosomes, *D,* located at the periphery of the cells. (**B** from Grant, D. A., Stern, I. B., and Everett, F. G.: Orban's periodontics, ed. 4, St. Louis, 1972, The C. V. Mosby Co.)

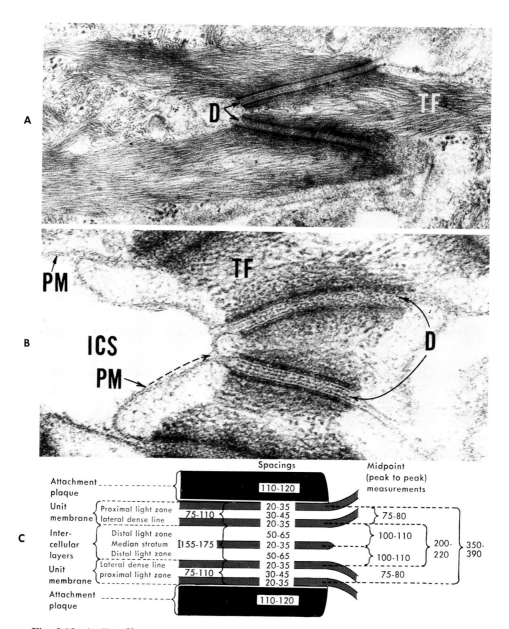

**Fig. 9-12. A,** Tonofilaments, *Tf*, extending to a series of desmosomes, *D*. Tonofilaments are sectioned in the long axis (human gingiva). **B,** Higher magnification of two desmosomes, *D*, showing substructure. Tonofilaments are cross sectioned. Intercellular space, *ICS*, is bounded by adjacent cell membranes, *PM*, whose unit membrane is clearly evident *(dashed arrow).* Unit membranes form part of substructure of desmosome. **C,** Diagrammatic cross-sectioned representation of desmosome and dimensions of various components. (From Stern, I. B.: Periodontics **3:**224, 1965.)

a single attachment plaque, the adjacent plasma membrane, and associated extracellular structure that appears to attach the epithelium to the connective tissue. The basal lamina is made up of a clear zone *(lamina lucida)* just below the epithelial cells and a dark zone *(lamina densa)* beyond the lamina lucida and adjacent to the connective tissue (Fig. 9-3).

The lateral borders of adjacent basal cells are closely apposed and connected by desmosomes (Fig. 9-11). These are specializations of the cell surface, consisting of adjacent cell membranes and a pair of denser regions (attachment plaques) as well as intervening extracellular structures (Fig. 9-12). The basal cells contain tonofilaments, which course toward, and in some way are attached to, the attachment plaques. There are also ribosomes and elements of rough-surfaced endoplasmic reticulum, indicative of protein-synthesizing activity.

The *spinous cells* (stratum spinosum) are irregularly polyhedral and larger

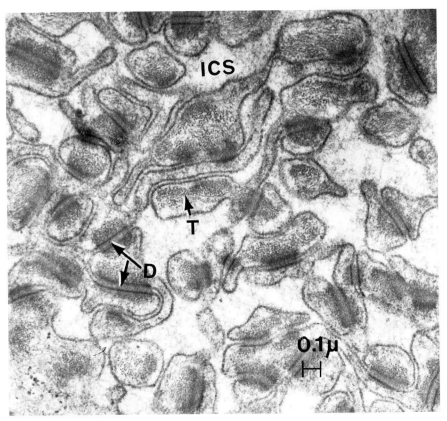

**Fig. 9-13.** Electron micrograph of prickle cell layer of human gingival epithelium showing intercellular bridges and tonofibrils. Here desmosomes are cut tangentially or "en face" as shown in the light micrograph Fig. 9-11, *A*. Note relatively close adaptation of cells at the processes ending in desmosomes, *D*. These processes contain tonofilaments, *T*, cut on end, which appear as fine dots. The relatively large intercellular space, *ICS*, contains material.

than the basal cells. On the basis of light microscopy, it appears that the cells are joined by "intercellular bridges" (Fig. 9-10, *A*). Tonofibrils seem to coarse from cell to cell across these bridges. Electron microscopic studies have shown that the "intercellular bridges" are desmosomes and the tonofibrils are bundles of tonofilaments (Fig. 9-13). The tonofilaments turn or loop adjacent to the attachment plaques and do not cross over into adjacent cells. It is suspected that an agglutinating material joins them to the attachment plaques. The tonofilament network and the desmosomes appear to make up a supporting system for the epithelium. The intercellular spaces of the spinous cells in keratinizing epithelia are large or distended; thus the desmosomes are made more prominent and these cells are given a prickly appearance. The spinous (prickle) cells resemble a cockleburr or sticker that has each spine ending at a desmosome. Of the four layers, the spinous cells are the most active in protein synthesis.

The next layer (*stratum granulosum*) contains flatter and wider cells. These are larger than the spinous cells. They contain basophilic keratohyalin granules (blue staining with hematoxylin-eosin) (Fig. 9-14, *A* to *C*). The nuclei show signs of degeneration and become pyknotic. This layer still synthesizes protein but at a diminished level. As the cell approaches the stratum corneum, the tonofilaments are more dense in quantity and are often seen associated with keratohyalin granules and ribosomes (Fig. 9-14, *D* to *F*). Sometimes, dense networks of tonofilaments and keratohyalin granules are evident. The cell surfaces become more regular and more closely applied to adjacent cell surfaces. The amount of intercellular material increases and presumably is discharged into the intercellular space by the cells.

The *stratum corneum* is made up of keratinized squamae, which are larger and flatter than the granular cells. Here all of the nuclei and other organelles such as ribosomes and mitochondria have disappeared (Fig. 9-14, *D*). The layer is acidophilic (stains red with hematoxylin-eosin) and is histologically amorphous. The keratohyalin granules have disappeared. The cells of the cornified layer are composed of densely packed filaments developed from the tonofilaments and presumably altered or coated by the protein of the keratohyalin granule. The cell has become compact and dehydrated and covers a greater surface area than does the basal cell from which it developed. It no longer synthesizes protein. It is closely applied to adjacent squamae. The cell surface and desmosomes are altered. The plasma membrane is denser and thicker than in the cells of deeper layers.

---

**Fig. 9-14. A,** Light micrograph of newborn rat skin showing basal cells, *B,* spinous cells, *S,* granular cells with numerous dense granules, *G,* and cornified cells, *C,* devoid of nuclei and other cellular structures except for the cornified (keratinized) components. **B** and **C,** Keratohyalin is formed as discrete spherical granules in some tissues or is formed as angular amorphous material in other tissues. **D** and **E,** The angular form is associated with tonofilaments primarily (*arrow*). **F,** Whereas the spherical form is surrounded by ribosomes (*arrow*) and may contain more than one material (*small arrows*).

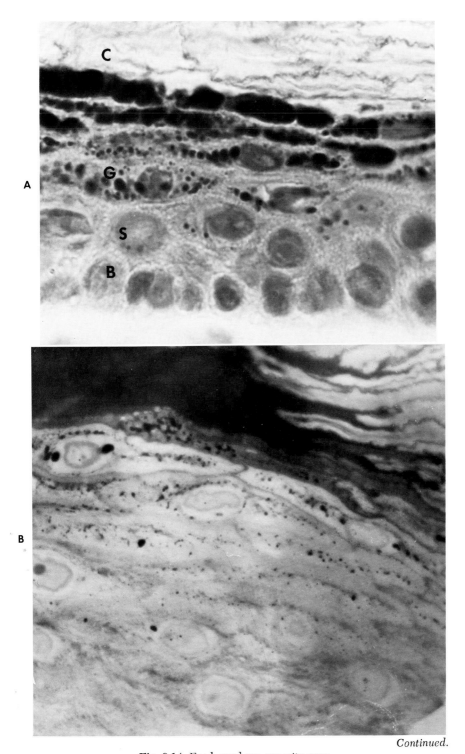

*Continued.*

**Fig. 9-14.** For legend see opposite page.

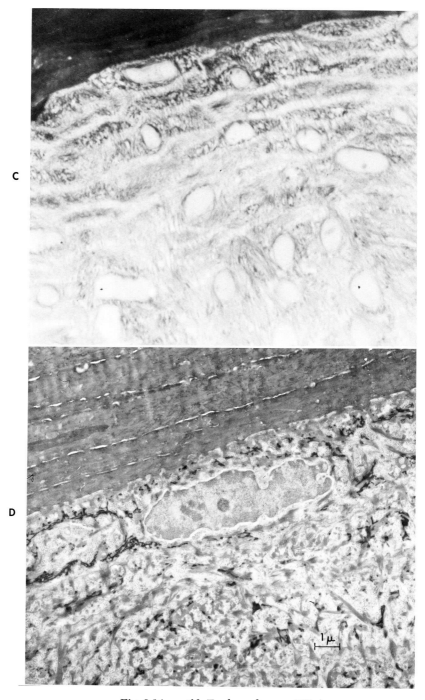

**Fig. 9-14, cont'd.** For legend see p. 268.

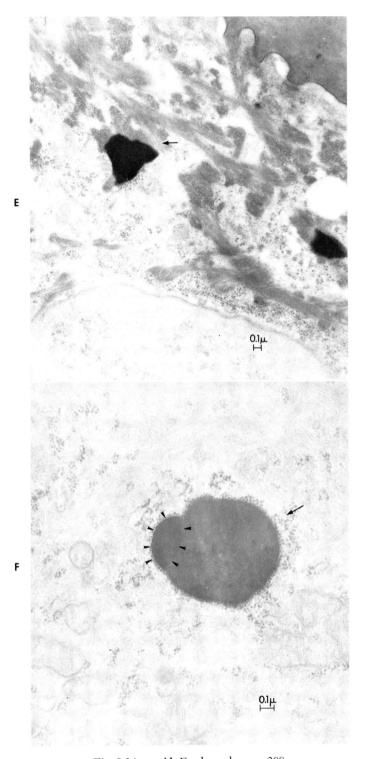

Fig. 9-14, cont'd. For legend see p. 268.

The Odland body (also known as a keratinosome or membrane-coating granule) is a small organelle that is found in the lower granular cells. It has an internal lamellated structure (Fig. 9-15, *A* and *B*). It is claimed by some that these structures are responsible for the thickening of the cell membrane that occurs during keratinization. Others claim that it discharges its contents into the intercellular space there, forming an intercellular agglutinating material. This much is known: The Odland bodies disappear as the cell moves upward in the stratum corneum. The inner unit of the cell membrane grows thicker at about this time and, in addition, a lamellate structure similar to that of the membrane-coating granule is found in the intercellular space (Fig. 9-15, *C*). Although either event may be attributable to the Odland bodies, the evidence seems to support the latter.

Epithelial cells that ultimately keratinize are called *keratocytes* or *keratinocytes*. Keratinocytes increase in volume in each successive layer from basal to granular. The cornified cells, however, are smaller in volume than the granular cells. The cells of each successive layer cover a larger area than do the cells of the layers immediately below. Nonkeratinizing epithelia differ from keratinizing epithelia primarily because they do not produce a cornified surface layer,

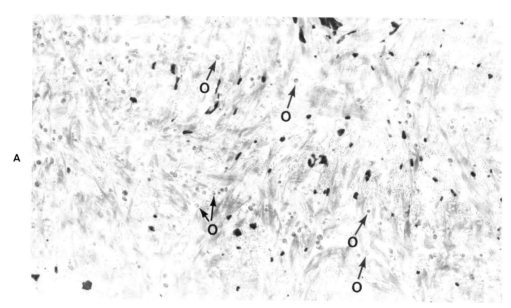

**Fig. 9-15. A,** Odland bodies, *O,* are found close to cell membrane *(arrows)* and desmosomes in granular cells. **B,** Odland bodies, *O,* lying close to plasma membrane *(arrows)* and in cells containing ribosome-associated keratohyalin granules. Note that some of the keratohyalin granules have two densities and perhaps two components. The Odland bodies contain an internal lamellar structure. **C,** Lamellar structure in intercelluar space *(arrows).* It is presumed that these lamellae are derived from Odland bodies that are no longer present.

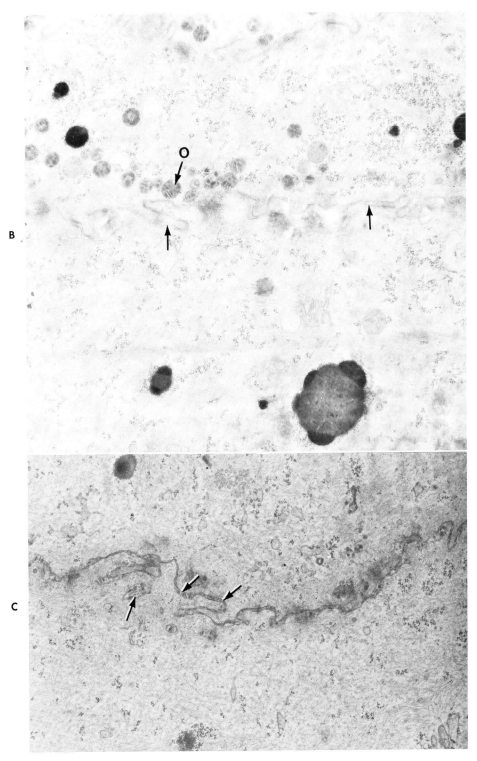

Fig. 9-15, cont'd. For legend see opposite page.

but there are other differences as well. The layers in nonkeratinizing epithelium are referred to as basal, intermediate, and superficial *(stratum basale, stratum intermedium, stratum superficiale)* (Fig. 9-9, *B*). The basal cells of both types are similar. The cells of the stratum intermedium are larger than cells of the stratum spinosum. The intercellular space is not obvious or distended and hence the cells do not have a prickly appearance. Nevertheless, the cells of the stratum intermedium often are referred to as spinous or prickle cells, even though they are not. They are attached by desmosomes and their cell surfaces are more closely applied than are spinous cells. There is no stratum granulosum, nor is there a stratum corneum. Nucleated cells exist at the surface (Fig. 9-16). These cells ultimately desquamate, as do the cornified squamae.

In *orthokeratinization,* keratinized squamae form as has been described. In *parakeratinization,* the cells retain pyknotic and condensed nuclei until they desquamate. There are signs of condensation of the superficial cells, which appear almost as if they were keratinizing. Tissues that are not keratinized at one stage of development may keratinize at another (Fig. 9-16). Similarly, tissues may be modulated from keratinized-parakeratinized and nonkeratinized variants in pathologic states. One frequently finds the terms "parakeratosis" and "keratosis" used in the literature. These terms refer to pathologic stages. When

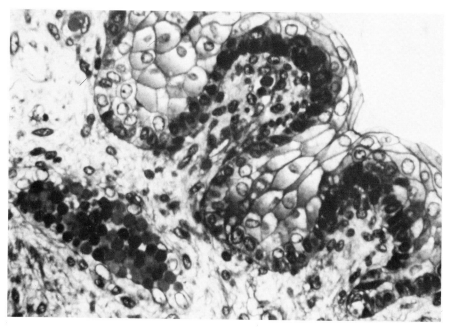

**Fig. 9-16.** Section of human fetal tongue showing the three cell strata of nonkeratinized epithelium.

keratinization is pathologic (i.e., occurring in normally nonkeratinized tissue), it is referred to as keratosis. When normally keratinizing tissue like the epidermis becomes parakeratinized, it is referred to as parakeratosis.

## SUBDIVISIONS OF ORAL MUCOSA

For descriptive purposes the oral mucosa may be divided into the following areas:

Keratinized areas
    Masticatory mucosa
    Vermilion border of lip
Nonkeratinized areas
    Lining mucosa
    Specialized mucosa

### Keratinized areas
### Masticatory mucosa ( gingiva and hard palate )

The masticatory mucosa is keratinized and is made up of the gingiva and the hard palate. They have similarities in thickness and keratinization of epithelium; in thickness, density, and firmness of lamina propria; and in being immovably attached. However, there are differences in their submucosa.

*Hard palate.* The mucous membrane of the hard palate is tightly fixed to the

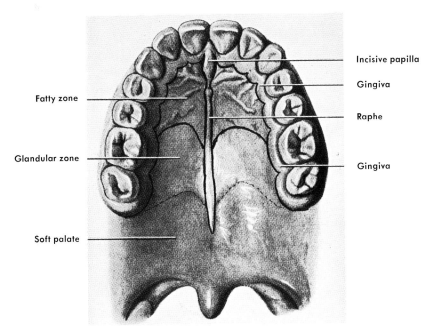

**Fig. 9-17.** Surface view of hard and soft palates. The different zones of palatine mucosa.

underlying periosteum and therefore immovable. Like the gingiva its color is pink. The epithelium is uniform in form with a rather well-keratinized surface. The lamina propria, a layer of dense connective tissue, is thicker in the anterior than in the posterior parts of the palate and has numerous long papillae. Various regions in the hard palate differ because of the varying structure of the submucous layer. The following zones can be distinguished (Fig. 9-17):

1. Gingival region, adjacent to the teeth
2. Palatine raphe, also known as the median area, extending from the incisive or palatine papilla posteriorly
3. Anterolateral area or fatty zone between the raphe and gingiva
4. Posterolateral or glandular zone between the raphe and gingiva

Except for narrow and specific zones, the palate has a distinct submucous layer. The zones that do not have a submucous layer occur peripherally where the palatine tissue is identical with the gingiva and along the midline for the entire length of the hard palate (the palatine raphe) (Fig. 9-17). The marginal area shows the same structure as the other regions of the gingiva. Only the lamina propria and periosteum are present below the epithelium (Fig. 9-18). Similarly, a submucosa is not found below the palatine raphe, or median area (Fig. 9-19). The lamina propria blends with the periosteum. If a palatine torus is present, the mucous membrane is thinner. The otherwise narrow raphe is widened and spreads over the entire torus.

The submucous layer occurs in wide regions extending between the palatine gingiva and palatine raphe. Despite this extensive submucosa, the mucous membrane is immovably attached to the periosteum of the maxillary and palatine bones. This attachment is formed by dense bands and trabeculae of fibrous connective tissue that join the lamina propria of the mucosa membrane to the periosteum. The submucous space is thus subdivided into irregular intercommunicating compartments of various sizes. These are filled with adipose tissue in the anterior part and with glands in the posterior part of the hard palate. The presence of fat or glands in the submucous layer acts as a cushion comparable to that which may be found in the subcutaneous tissue of the palm of the hand and the sole of the foot.

When the submucosa of hard palate and of gingiva are compared, there are pronounced differences. The dense connective tissue that makes up the lamina propria of gingiva is bound to the periosteum of the alveolar process or to the cervical region of the tooth. A submucus layer, as such, cannot generally be recognized. In the lateral areas of the hard palate (Fig. 9-19), in both fatty and glandular zones, the lamina propria is fixed to the periosteum by bands of dense fibrous connective tissue. These bands are arranged at right angles to the surface and divide the submucous layer into irregularly shaped spaces. The distance between lamina propria and periosteum is smaller in the anterior than in the posterior parts. In the anterior zone the connective tissue contains fat (Fig. 9-20), whereas in the posterior part it contains mucous glands (Fig.

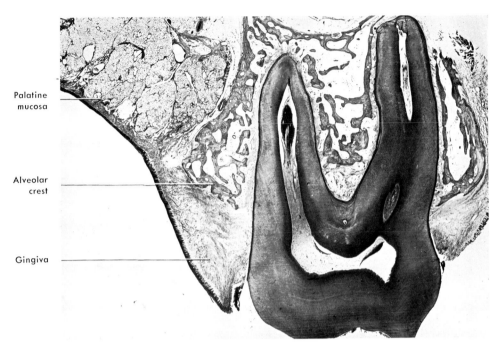

Palatine
mucosa

Alveolar
crest

Gingiva

Fig. 9-18. Structural differences between gingiva and palatine mucosa. Region of first molar.

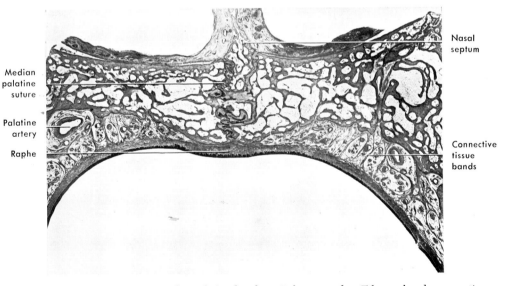

Nasal
septum

Median
palatine
suture

Palatine
artery

Raphe

Connective
tissue
bands

Fig. 9-19. Transverse section through hard palate. Palatine raphe. Fibrous bands connecting mucosa and periosteum in lateral areas. Palatine vessels. (From Pendleton, E. C.: J. Am. Dent. Assoc. **21**:488, 1934.)

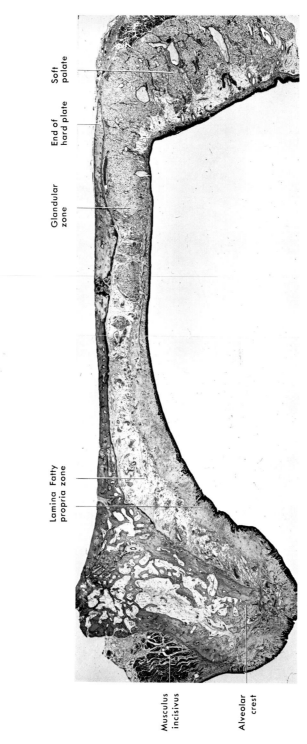

**Fig. 9-20.** Longitudinal section through the hard and soft palates lateral to midline. Fatty and glandular zones of hard palate.

9-20). The glandular layers of the hard palate and of the soft palate are continuous.

At the juncture between the alveolar process and the horizontal plate of the hard palate, the anterior palatine vessels and nerves course surrounded by loose connective tissue. This wedge-shaped area (Fig. 9-21) is large in the posterior part of the palate and smaller in size in the anterior. It is important for oral surgeons and periodontists to know the distribution of these vessels.

*Incisive papilla.* The oval incisive (palatine) papilla is formed of dense connective tissue. It contains the oral parts of the vestigial nasopalatine ducts. They are blind ducts of varying length lined by simple or pseudostratified columnar epithelium, rich in goblet cells. Small mucous glands open into the lumen of the ducts. These ducts sometimes become cystic in man. Frequently the ducts are surrounded by small, irregular islands of hyaline cartilage, which are the vestigial extensions of the paraseptal cartilages. In most mammals the nasopalatine ducts are patent and, together with Jacobson's organ, are considered as auxiliary olfactory sense organs. Jacobson's organ (the vomeronasal organ) is a small ellipsoid (cigar-shaped) structure lined with olfactory epithelium that extends from the nose to the oral cavity. In man cartilage is sometimes found in the anterior parts of the papilla and in this location bears no relation to the nasopalatine ducts (Fig. 9-22).

*Palatine rugae (transverse palatine ridges).* The palatine rugae, irregular and often asymmetric in man, are ridges of mucous membrane extending laterally

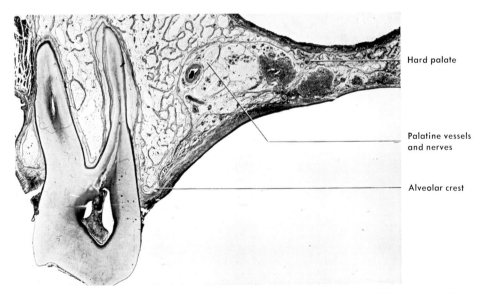

Hard palate

Palatine vessels and nerves

Alveolar crest

**Fig. 9-21.** Transverse section through posterior part of hard palate, region of the second molar. Loose connective tissue in groove between alveolar process and hard palate around palatine vessels and nerves.

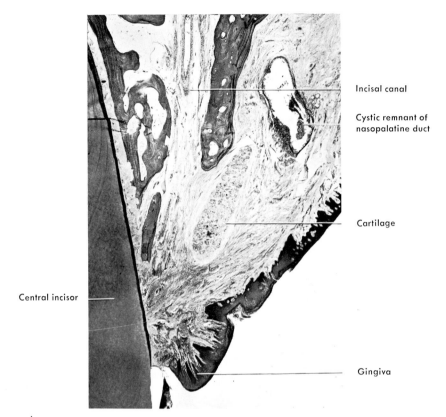

Central incisor

Incisal canal

Cystic remnant of
nasopalatine duct

Cartilage

Gingiva

Fig. 9-22. Sagittal section through palatine papilla and anterior palatine canal. Note cartilage in papilla.

from the incisive papilla and the anterior part of the raphe. Their core is made of a dense connective tissue layer with fine interwoven fibers.

*Epithelial pearls.* In the midline, especially in the region of the incisive papilla, epithelial pearls may be found in the lamina propria. They consist of concentrically arranged epithelial cells that are frequently keratinized. They are remnants of the epithelium formed in the line of fusion between the palatine processes (Chapter 1).

*Gingiva.* The gingiva extends from the dentogingival junction to the alveolar mucosa. The gingiva is subject to friction and pressure in the process of mastication. The morphology of both the epithelium and connective tissues indicates that it is adapted to these forces. It is made up of stratified squamous epithelium, which may be keratinized or nonkeratinized but most often is parakeratinized. The epithelium covers a dense lamina propria. The collagen fibers of the lamina propria may either insert into the alveolar bone and the cementum or blend with the periosteum.

The gingiva is limited on the outer surface of both jaws by the mucogingival junction which separates it from the alveolar mucosa (Fig. 9-23). The alveolar

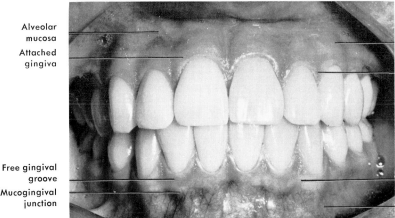

Alveolar mucosa

Attached gingiva

Mucogingival junction

Interdental papilla

Free gingival groove

Mucogingival junction

Attached gingiva

Alveolar mucosa

**Fig. 9-23.** Vestibular surface of gingiva of young adult. (Courtesy Dr. A. Ogilvie, Seattle, Wash.)

mucosa is red and contains numerous small vessels close to the surface. On the inner surface of the lower jaw a line of demarcation is found between the gingiva and the mucosa on the floor of the mouth. On the palate the distinction between the gingiva and the peripheral palatal mucosa is not so sharp.*

The gingiva can be divided into the *free gingiva,* the *attached gingiva* (Fig. 9-24), and the *interdental papilla.* The dividing line between the free and the attached gingiva is the *free gingival groove,* which runs parallel to the margin of the gingiva at a distance of 0.5 to 1.5 mm. The free gingival groove, not always visible microscopically, appears in histologic sections (Fig. 9-25, A) as a shallow V-shaped notch corresponding to the heavy epithelial ridge that divides the free and the attached gingiva. The free gingival groove develops at the level of, or somewhat apical to, the bottom of the gingival sulcus. In some cases the free gingival groove is not so well defined as in others, and then the division between the free and the attached gingiva is not clear. The free gingival groove and the epithelial ridge are probably caused by functional impacts upon the free gingiva.

---

*These surfaces are frequently referred to as buccal or labial, lingual or palatal. The oral cavity can be divided into two parts: the vestibulum oris (vestibule) and the cavum oris proprium (oral cavity proper). The term *vestibular* is used to describe those surfaces that face the vestibule, thus the need of differentiating between buccal and labial is eliminated. This tends to simplify descriptions and coincides with proper anatomic usage. The vestibular cavity is bounded anterolaterally by the mucous membranes of the lips and cheeks and internally by the teeth and gingiva. Vestibular would therefore apply to any tooth surface facing the vestibular cavity. Similarly the term *oral* describes the palatal and lingual. The oral cavity proper is bounded anterolaterally by the teeth and gingiva, superiorly by the soft and hard palate, inferiorly by the tongue and mucous membranes of the floor of the mouth, and posteriorly by the pillars of the fauces, the opening into the oral pharynx.

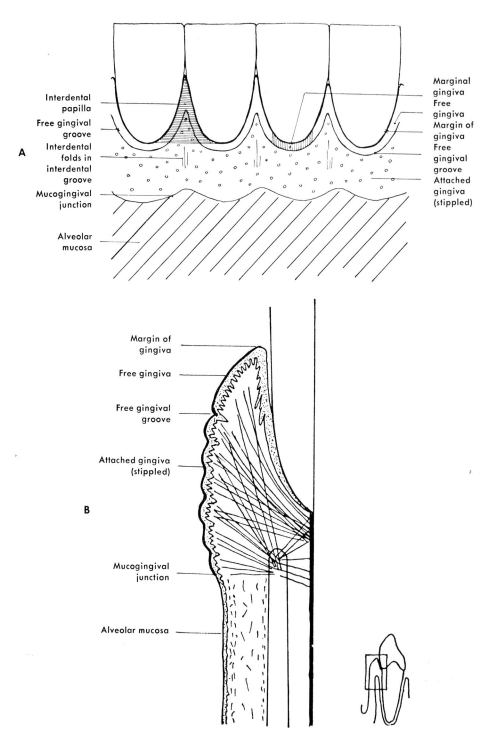

Fig. 9-24. **A,** Diagram illustrating surface characteristics of gingiva. **B,** Diagram illustrating difference between free gingiva, attached gingiva, and alveolar mucosa.

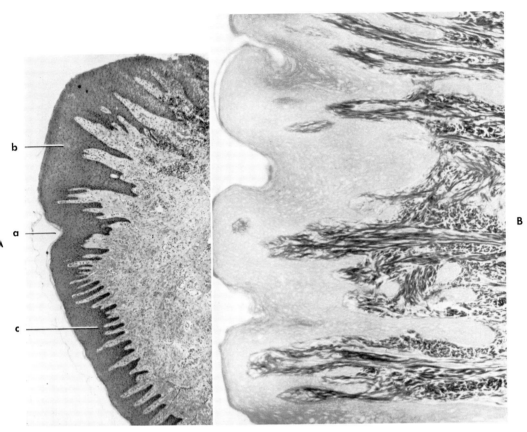

**Fig. 9-25. A,** Biopsy specimen of gingiva showing free gingival groove, *a,* and corresponding heavy epithelial ridge; *b,* free gingiva; *c,* attached gingiva. **B,** Gingival specimen showing stippling. Note relation of connective tissue fiber bundles to stippled surface. (Mallory stain.) (From Grant, D. A., Stern, I. B., and Everett, F. G.: Orban's periodontics, ed. 4, St. Louis, 1972, The C. V. Mosby Co.)

The attached gingiva is characterized by a surface that appears stippled (Fig. 9-25, *B*). Portions at the epithelium appear to be elevated, and between the elevations there are shallow depressions, the net result of which is stippling. The depressions correspond to the center of heavier epithelial ridges and show signs of degeneration and keratinization at their depth. There may be protuberances of the epithelium as well as stippling. They probably are functional adaptations to mechanical impacts. The disappearance of stippling is an indication of edema, an expression of an involvement of the attached gingiva in a progressing gingivitis.

Although the degree of stippling (Fig. 9-23) and the texture of the collagenous fibers vary with different individuals, there are also differences according to age and sex. In younger females the connective tissue is more finely textured than that of the male. However, with increasing age, the collagenous fiber bundles

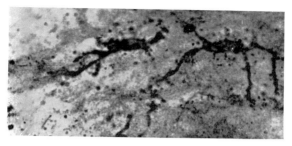

**Fig. 9-26.** Macrophages in normal gingiva. (Rio Hortega stain; ×1000.) (From Aprile, E. C. de: Arch. Hist. Normal Pat. 3:473, 1947.)

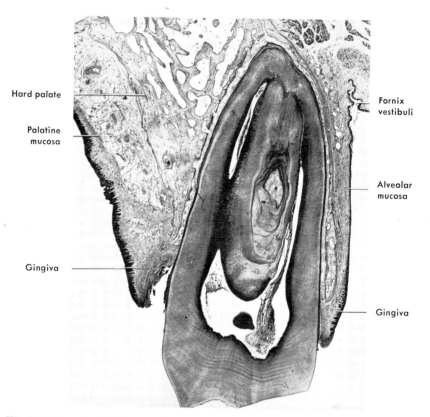

Hard palate

Palatine mucosa

Gingiva

Fornix vestibuli

Alveolar mucosa

Gingiva

**Fig. 9-27.** Structural differences between gingiva and alveolar mucosa. Upper premolar.

become more coarse in both sexes. Males tend to have more heavily stippled gingivae than do females. Like the human epidermis, the cells of the oral epithelium show another sex difference. In females the majority of the nuclei contain a large chromatin particle adjacent to the nuclear membrane.

The attached gingiva appears slightly depressed between adjacent teeth, corresponding to the depression on the alveolar process between eminences of the sockets. In these depressions the attached gingiva often forms slight vertical folds called interdental grooves.

The interdental papilla is that part of the gingiva that fills the space between two adjacent teeth. When viewed from the oral or vestibular, the surface of the interdental papilla is triangular. In a three-dimensional view the interdental papilla of the posterior teeth is tentshaped, whereas it is pyramidal between the anterior teeth. When the interdental papilla is tent shaped, the oral and the vestibular corners are high, whereas the central part is like a valley. The central concave area fits below the contact point, and this depressed part of the interdental papilla is called the *col*. The col is covered by thin nonkeratinized epithelium, and it has been suggested that the col (the nonkeratinized epithelium) is more vulnerable to periodontal disease.

The lamina propria of the gingiva consists of a dense connective tissue that does not contain large vessels. Small numbers of lymphocytes, plasma cells, and macrophages are present in the connective tissue of normal gingiva (Fig. 9-26) subjacent to the sulcus and are involved in defense and repair. The papillae of the connective tissue are characteristically long, slender, and numerous. The presence of these high papillae makes for ease in the histologic differentiation of gingiva and alveolar mucosa, in which the papillae are quite low (Fig. 9-27). The tissue of the lamina propria contains only few elastic fibers and for the most part they are confined to the walls of the blood vessels. Other elastic fibers known as oxytalan fibers (because of special staining qualities) are also present. On the other hand, the alveolar mucosa and the submucosa contain numerous elastic fibers. These fibers are thickest in the submucosa.

The gingival fibers of the periodontal ligament enter into the lamina propria, attaching the gingiva firmly to the teeth (Chapter 7). The gingiva is also immovably and firmly attached to the periosteum of the alveolar bone. Because of this arrangement it is often referred to as mucoperiosteum. Here a dense connective tissue, consisting of coarse collagen bundles (Fig. 9-28, *A*), extends from the bone to the lamina propria. In contrast, the submucosa underlying the alveolar mucous membrane is loosely textured (Fig. 9-28, *B*). The fiber bundles of the lamina propria of the alveolar mucosa are thin and regularly interwoven.

The gingiva contains dense fibers of collagen sometimes referred to as the gingival ligament which are divided into the following major groups:

1. *Dentogingival.* Extends from the cervical cementum into the lamina propria of the gingiva. The fibers of the gingival ligament constitute the most numerous group of gingival fibers.
2. *Alveologingival.* The fibers arise from the alveolar crest and extend into the lamina propria.
3. *Circular.* A small group of fibers that circle the tooth and interlace with the other fibers.
4. *Dentoperiosteal.* These fibers can be followed from the cementum into the periosteum of the alveolar crest and of the vestibular and oral surfaces of the alveolar bone.

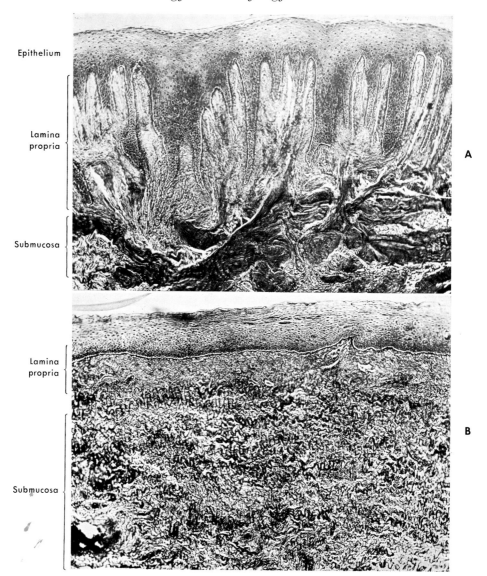

Epithelium

Lamina propria

A

Submucosa

Lamina propria

B

Submucosa

**Fig. 9-28.** Differences between gingiva, **A,** and alveolar mucosa, **B.** Silver impregnation of collagenous fibers. Note coarse bundles of fibers in gingiva and finer fibers in alveolar mucosa.

There are also accessory fibers that extend interproximally between adjacent teeth and are also referred to as transseptal fibers. These fibers comprise the *interdental ligament.*

The gingiva is normally pink but may sometimes have a grayish tint. The color depends in part on the type (keratinized or not) and thickness of the surface layer and in part upon pigmentation. The surface may be translucent or transparent, permitting the color of the underlying tissues to be seen. The

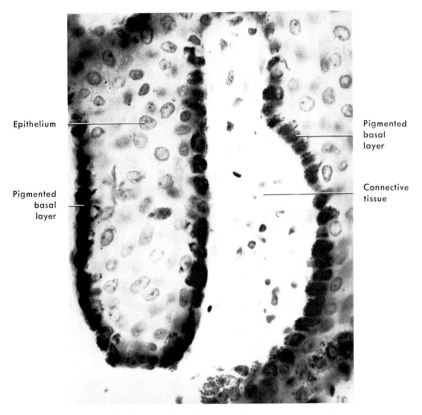

Epithelium

Pigmented basal layer

Pigmented basal layer

Connective tissue

**Fig. 9-29.** Basal cells of gingiva showing pigmentation.

reddish or pinkish tint is attributable to the color given the underlying tissue by the blood vessels and the circulating blood.

The presence of melanin pigment in the epithelium may give it a brown to black coloration. Pigmentation is most abundant at the base of the interdental papilla. It may increase considerably in a number of pathologic stages. Melanin is stored by the basal cells in the form of melanosomes, but these cells do not produce the pigment (Fig. 9-29). Melanin is elaborated by specific cells, *melanocytes*, residing in the basal layer and is transferred to the basal cells. The melanocytes are derived from the embryologic neural crest and migrate into the epithelium (Fig. 9-30). Oral pigmentation can be studied by use of either the dopa reaction or silver-staining techniques. In the dopa reaction the cells containing tyrosinase enzyme appear dark. Therefore the melanin-producing cells, which contain tyrosinase (dopa oxidase), are demonstrated. Silver stains also dye the melanin pigment. The dopa reaction is also found in certain connective tissue cells of the lamina propria that contain melanin (melanophages). These cells obtain the pigment from the melanocytes. Melanocytes appear as clear

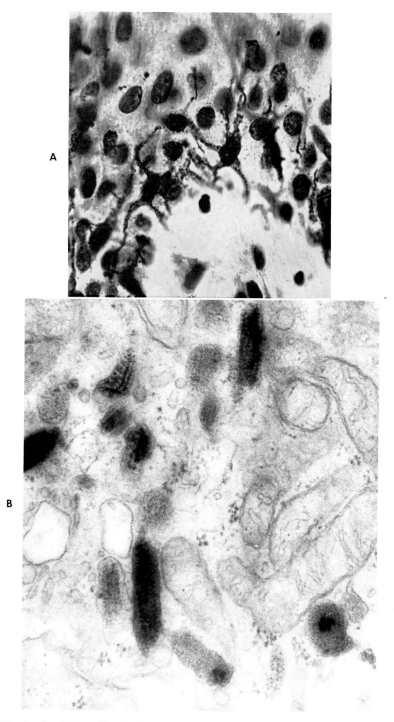

**Fig. 9-30. A,** Dendritic cells (melanocytes) in basal layer of epithelium. Biopsy of normal gingiva. **B,** Ultrastructural photographs of melanosomes from human gingiva showing substructural form. It is believed that tyrosinase associated with these structures is responsible for melanization and when melanosomes become fully melanized they are transferred to keratinocytes. (×1000.) (**A,** from Aprile, E. C. de: Arch. Hist. Normal Pat. 3:473, 1947.)

cells in hematoxylin sections. Silver stains reveal a spiderlike (dendritic) appearance. Thus melanocytes are referred to as "clear cells" or "dendritic cells." The number of melanocytes per square millimeter is quite constant for any particular region and no difference in their numbers is found in the mucosa of blacks and whites.

The following are three types of epithelial surface layers that are the result from differences in differentiation (Fig. 9-9):

1. *Keratinization,* in which the superficial cells form scales of keratin and lose their nuclei. A stratum granulosum is present.
2. *Parakeratinization,* in which the superficial cells retain pyknotic nuclei and show some signs of being keratinized; however, the stratum granulosum is generally absent.
3. *Nonkeratinization,* in which the surface cells are nucleated and show no signs of keratinization.

The gingiva is parakeratinized 75%, keratinized 15%, and nonkeratinized 10% of the time. It has been suggested that inflammation, which is seen in almost all gingival specimens, interferes with keratinization. The more highly keratinized the tissue, the whiter and less translucent is the tissue.

The Langerhans cell is another clear cell or dendritic cell found in the upper layers of the skin and the mucosal epithelium. This cell is free of melanin and does not give a dopa reaction. It stains with gold chloride. The nature of this cell is as yet unknown. Neither the Langerhans cell nor the melanocyte forms desmosomal attachments to the epithelial cells.

There is still another cell found among the basal cells. This cell called the *Merkel cell* has nerve tissue immediately subjacent and is presumed to be a pressure-sensitive (touch) cell. Thus the oral epithelium not only contains the normal population of keratinocytes arranged in strata according to degree of differentiation, it also contains as normal residents three types of cells, the *melanocytes,* the *Langerhans* cells, and the *Merkel cells.*

Other cells such as lymphocytes and polymorphonuclear leukocytes are also found at various levels of the epithelium. These cells are transients and can pass through the epithelium to the surface.

*Blood and nerve supply.* The blood supply of the gingiva is derived chiefly from the branches of the alveolar arteries that pass upward through the interdental septa. The interdental alveolar arteries perforate the alveolar crest in the interdental space and end in the interdental papilla, supplying it and the adjacent areas of the buccal and lingual gingiva. In the gingiva these branches anastomose with superficial branches of arteries that supply the oral and vestibular mucosa and marginal gingiva, for instance, with branches of the lingual, buccal, mental, and palatine arteries. The numerous lymph vessels of the gingiva lead to submental and submandibular lymph nodes.

The gingiva is well innervated. Different types of nerve endings can be observed, such as the Meissner or Krause corpuscles, end bulbs, loops, or fine fibers that enter the epithelium as "ultraterminal" fibers (Fig. 9-8).

### Vermilion border of lip

The transitional zone between the skin of the lip and the mucous membrane of the lip is the red zone, or the vermilion border. It is found only in man (Fig. 9-31). The skin on the outer surface of the lip is covered by a moderately thick, keratinized epithelium with a rather thick stratum corneum. The papillae of the connective tissue are few and short. Many sebaceous glands are found in connection with the hair follicles. Sweat glands occur between them.

The boundary between the red zone and the mucous membrane of the inner surface of the lip occurs where the keratinization of the transitional zone ends. The epithelium of the mucous membrane of the lip is not keratinized.

The transitional region is characterized by numerous, densely arranged, long papillae of the lamina propria, reaching deep into the epithelium and carrying large capillary loops close to the surface. Thus blood is visible through the thin parts of the translucent epithelium and gives the red color to the lips. Because this transitional zone contains only occasional sebaceous glands, it is subject to drying and therefore requires moistening by the tongue.

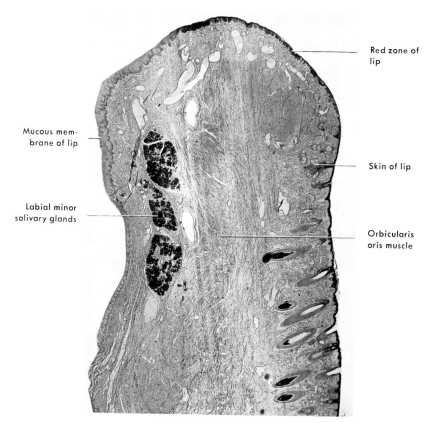

Red zone of lip

Mucous membrane of lip

Skin of lip

Labial minor salivary glands

Orbicularis oris muscle

**Fig. 9-31.** Section through the lip.

## Nonkeratinized areas

### Lining mucosa

Lining mucosa is found on the lip, cheek, vestibular fornix, and alveolar mucosa. All the zones of the lining mucosa are characterized by having a relatively thick nonkeratinized epithelium and a thin lamina propria. Different zones of lining mucosa vary from one another in the structure of their submucosa. Where the lining mucosa reflects from the movable lips, cheeks, and tongue to the alveolar bone, the submucosa is loosely textured. The reflectory mucosa found in the fornix vestibuli and in the sublingual sulcus at the floor of the oral cavity has a submucosa that is loose and of considerable volume. The mucous membrane is movably attached to the deep structures and does not restrict the movement of lips and cheeks and the tongue.

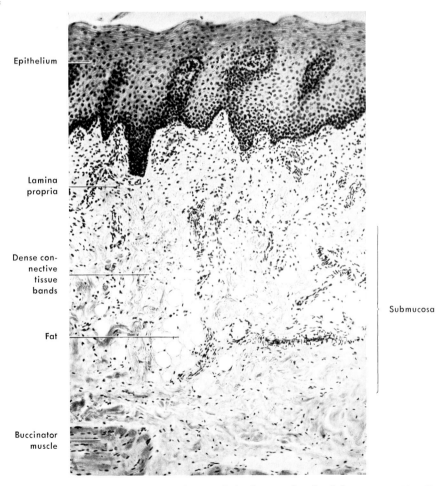

Fig. 9-32. Section through mucous membrane of cheek. Note bands of dense connective tissue attaching lamina propria to fascia of buccinator muscle.

Where lining mucosa covers muscle as on the lips, cheeks, and underside of the tongue, the mucosa is fixed to the epimysium or fascia. In these regions the mucosa is also highly elastic. These two characteristics permit the mucosa to maintain a relatively smooth surface during muscular movement. Thus heavy folding, which could lead to injury during chewing if such folds were caught between the teeth, does not occur.

The mucosa of the soft palate is intermediate between this type of lining mucosa and the reflecting mucosa.

*Lip and cheek.* The epithelium of the mucosa of the lips (Fig. 9-31) and of the cheek (Fig. 9-32) is stratified squamous nonkeratinized epithelium. The lamina propria of the labial and buccal mucosa consists of dense connective tissue and has short, irregular papillae.

The submucous layer connects the lamina propria to the thin fascia of the muscles and consist of strands of densely grouped collagen fibers. There is loose connective tissue containing fat and small mixed glands between these strands. The strands of dense connective tissue limit the mobility of the mucous membrane, holding it to the musculature and preventing its elevation into folds. This prevents the mucous membrane of the lips and cheeks from lodging between the biting surfaces of the teeth during mastication. The mixed minor salivary glands of the lips are situated in the submucosa, whereas in the cheek the glands are larger and are usually found between the bundles of the buccinator muscle and sometimes on its outer surface. The cheek, lateral to the corner of the mouth, may contain isolated sebaceous glands called Fordyce's spots (Fig. 9-33). There may occur lateral to the corner of the mouth and are often seen opposite the molars.

A comparison of masticatory and buccal mucosa shows that in the keratinized tissue the epithelium is thinner. It has a granular layer, the basal cells are larger but the average cell size is smaller, and the cells have an angular shape. Further,

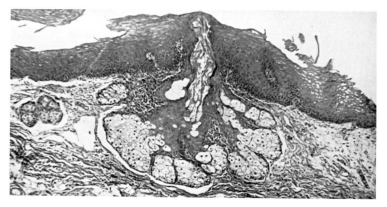

**Fig. 9-33.** Sebaceous gland in cheek (Fordyce spot).

it is characterized by having many tonofibrils, wider intercellular spaces, and "prickles" that form "intercellular bridges." Even the lamina propria of the two differ. In masticatory mucosa the basement membrane contains more reticular fibers, and its papillae are high and more closely spaced.

*Vestibular fornix and alveolar mucosa.* The mucosa of the lips and cheeks reflects from the vestibular fornix to the alveolar mucosa covering the bone. The mucous membrane of the cheeks and lips is attached firmly to the buccinator muscle in the cheeks and the orbicularis oris muscle in the lips. In the fornix the mucosa is loosely connected to the underlying structures, and so the necessary movements of the lips and cheeks are permitted. The mucous membrane covering the outer surface of the alveolar process (alveolar mucosa) is attached loosely to the periosteum. It is continuous with, but different from, the gingiva, which is firmly attached to the periosteum of the alveolar crest and to the teeth.

The median and lateral labial frenula are folds of the mucous membrane containing loose connective tissue. No muscle fibers are found in these folds.

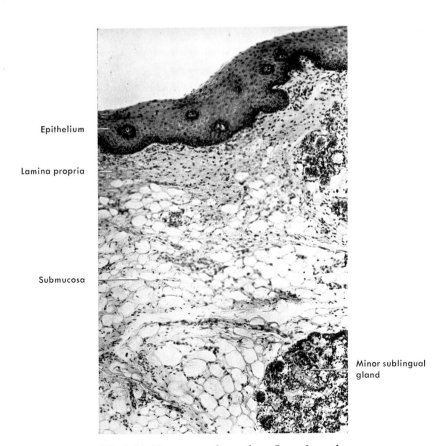

Epithelium

Lamina propria

Submucosa

Minor sublingual gland

Fig. 9-34. Mucous membrane from floor of mouth.

Gingiva and alveolar mucosa are separated by the mucogingival junction. The attached gingiva is stippled, firm, and thick, lacks a separate submucous layer, is immovably attached to bone and teeth by course collagen fibers, and has no glands. The gingival epithelium is thick and mostly parakeratinized or keratinized. The epithelial ridges and the papillae of the lamina propria are high. The alveolar mucosa is thin and loosely attached to the periosteum by a well-defined submucous layer of loose connective tissue (Fig. 9-28, *B*), and it may contain small mixed glands. The epithelium is thin and nonkeratinized, and the epithelial ridges and papillae are low and often entirely missing. These differences cause the variation in color between the pale pink gingiva and the red lining mucosa.

*Inferior surface of tongue; floor of oral cavity.* The mucous membrane on the floor of the oral cavity is thin and loosely attached to the underlying structures to allow for the free mobility of the tongue. The epithelium is nonkeratinized and the papillae of the lamina propria are short (Fig. 9-34). The submucosa contains adipose tissue. The sublingual glands lie close to the covering mucosa in the sublingual fold. The sublingual mucosa and the lingual gingiva have a junction corresponding to the mucogingival junction on the vestibular surface. The sublingual mucosa reflects onto the lower surface of the tongue and continues as the ventrolingual mucosa.

The mucous membrane of the inferior surface of the tongue is smooth and relatively thin (Fig. 9-35). The epithelium is nonkeratinized. The papillae of the connective tissue are numerous but short. Here the submucosa cannot be identified as a separate layer. It binds the mucosa membrane tightly to the connective tissue surrounding the bundles of the muscles of the tongue.

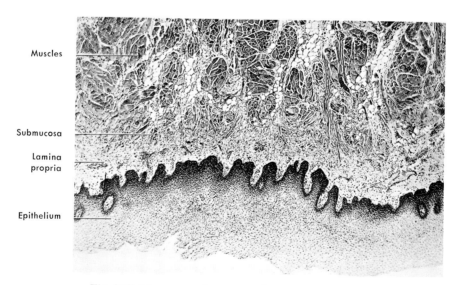

Muscles

Submucosa

Lamina propria

Epithelium

**Fig. 9-35.** Mucous membrane on inferior surface of tongue.

*Soft palate.* The mucous membrane on the oral surface of the soft palate is highly vascularized and reddish in color, noticeably differing from the pale color of the hard palate. The papillae of the connective tissue are few and short. The stratified squamous epithelium is nonkeratinized (Fig. 9-36). The lamina propria shows a distinct layer of elastic fibers separating it from the submucosa. The latter is relatively loose and contains an almost continuous layer of mucous glands. It also contains taste buds. Typical oral mucosa continues around the free border of the soft palate for a variable distance and is then replaced by nasal mucosa with its pseudostratified, ciliated columnar epithelium.

### Specialized mucosa

*Dorsal lingual mucosa.* The superior surface of the tongue is rough and irregular (Fig. 9-37). A V-shaped line divides it into an anterior part, or body, and a posterior part, or base. The former comprises about two thirds of the length of the organ, and the latter forms the posterior one third. The fact that these two parts develop embryologically from different visceral arches (Chapter 1) accounts for the different source of nerves of the general senses: the anterior

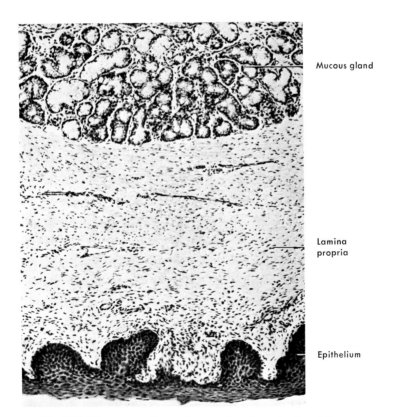

Mucous gland

Lamina propria

Epithelium

Fig. 9-36. Mucous membrane from oral surface of soft palate.

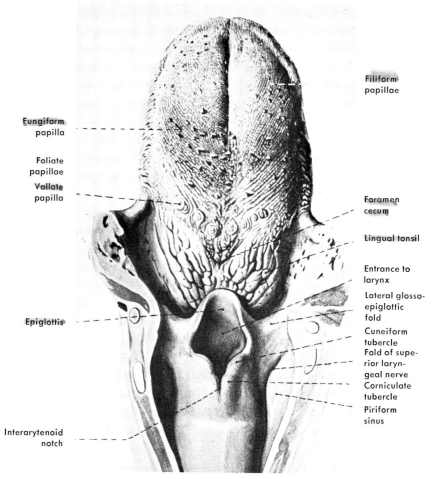

Fungiform
papilla

Foliate
papillae

Vallate
papilla

Filiform
papillae

Foramen
cecum

Lingual tonsil

Entrance to
larynx

Lateral glosso-
epiglottic
fold

Epiglottis

Cuneiform
tubercle
Fold of supe-
rior laryn-
geal nerve
Corniculate
tubercle
Piriform
sinus

Interarytenoid
notch

**Fig. 9-37.** Surface view of human tongue. (From Sicher, H., and Tandler, J.: Anatomie für Zahnärzte [Anatomy for dentists], Vienna, 1928, Julius Springer Verlag.)

two thirds are supplied by the trigeminal nerve through its lingual branch and the posterior one third by the glossopharyngeal nerve.

The body and the base of the tongue differ widely in the structure of the mucous membrane. The anterior part can be termed the papillary and the posterior part the lymphatic portion of the dorsolingual mucosa. On the anterior part are found numerous fine-pointed, cone-shaped papillae that give it a velvet-like appearance. These projections, the filiform (thread-shaped) papillae are epithelial structures containing a core of connective tissue from which secondary papillae protude toward the epithelium (Fig. 9-38, *A*). The covering epithelium is keratinized and forms tufts at the apex of the dermal papilla. The filiform papillae do not contain taste buds.

Interspersed between the filiform papillae are the isolated fungiform (mush-

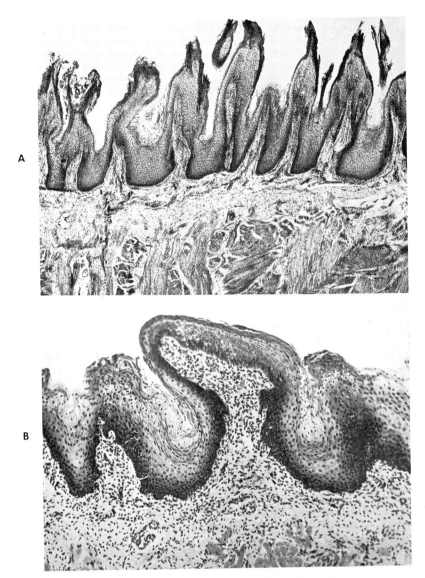

Fig. 9-38. Filiform, **A**, and fungiform, **B**, papillae.

room-shaped) papillae (Fig. 9-38, *B*), which are round, reddish prominences. Their color is derived from a rich capillary network visible through the relatively thin epithelium. Fungiform papillae contain a few (one to three) taste buds found only on their dorsal surface.

In front of the dividing V-shaped terminal sulcus, between the body and the base of the tongue, are eight to ten vallate (walled) papillae (Fig. 9-39). They do not protrude above the surface of the tongue but are bounded by a deep circular furrow so that their only connection to the substance of the tongue is

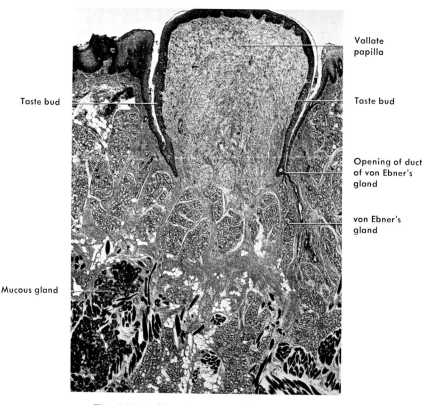

Vallate
papilla

Taste bud

Taste bud

Opening of duct
of von Ebner's
gland

von Ebner's
gland

Mucous gland

**Fig. 9-39.** Vallate (or circumvallate) papilla.

at their narrow base. Their free surface shows numerous secondary papillae that are covered by a thin, smooth epithelium. On the lateral surface of the vallate papillae, the epithelium contains numerous taste buds. The ducts of small serous glands called von Ebner's glands open into the trough. They may serve to wash out the soluble elements of food and are the main source of salivary lipase.

On the lateral border of the posterior parts of the tongue, sharp parallel clefts of varying length can often be observed. They bound narrow folds of the mucous membrane and are the vestige of the large foliate papillae found in many mammals. They contain taste buds.

*Taste buds.* Taste buds are small ovoid or barrel-shaped intraepithelial organs about 80 microns high and 40 microns thick (Fig. 9-40). They extend from the basal lamina to the surface of the epithelium. Their outer surface is almost covered by a few flat epithelial cells, which surround a small opening, the *taste pore* (a taste bud may have more than one taste pore). It leads into a narrow space lined by the supporting cells of the taste bud. The outer supporting cells are arranged like the staves of a barrel. The inner and shorter ones are spindle shaped. Between the latter are arranged ten to twelve neuroepithelial cells, the receptors of taste stimuli. They are slender, dark-staining cells that carry a finger-

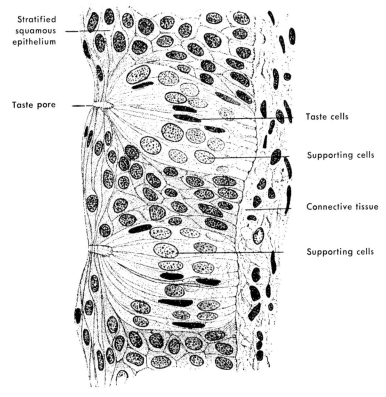

Stratified
squamous
epithelium

Taste pore

Taste cells

Supporting cells

Connective tissue

Supporting cells

**Fig. 9-40.** Taste buds from slope of vallate papilla. (From Schaffer, J.: Lehrbuch der Histologie und Histogenese [Textbook of histology and histogenesis], ed. 2, Leipzig, 1922, Wilhelm Engelmann.)

like processes at their superficial end. The fingerlike processes are visable at the ultrastructural level and resemble hairs at the light microscope level. The hairs reach into the space beneath the taste pore.

A rich plexus of nerves is found below the taste buds. Some fibers enter the epithelium and end in contact with the sensory cells of the taste bud.

Taste buds are numerous on the inner wall of the trough surrounding the vallate papillae, in the folds of the foliate papillae, on the posterior surface of the epiglottis, and on some of the fungiform papillae at the tip and the lateral borders of the tongue (Fig. 9-41).

The classical view maintains that the primary taste sensations, i.e., sweet, salty, bitter, and sour, are perceived in different regions of the tongue and on the palate. Sweet is tasted at the tip and salty at the lateral border of the body of the tongue. Bitter and sour are recognized on the palate but may also be recognized in the posterior part of the tongue, bitter in the middle and sour in the lateral areas. The distribution of the receptors for primary taste qualities can be correlated diagrammatically and somewhat arbitrarily to the different types of papillae. The vallate

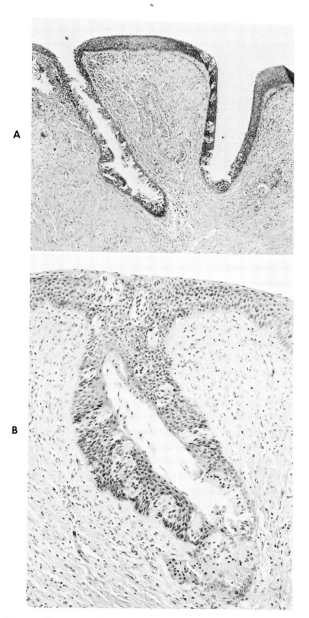

**Fig. 9-41. A,** Circumvallate papilla showing trough and numerous taste buds *(light areas).* **B,** Higher magnification of trough and taste buds. (From Bhaskar, S. N.: Synopsis of oral histology, St. Louis, 1962, The C. V. Mosby Co.)

papillae recognize bitter taste; the foliate papillae recognize sour taste. The taste buds on the fungiform papillae at the tip of the tongue are receptors for sweet taste and those at the borders are for salty taste. Bitter and sour taste sensations are mediated by the glossopharyngeal nerve and sweet and salty taste, by the intermediofacial nerve by the chorda tympani.

On the other hand, many authorities believe that taste cannot be broken down into these four primaries, sweet, sour, salty, and bitter, but that taste consists of a range of stimuli that form a spectrum of sensations making up all taste senses. Taste occurs when a chemical substance contacts a receptor cell in the taste bud. Each taste bud is innervated by many fibers. The reception of a chemical substance fires the nerve. Whether the nerve responds to one stimulus or to differing stimuli has not yet been resolved; so taste may be a continuum or a composite of the primaries.

At the angle of the V-shaped terminal groove on the tongue is located the foramen cecum, which represents the remnant of the thyroglossal duct (Chapter 1). Posterior to the terminal sulcus, the surface of the tongue is irregularly studded with round or oval prominences, the lingual follicles. Each of these shows one or more lymph nodules, sometimes containing a germinal center (Fig. 9-42). Most of these prominences have a small pit at the center, the lingual crypt, which is lined with stratified squamous epithelium. Innumerable lymphocytes migrate into the crypts through the epithelium. Ducts of the small posterior lingual mucous glands open into the crypts. Together the lingual follicles form the lingual tonsil.

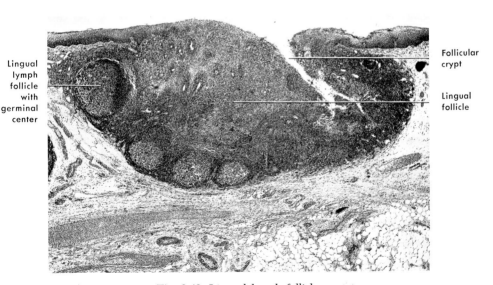

**Fig. 9-42.** Lingual lymph follicle.

## GINGIVAL SULCUS AND DENTOGINGIVAL JUNCTION
### Gingival sulcus

The gingival sulcus or crevice is the name given to the invagination made by the gingiva as it joins with the tooth surface. The gingiva does not join the tooth at the gingival margin. It forms a small infolding known as the *sulcus*. The sulcus extends from the free gingival margin to the dentogingival junction. In health its depth is at the approximate level of the free gingival groove on the outer surface of the gingiva. The sulcus may be responsible for the formation of the groove since it leaves the gingival margin without firm support. The groove is believed to be formed by the functional folding of the free gingival margin during mastication. The sulcular (crevicular) epithelium is nonkeratinized in man. It lacks epithelial ridges and so forms a smooth interface with the lamina propria. It is thinner than the epithelium of the gingiva. The sulcular epithelium is continuous with the gingival epithelium and the attachment epithelium. These three epithelia have a continuous and coextensive basal lamina.

### Dentogingival junction

The junction of the gingiva and the tooth is of great physiologic and clinical importance. This union is unique in many ways and may be a point of lessened resistance to mechanical forces and bacterial attack. The gingiva consists of two tissues in maintaining the junction intact. Their biology differs. The dense, resilient lamina propria takes up impacts produced during mastication. In a similar sense so does the keratinized or parakeratinized surface of the gingiva. When the epithelium is injured, the turnover of cells and their ability to migrate repairs the wound. When the connective tissue is injured, ribosomes within the fibroblasts form molecules of the precursor protein of collagen (procollagen) and ground substances as well, contributing to repair.

Defense against bacterial injury is a function of the defense mechanism of the body. Macrophages, lymphocytes, plasma cells, and white blood cells protect against invasion and form antibodies against bacterial antigens.

Both epithelium and connective tissue are attached to the tooth, and in health each contributes to the integrity of the dentogingival junction. Again, the firmness of this junction is maintained by the gingival division of the periodontal ligament. It is weakened by any situation that causes the collagen to break down (collagenolysis). The adherence of epithelium to the tooth is a function of the attachment (junctional) epithelium. It is weakened by any cause that injures the epithelium.

*Development of junctional (attachment) epithelium.* When the ameloblasts finish formation of the enamel matrix, they leave a thin membrane on the surface of the enamel, the *primary enamel cuticle.* This cuticle may be connected with the interprismatic enamel substance and the ameloblasts. The ameloblasts shorten after the primary enamel cuticle has been formed, and the epithelial

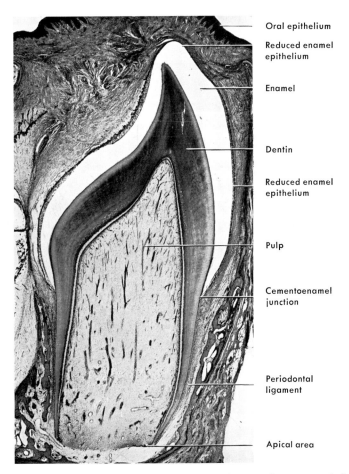

Oral epithelium

Reduced enamel
epithelium

Enamel

Dentin

Reduced enamel
epithelium

Pulp

Cementoenamel
junction

Periodontal
ligament

Apical area

**Fig. 9-43.** Human permanent incisor. Entire surface of enamel is covered by reduced enamel epithelium. Mature enamel is lost by decalcification. (From Gottlieb, B., and Orban, B.: Biology of the investing structures of the teeth. In Gordon, S. M., editor: Dental science and dental art, Philadelphia, 1938, Lea & Febiger.)

enamel organ is reduced to a few layers of flat cuboid cells, which are then called *reduced enamel epithelium*. Under normal conditions it covers the entire enamel surface, extending to the cementoenamel junction (Fig. 9-43), and remains attached to the primary enamel cuticle. During eruption, the tip of the tooth approaches the oral mucosa, and the reduced enamel epithelium and the oral epithelium meet and fuse (Fig. 9-44). The remnant of the primary enamel cuticle after eruption is referred to as Nasmyth's membrane.

The epithelium that covers the tip of the crown degenerates in its center, and the crown emerges through this perforation into the oral cavity (Fig. 9-45). The reduced enamel epithelium remains organically attached to the part of the enamel that has not yet erupted. Once the tip of the crown has emerged, the

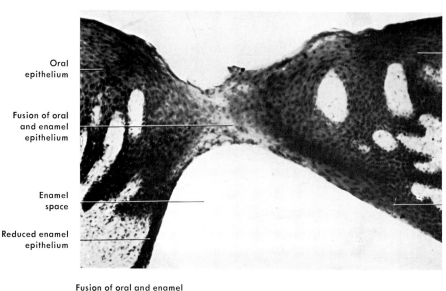

Oral epithelium

Fusion of oral and enamel epithelium

Enamel space

Reduced enamel epithelium

Oral epithelium

Reduced enamel epithelium

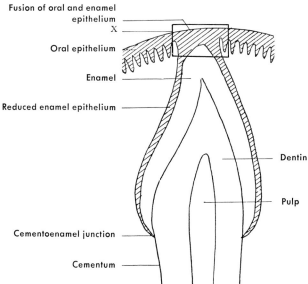

Fusion of oral and enamel epithelium
X

Oral epithelium

Enamel

Reduced enamel epithelium

Dentin

Pulp

Cementoenamel junction

Cementum

**Fig. 9-44.** Reduced enamel epithelium fuses with oral epithelium. x in diagram indicates area from which photomicrograph was taken.

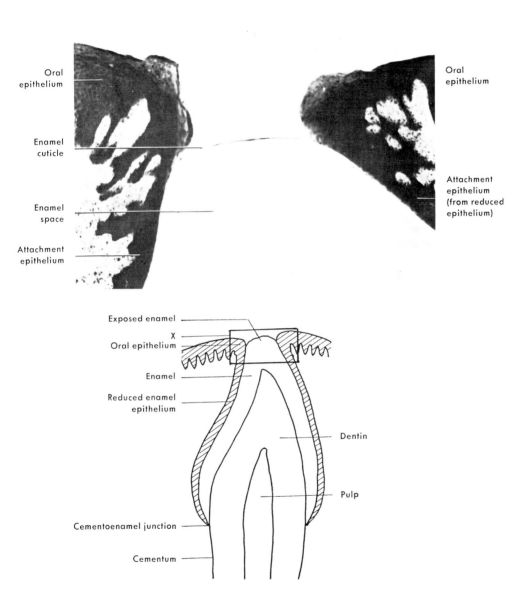

**Fig. 9-45.** Tooth emerges through a perforation in fused epithelia. X in diagram indicates area from which photomicrograph was taken.

reduced enamel epithelium is termed the primary *attachment epithelium*.* At the margin of the gingiva the attachment epithelium is continuous with the oral epithelium (Fig. 9-46). As the tooth erupts, the reduced enamel epithelium grows gradually shorter. The shallow groove that develops between the gingiva and the surface of the tooth and extends around its circumference is the *gingival sulcus* (Fig. 9-46). It is continuous with the attachment epithelium on one side and by the gingival margin on the other side. The part of the gingiva encompassing the sulcus and the equivalent amount of outer gingival surface is the free or *marginal gingiva*.

Although the firmness and mechanical strength of the dentogingival junction is mainly attributable to the connective tissue attachment, the attachment of the epithelium to the enamel is by no means loose or weak. This can be demonstrated with ground histologic sections of frozen specimens where enamel and soft tissues

*Some confusion may result if the student refers to the older literature in which the attachment epithelium is referred to as the epithelial attachment. It was first named the epithelial attachment (*Epithelansatz*) by Gottlieb, but after it was examined electron microscopically it was renamed the junctional or attachment epithelium by Stern. This epithelium synthesizes the material that attaches it to the tooth. This material, its morphology, mode, and mechanism of function, is what is now called the epithelial attachment. Thus the cellular structure is referred to as junctional or attachment epithelium and its extracellular tooth-attaching substance is referred to as the epithelial attachment.

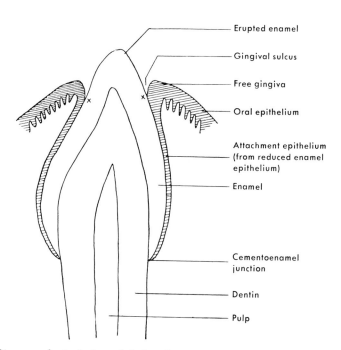

**Fig. 9-46.** Diagram of attached epithelial cuff and gingival sulcus at an early stage of tooth eruption. Bottom of the sulcus at X.

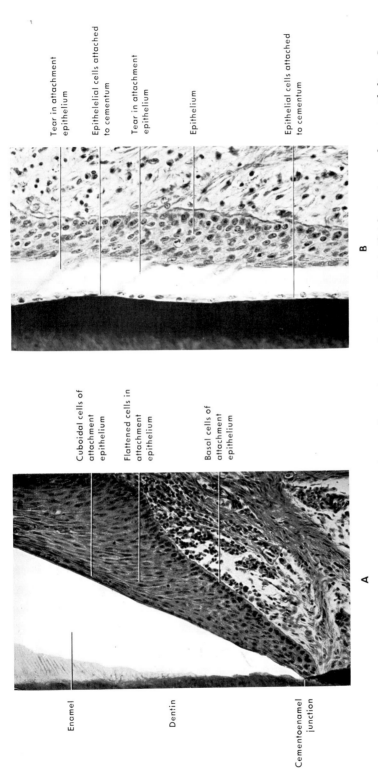

**Fig. 9-47.** *A*, Arrangement of cells in attachment epithelium indicates functional influences. *B*, Artificial tear in attachment epithelium. Some cells remain attached to cementum, while others bridge the tear. (*A* from Orban, B.: J. Am. Dent. Assoc. **16**:1206, 1929.)

Labels for A:
Enamel
Dentin
Cementoenamel junction
Cuboidal cells of attachment epithelium
Flattened cells in attachment epithelium
Basal cells of attachment epithelium

Labels for B:
Tear in attachment epithelium
Epithelelial cells attached to cementum
Tear in attachment epithelium
Epithelium
Epithelial cells attached to cementum

are retained in their normal relation. When an attempt is made to detach the gingiva from the tooth in these preparations, the epithelium tears, but does not peel off from the enamel surface (Fig. 9-47). Similar results are obtained surgically when gingival flaps are pulled away from teeth.

**Shift of dentogingival junction.** The position of the gingiva on the surface of the tooth changes with time. When the tip of the enamel first emerges through the mucous membrane of the oral cavity, the epithelium covers almost the entire enamel (Fig. 9-48). The tooth erupts until it reaches the plane of occlusion (Chapter 11). The attachment epithelium separates from the enamel surface gradually while the crown emerges into the oral cavity. When the tooth first reaches the plane of occlusion, one third to one fourth of the enamel still remains covered by the gingiva (Fig. 9-49). A gradual exposure of the crown follows. The actual movement of the teeth toward the occlusal plane is termed *active eruption.* This applies to the preclinical phase of eruption also. The separation of the primary attachment epithelium from the enamel is termed *passive eruption.*

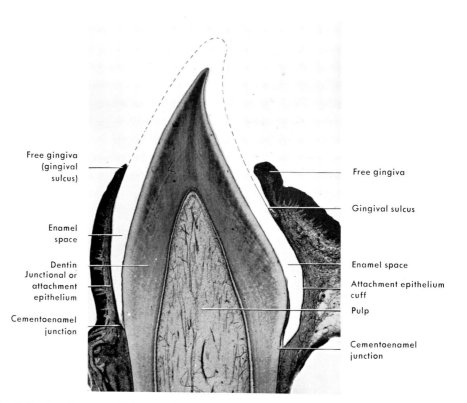

Free gingiva (gingival sulcus)

Enamel space

Dentin
Junctional or attachment epithelium

Cementoenamel junction

Free gingiva

Gingival sulcus

Enamel space

Attachment epithelium cuff

Pulp

Cementoenamel junction

**Fig. 9-48.** Attachment epithelium and gingival sulcus in erupting tooth. *Dotted line,* Erupted part of enamel. Enamel is lost in decalcification. (From Kronfeld, R.: J. Am. Dent. Assoc. **18:**382, 1936.)

Further recession exposing the cementum may ultimately occur. At that stage the reduced enamel epithelium has disappeared and the primary attachment epithelium is replaced by a *secondary attachment epithelium* derived from the gingival epithelium.

There is a conceptual construct, called passive exposure, that may be useful in describing the various levels of attachment that may occur as the gingiva recedes onto the cementum. Some people believe passive eruption to be a normal occurrence with aging. The belief that this is a "normal" occurrence may not be correct. Crown exposure involving passive eruption and further recession is a continuous occurrence and has been described in four stages. The first two may be physiologic. Many conceive of the last two as normal also, but there is a strong possibility that they are pathologic.

*First stage.* The bottom of the gingival sulcus remains in the region of the enamel-covered crown for some time, and the apical end of the attachment epithelium (reduced enamel epithelium) stays at the cementoenamel junction

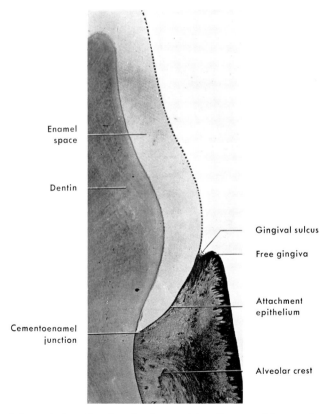

**Fig. 9-49.** Tooth in occlusion. One fourth of enamel is still covered by attachment epithelium. (From Kronfeld, R.: J. Am. Dent. Assoc. **18**:382, 1936.)

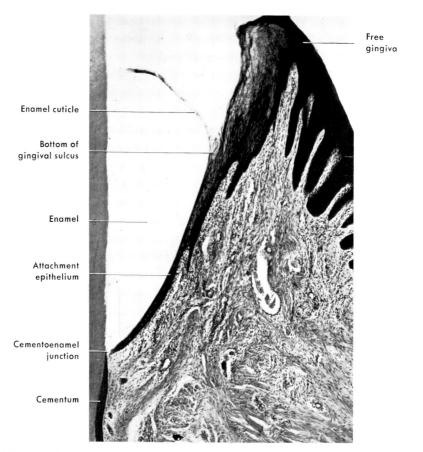

Fig. 9-50. Attachment epithelium on enamel. First stage of crown exposure. (From Gottlieb, B., and Orban, B.: Biology and pathology of the tooth [translated by M. Diamond], New York, 1938, The Macmillan Co.)

(Fig. 9-50). This relation persists in primary teeth almost up to 1 year of age before shedding and, in permanent teeth, usually to the age of 20 or 30 years. However, this relation is subject to a wide range of variation (Fig. 9-51).

*Second stage.* The bottom of the gingival sulcus is still on the enamel and the apical end of the attachment epithelium has shifted to the surface of the cementum (Fig. 9-52).

The downgrowth of the attachment epithelial along the cementum is but one facet of the shift of the dentogingival junction. This entails dissolution of fiber bundles that were anchored in the cervical parts of the cementum, now covered by the epithelium, and an apical shift of the gingival and transseptal fibers. It may be that destruction of the fibers is caused by enzymes formed by the epithelial cells. It may be that the step is a manifestation of periodontal disease. This stage of tooth exposure may persist to the age of 40 years or later.

*Third stage.* When the bottom of the gingival sulcus is at the cementoenamel

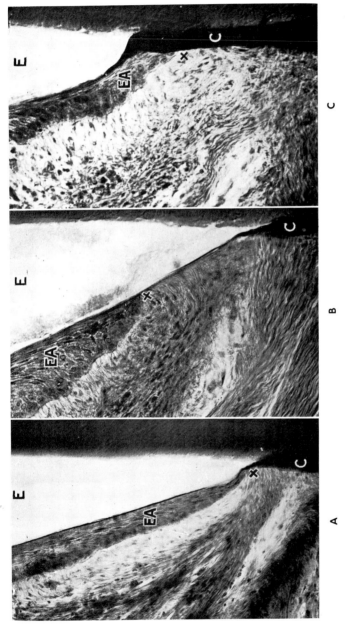

**Fig. 9-51.** Three sections of same tooth showing different relations of tissues at cementoenamel junction. **A,** Attachment epithelium reaching to cementoenamel junction. **B,** Attachment epithelium ends coronally to cementoenamel junction. **C,** Attachment epithelium covers part of cementum. Cementum overlaps edge of enamel. *C,* Cementum; *E,* enamel (lost in decalcification); *EA,* attachment epithelium; *x,* end of attachment epithelium. (From Orban, B.: J. Am. Dent. Assoc. **17:**1977, 1930.)

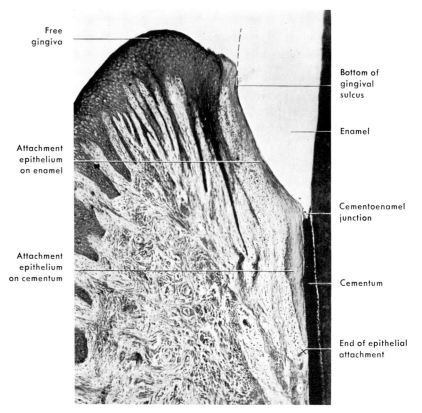

Free
gingiva

Bottom of
gingival
sulcus

Enamel

Attachment
epithelium
on enamel

Cementoenamel
junction

Attachment
epithelium
on cementum

Cementum

End of epithelial
attachment

**Fig. 9-52.** Attachment epithelium partly on enamel and partly on cementum. Second stage of passive tooth exposure. (From Gottlieb, B., and Orban, B.: Biology and pathology of the tooth [translated by M. Diamond], New York, 1938, The Macmillan Co.)

junction, the epithelium attachment is entirely on the cementum, and the enamel-covered crown is fully exposed (Fig. 9-53). This stage in the exposure of a tooth no longer is a passive manifestation. The epithelium shifts gradually along the surface of the tooth and does not remain at the cementoenamel junction. This more or less continuous, but slow, process is regarded as the body's attempt to maintain an intact dentogingival junction in the face of factors that cause its deterioration.

*Fourth stage.* This stage represents recession of the gingiva. When the entire attachment is on cementum, the gingiva may appear normal but the process is regarded as pathologic (Figs. 9-54 and 9-55). It may occur without perceptible evidence of inflammatory periodontal disease.

The rates of crown exposure and recession vary in different persons. In some cases the fourth stage is observed in persons during their twenties. In others, even at 50 years of age or older the teeth are still in the first or second stage. The rate varies also in different teeth of the same jaw and on different surfaces

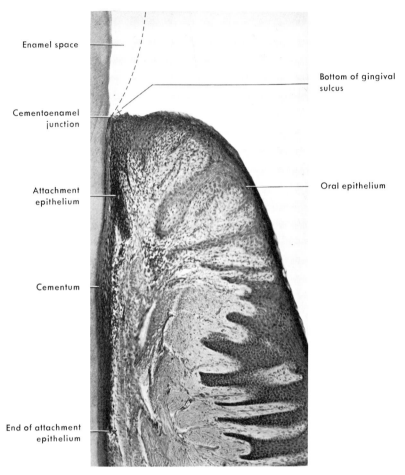

Enamel space

Bottom of gingival sulcus

Cementoenamel junction

Attachment epithelium

Oral epithelium

Cementum

End of attachment epithelium

**Fig. 9-53.** Recession is at bottom of gingival sulcus at cementoenamel junction, and attachment epithelium is on cementum. (From Gottlieb, B.: J. Am. Dent. Assoc. **14**:2178, 1972.)

of the same tooth. One side may be in the first stage and the other in the second or even the fourth stage (Fig. 9-55).

Gradual exposure of the tooth makes it necessary to distinguish between the anatomic and the clinical crowns of the tooth (Fig. 9-56). That part of the tooth covered by enamel is the anatomic crown. The clinical crown is the part of the tooth exposed in the oral cavity. In the first and second stages the clinical crown is smaller than the anatomic crown. With recession (third stage) the entire enamel-covered part of the tooth is exposed, and the clinical crown is equal to the anatomic crown. Later the clinical crown is larger than the anatomic crown because parts of the root have been exposed (fourth stage). This type of crown exposure is to be differentiated from crown exposure that is produced by pocket formation.

***Sulcus and cuticles.*** For a long time the epithelium was believed only to contact

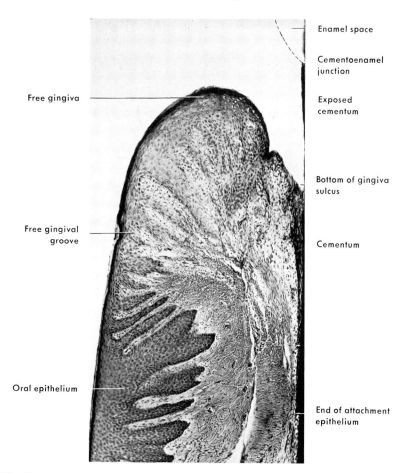

Free gingiva

Enamel space

Cementoenamel junction

Exposed cementum

Bottom of gingiva sulcus

Free gingival groove

Cementum

Oral epithelium

End of attachment epithelium

**Fig. 9-54.** Recession. Bottom of gingival sulcus and attachment epithelium both on the cementum. Continued recession reduces the width of the gingiva. (From Gottlieb, B.: J. Am. Dent. Assoc. 14:2178, 1927.)

but not attach to the enamel. The contact was supposed to be maintained by the turgor of the connective tissue elements of the gingiva. Thus a capillary space was supposed to exist between the gingiva and enamel to the cementoenamel junction. Gottlieb and Orban demonstrated the presence of an organic attachment, which they termed the epithelial attachment. The mode or mechanism of the epithelial attachment is very important. The classical view proposed by Gottlieb and Orban involves the primary cuticle mediating an organic union between ameloblasts and the enamel. When the ameloblasts are replaced by the oral epithelium, a secondary cuticle is formed. When the epithelium proliferates beyond the cementoenamel junction, the cuticle extends along the cementum (Figs. 9-57 and 9-58). Secondary enamel cuticle and the cemental cuticle are referred to as dental cuticle. These cuticles are microscopically evident as an amorphous material between the attachment epithelium and the tooth.

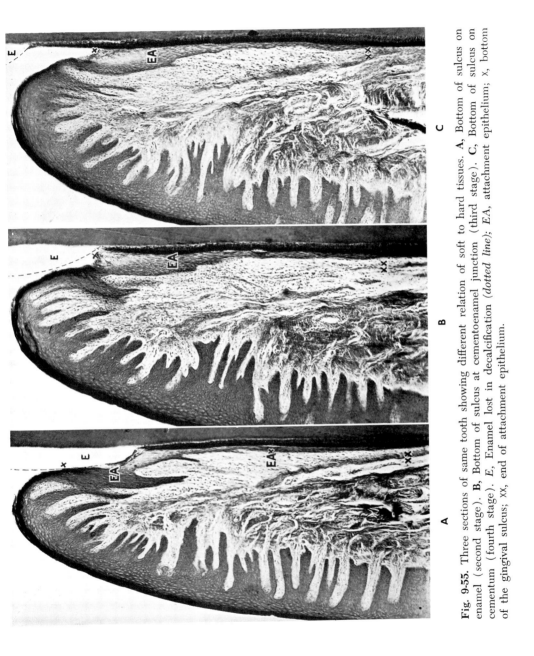

**Fig. 9-55.** Three sections of same tooth showing different relation of soft to hard tissues. **A,** Bottom of sulcus on enamel (second stage). **B,** Bottom of sulcus at cementoenamel junction (third stage). **C,** Bottom of sulcus on cementum (fourth stage). *E,* Enamel lost in decalcification (*dotted line*); *EA,* attachment epithelium; x, bottom of the gingival sulcus; XX, end of attachment epithelium.

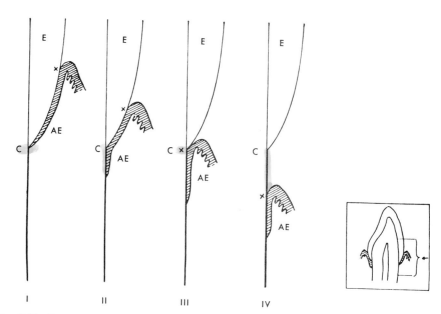

**Fig. 9-56.** Diagram of the four stages in eruption. In stages I and II (passive eruption), anatomic crown is larger than clinical crown. III and IV represent recession. In stage III, anatomic and clinical crowns are equal. In stage IV, clinical crown is larger than anatomic crown. *Arrow* in small diagram indicates area from which the drawings were made. *C*, Cementoenamel junction; *E*, enamel; *AE*, attachment epithelium; x, bottom of gingival sulcus.

***Deepening of sulcus (pocket formation).*** The gingival sulcus forms when the tip of the crown emerges through the oral mucosa. It deepens as a result of separation of the reduced dental epithelium from the actively erupting tooth. At first after the tip of the crown has appeared in the oral cavity the epithelium separates rapidly from the surface of the tooth. Later, when the tooth comes to occlude with its antagonist, the separation of the attachment from the surface of the tooth slows down.

The formation and relative depth of the gingival sulcus at different ages is still a controversial subject. At one time, it was believed that from the time the tip of the crown had pierced the oral mucosa the gingival sulcus extended to the cementoenamel junction (Fig. 9-59, I). It was assumed that the attachment of the gingival epithelium to the tooth occurred only at the cementoenamel junction. The concept of an epithelial attachment introduced by Gottlieb and Orban showed that no cleft existed between epithelium and enamel and that these tissues were organically connected. The gingival sulcus was shown to be a shallow groove, the bottom of which is at the point of separation of attached epithelium from the tooth (Fig. 9-59, II).

Some investigators contended that the deepening of the gingival sulcus was caused by a tear in the attached epithelium (Fig. 9-59, III). Others believed, however, deepening occurred as a result of the downgrowth of the oral epithe-

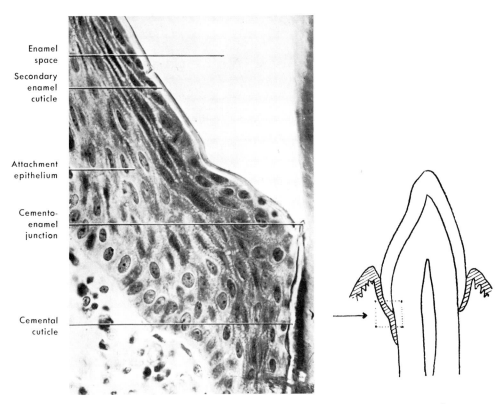

Enamel
space

Secondary
enamel
cuticle

Attachment
epithelium

Cemento-
enamel
junction

Cemental
cuticle

**Fig. 9-57.** "Secondary enamel cuticle" follows the attachment epithelium to cementum forming the dental cuticle. *Arrow* in the diagram indicates area from which photomicrograph was taken.

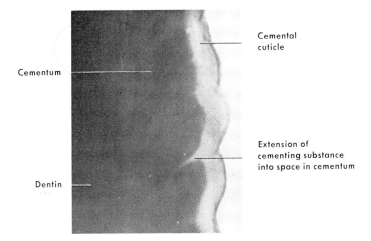

Cemental
cuticle

Cementum

Extension of
cementing substance
into space in cementum

Dentin

**Fig. 9-58.** Cemental cuticle extending into cementum. (From Gottlieb, B., and Orban, B.: Biology and pathology of the tooth [translated by M. Diamond], New York, 1938, The Macmillan Co.)

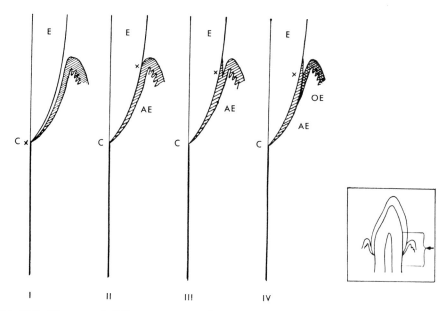

**Fig. 9-59.** Diagram of different views on formation of gingival sulcus as discussed in text. *Arrow* in small diagram indicates area from which drawings were made.

lium alongside the reduced enamel epithelium (primary attachment epithelium), as shown in Fig. 9-59, IV.

What the depth of a normal gingival sulcus should be has been a frequent source of argument. Under normal conditions the depth of the sulcus is variable; 45% of all measured sulci are below 0.5 mm. The average sulcus is 1.8 mm. The more shallow a sulcus, the more likely that the gingival margin is not inflamed.

Lymphocytes and plasma cells are routinely seen in the connective tissue at the bottom of the gingival sulcus and below the attachment epithelium. This is a defense reaction to the bacteria in the gingival sulcus and constitutes a barrier against the invasion of bacteria and the penetration of toxins. Whether there is a direct or indirect effect of the bacterial products is now under active investigation.

*Epithelial attachment.* In the past decade the ultrastructural attachment of the ameloblasts (primary attachment epithelium) to the tooth was first shown by Stern and confirmed by Listgarten and Schroeder, among others, to be basal lamina to which hemidesmosomes are attached (Fig. 9-6, *A*). This mode of attachment is referred to as the *epithelial attachment.* The secondary attachment epithelium composed of cells derived from the oral epithelium forms an epithelial attachment identical with that of the primary attachment epithelium, i.e., a basal lamina and hemidesmosomes. Both reduced ameloblasts and gingival epithelial cells have been shown to form an electron-microscopic basal lamina on enamel and cementum. Hemidesmosomes of these cells attach to the basal lamina in the

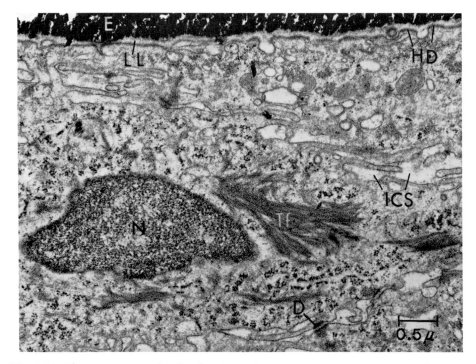

**Fig. 9-60.** Electron micrograph of cells of attachment epithelium of rat incisor adjacent to enamel, *E*. Hemidesmosomes, *HD*, abut on and attach to lamina lucida, *LL*. Lamina densa is fully calcified and cannot be demonstrated in this calcified specimen. Lamina lucida is approximately 400 Å wide. Note that intercellular space, *ICS*, is wider than lamina lucida. Cells are attached to each other by desmosomes, *D. N*, Nucleus; *Tf*, a bundle of tonofilaments. (From Grant, D. A., Stern, I. B., and Everett, F. G.: Orban's periodontics, ed. 4, St. Louis, 1972, The C. V. Mosby Co.)

same manner as all basal cells. Thus there is an epithelial attachment. It is submicroscopic, approximately 400 Å wide, and formed by the attachment epithelium. Its exact biochemical nature is unknown, but some of its constituents have been grossly identified. Apparently these constituents are produced by the epithelium. The adhesive forces in this zone are molecular in nature and act across a distance smaller than 400 Å.

*Migration of attachment epithelium.* The epithelial attachment resembles an electron-microscopic basal lamina. The cells of the attachment epithelium are held to this structure by hemidesmosomes (Fig. 9-60).

Can it be that the cells adjacent to the tooth are basal cells? Mitotic figures have been observed in such cells. When tritiated thymidine is administered to experimental animals, those cells about to undergo DNA synthesis pick up radioactive thymidine. The radioactivity can be detected in histologic sections by the use of photographic emulsion. After the administration of the tritiated thymidine, labeled cells are found in the attachment epithelium.

When cells leave the stratum germinativum, they become specialized and no longer divide. For instance, in oral epithelium, cells specialize to form keratin. In attachment epithelium, the cells specialize and synthesize the epithelial attachment. They then migrate over it, with their attachment being maintained by the hemidesmosomes.

The time it takes for labeled attachment epithelial cells to migrate and

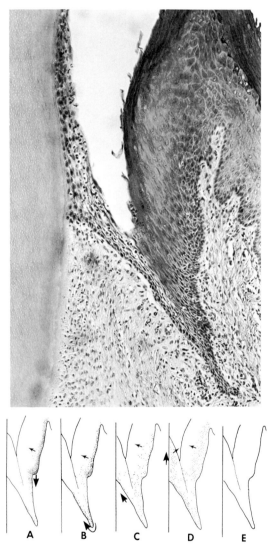

**Fig. 9-61.** Composite of labeled cells and their positions, **A,** ½ hour; **B,** 6 hours; **C,** 24 hours; **D,** 72 hours; and **E,** 144 hours after administration of tritiated thymidine to rats. Diagram of the morphology of attachment epithelium and adjacent tissues is representative of gingiva on cemental (oral) surface of the continuously growing rat incisor. *Large arrows,* Migration of attachment (junctional) epithelium toward and along tooth surface. *Small arrows,* Migration of cells toward sulcus. (From Anderson, G. C., and Stern, I. B.: Periodontics 4:115, 1966.)

desquamate is called transit time. It is less than 144 hours for the continuously growing incisor of rodents (Fig. 9-61), in the vicinity of 72 to 120 hours for primates, and presumably much the same for man.

How can the cells be attached to the tooth if they are actively migrating? The same mechanism is present at the epidermis–connective tissue junction. The

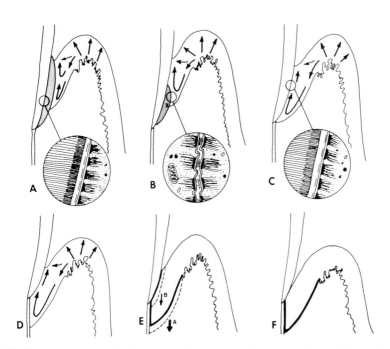

**Fig. 9-62.** Current concept of dynamics of migration of junctional epithelium. **A,** Primary junctional epithelium consists of reduced ameloblasts attached by hemidesmosomes to the lamina lucida, an electron microscopic structure. The gingival epithelial cells migrate either to the gingival surface and keratinize or (*arrows*) toward the reduced enamel epithelium, to which they attach. **B,** Primary junctional epithelium gradually degenerates and is replaced by the secondary junctional epithelium. Cells of the two tissues are joined by desmosomes and by tight junctions. At the point of fusion of the two tissues, x, mitotic activity is increased. Here the cells of the outer enamel epithelium and possibly the stratum intermedium join the cells of the gingival epithelium in forming a locus of proliferation. **C,** With the complete degeneration of the primary attachment epithelium, the secondary attachment epithelium contacts the enamel and attachs by the same mechanism as shown in **A. D,** In time, the secondary junctional epithelium may be found attaching to both the enamel and the cementum. How did this apical migration occur? **E,** Secondary junctional epithelium renews itself in a matter of days, as does the gingival epithelium. Cells migrate in the pathways denoted by the *arrows* in **D.** The cells of the junctional epithelium travel along the electron microscopic basal lamina lucida–lamina densa complex, which forms the epithelial attachment (*heavy line*). When the basal cells at **A** migrate apically, they form a new attachment. Junctional cells at **B** may also migrate apically, with either the resultant deepening of the sulcus or the processive exposure of the clinical crown (recession). **F,** When the junctional epithelium has completely migrated into the cementum, the attachment is mediated by the lamina lucida and by hemidesmosomes, as it was on the enamel. (From Grant, D. A., Stern, I. B., and Everett, F. G.: *Orban's periodontics*, ed. 4, St. Louis, 1972, The C. V. Mosby Co.)

epithelial cells are affixed to the connective tissue through the basal lamina, yet they can detach from it and migrate toward the surface. Similarly in healing wounds the epithelial cells form a basal lamina on the connective tissue and migrate over it to epithelize the wound. At no time is the epithelium loose from the connective tissue. The two issues are in intimate connection. Picture the epithelial attachment as the basal lamina of the attachment (junctional) epithelium. It turns about the most apical cell and extends up along the tooth surface. The cells can then migrate along this basement membrane (Fig. 9-61). The hemidesmosomes hold the cells to this structure so that the strength of the attachment is not diminished despite the migration. The physical integrity of the attachment is maintained during the four stages of tooth exposure by this same biologic mechanism.

The reduced ameloblasts do not divide; on the other hand, basal cells adjacent to the tooth do divide and then migrate up and along the tooth, desquamating in 4 to 6 days. They seem to migrate from a locus of proliferation in the basal layer at the junction of the oral and the attachment epithelia. While the reduced ameloblasts are still present, the cells of the oral epithelium join them by forming desmosomes. Gradually the reduced enamel epithelium is lost and the cells of the oral epithelium contact the tooth surface, there forming hemidesmosomes and a lamina lucida, by means of which the cells attach themselves to the tooth. The apical migration of the sulcus is the result of a detachment of basal cells and a reestablishment of their epithelial attachment at a more apical level. It is not the result of a degeneration and peeling off of the most coronal cells of the attachment epithelium. The mechanism of sulcus deepening by the deepening of splits and so forth (Fig. 9-61) is not accurate, since the attachment is formed by the more deeply located basal cells (Fig. 9-62). Perhaps toxic or inflammatory influences diminish the ability of the basal cells to synthesize DNA or otherwise interfere with the physiology of these cells. Perhaps collagenolysis destroys the subjacent collagen fibers, permitting the epithelium to migrate apically. Perhaps immunologically competent cells or antibody complexes produce tissue damage and permit the epithelium to migrate apically. In any event the junctional epithelium moves apically and reestablishes the epithelial attachment. If this results in a deepening of the sulcus, as gauged by a difference in the position of the top of the epithelial attachment relative to the marginal gingiva, a pocket will have formed.

## CLINICAL CONSIDERATIONS

It is essential to be thoroughly familiar with the structure and biologic interrelations of the various periodontal tissues in order to understand the pathogenesis of periodontal disease. Periodontal disturbances have their origin in the region of the gingival sulcus with the formation of a deepened gingival pocket, which results in response to plaque toxins. Reduction in pocket depth is the primary objective of treatment. Treatment methods should be judged by their ability to accomplish this end.

The level of the gingival attachment to the tooth plays an important role in restorative dentistry. In young persons the clinical crown is smaller than the anatomic crown. It is therefore very difficult to prepare a tooth properly for an abutment or crown in young individuals. Moreover, when recession occurs at a later time, the restoration may require replacement.

When the root is exposed by recession and a restoration is to be placed, the preparation need not extend to the gingiva. The first requirement is that the restoration be adapted to mechanical needs. In extension of the gingival margin of any restoration the following rules should be observed. If the gingiva is still on the enamel and the gingival papilla fills the entire interdental space, the gingival margin of a cavity should be placed in the sulcus or below the marginal gingiva. Special care should be taken to avoid injury to the gingiva and the dentogingival junction and to prevent premature recession of the gingiva. When periodontal disease is present, treatment should precede the placing of a restoration. If the gingiva has receded to the cementum and the gingival papilla does not fill the interdental space, the margin of a cavity need not necessarily be carried below the free margin of the gingiva.

With gingival recession and exposure of the cervical part of the anatomic root, cemental caries or abrasion may occur. Improperly constructed clasps, overzealous scaling, and strongly abrasive dentrifrices may result in pronounced abrasion. After loss of the cementum, the dentin may be extremely sensitive to thermal or chemical stimuli. Desensitizing drugs, judiciously applied, may be used to accelerate sclerosis of the tubules and reparative dentin formation.

The difference in the structure of the submucosa in various regions of the oral cavity is of great clinical importance. Whenever the submucosa consists of a layer of loose connective tissue, edema or hemorrhage can cause much swelling, and infection can spread speedily and extensively. As a rule, inflammatory infiltrations in such parts are not very painful. If possible, injections should be made into loose submucous connective tissue (i.e., the fornix and the alveolar mucosa). The only place in the palate where larger amounts of fluid can be injected without damaging the tissues is the loose connective tissue in the furrow between the palatal and the alveolar processes (Fig. 9-21).

The gingiva is exposed to heavy mechanical stresses during mastication. Moreover, the epithelial attachment to the tooth is relatively weak, and injuries or infections can cause permanent damage. Keratinization of the gingiva may afford relative protection. Therefore steps taken to increase keratinization can be considered preventive measures. One of the methods of inducing keratinization is mechanical stimulation such as massage or brushing.

Unfavorable mechanical irritation of the gingiva may ensue from sharp edges of carious cavities, overhanging fillings or crowns, and accumulation of plaque calculus. These may cause chronic inflammation of the gingival tissue.

Many systemic diseases cause characteristic changes in the oral mucosa. For instance, metal poisoning (lead, bismuth) causes characteristic discoloration of the gingival margin. Leukemia, pernicious anemia, and other blood dyscrasias can be diagnosed by characteristic infiltrations of the oral mucosa. In the first stages of measles, small red spots with bluish white centers can be seen in the mucous membrane of the cheeks, even before the skin rash appears. They are known as Koplik's spots. Endocrine disturbances, including those of the sex hormones and of the pancreas, may be reflected in the oral mucosa.

Changes of the tongue are sometimes diagnostically significant. In scarlet fever the atrophy of the lingual mucosa causes the peculiar redness of the straw-berry tongue. Systemic diseases such as pernicious anemia and vitamin deficiencies, especially vitamin B-complex deficiency, lead to characteristic changes, such as magenta tongue and beefy red tongue.

In denture construction it is important to observe the firmness or looseness of the mucous membrane. In denture-bearing areas the mucosa should be firm.

In old age the mucous membrane of the mouth may atrophy. It is then thin and parchmentlike. The atrophy of the lingual papillae leaves the upper surface of the tongue smooth, shiny, and varnished in appearance. Atrophy of the major and minor salivary glands may lead to xerostomia (dry mouth) and sometimes to a secondary atrophy of the mucous membrane. In a large percentage of individuals the sebaceous glands of the cheek are visible as fairly large, yellowish patches called Fordyce's spots. They do not represent a pathologic change (Fig. 9-33).

### REFERENCES

Adams, D.: Surface coatings of cells in the oral epithelium of the human fetus, J. Anat. **118**:61, 1974.

Ainamo, J., and Löe, H.: Anatomical characteristics of gingiva. A clinical and microscopic study of the free and attached gingiva, J. Periodontol. **37**:5, 1966.

Anderson, G. S., and Stern, I. B.: The proliferation and migration of the attachment epithelium on the cemental surface of the rat incisor, Periodontics **4**:115, 1966.

Barker, D. S.: The dendritic cell system in human gingival epithelium, Arch. Oral Biol. **12**:203, 1967.

Barnett, M. L., and Szabó, G.: Gap junctions in human gingival keratinized epithelium, J. Periodont. Res. **8**:117, 1973.

Barnett, M. L.: Mast cells in the epithelial layer of human gingiva, J. Ultrastructure Res. **43**:247, 1973.

Baume, L. J.: The structure of the epithelial attachment revealed by phase contrast microscopy, J. Periodontol. **24**:99, 1953.

Beagrie, G. S., and Skougaard, M. R.: Observations in the life cycle of the gingival epithelial cells of mice as revealed by autoradiography, Acta Odontol. Scand. **20**:15, 1962.

Beidler, L. N., and Smallman, R. L. S.: Renewal of cells within taste buds, J. Cell Biol. **27**:263, 1965.

Bolden, T. E.: Histology of oral pigmentation, J. Periodontol. **31**:361, 1960.

Bradley, R. M., and Stern, I. B.: The development of the human taste bud during the foetal period, J. Anat. [London] **101**:743, 1967.

Bradley, R. M., and Mistretta, C. M.: The morphological and functional development of fetal gustatory receptors. In Emmelin, N., and Zotterman, Y., editors: Oral physiology, Oxford, 1972, Pergamon Press, Ltd., pp. 239-253.

Buck, D.: The uptake of $H^3$ proline in the guinea pig gingiva and palate, J. Periodontol. **4**:94, 1969.

Cleaton-Jones, P., and Fleisch, L.: A comparative study of the surface of keratinized and non-keratinized oral epithelia, J. Periodont. Res. **8**:366, 1973.

Dale, B. A., and Stern, I. B.: SDS polyacrylamide electrophoresis of proteins of newborn rat skin. I. Cell strata and nuclear proteins, J. Invest. Dermatol. **65**:220, August 1975.

Dale, B. A., and Stern, I. B.: SDS polyacrylamide electrophoresis of proteins of newborn rat skin. II. Keratohyalin and stratum corneum proteins. J. Invest. Dermatol. **65:**223, August 1975.

DeHan, R., and Graziadei, P. P. C.: Functional anatomy of frog's taste organs, Experientia **27:**823, 1971.

Egelberg, J.: The blood vessels of the dento-gingival junction, J. Periodont. Res. **1:**163, 1966.

El-Labban, N. G., and Kramer, I. R. H.: On the so-called microgranules in the non-keratinized buccal epithelium, J. Ultrastruct. Res. **48:**377, 1974.

Emslie, R. D., and Weinmann, J. P.: The architectural pattern of the boundary between epithelium and connective tissue of the gingiva in the rhesus monkey, Anat. Rec. **105:**35, 1949.

Farbman, A. I.: Electron microscope study of a small cytoplasmic structure in rat oral epithelium, J. Cell Biol. **21:**491-495, 1964.

Farbman, A. I.: Electron microscope study of the developing taste bud in rat fungiform papillae, Dev. Biol. **11:**110, 1965.

Farbman, A. I.: Plasma membrane changes during keratinization, Anat. Rec. **156:**269-282, 1966.

Farbman, A. I.: Structure of chemoreceptors. In Symposium on foods. Chemistry and Physiology of Flavors, Westport, Conn., 1967, Avi Publishing Co., pp. 25-51.

Frank, R. M., and Cimasoni, G.: Electron microscopic study of the human epithelial attachment, J. Dent. Res. **49:**691, 1970.

Frank, R. M., and Cimasoni, G.: Ultrastructure de l'épithélium cliniquement normal du sillon et de la jonction gingivo-dentaires, Z. Zellforsch. Mikrosk. Anat. **109:**356, 1970.

Frithiof, L.: Ultrastructural changes in the plasma membrane in human oral epithelium, J. Ultrastruct. Res. **32:**1, 1970.

Frithiof, L., and Wersall, J.: A highly ordered structure in keratinizing human oral epithelium, J. Ultrastruct. Res. **12:**371-379, 1965.

Gavin, J. B.: The ultrastructure of the crevicular epithelium of cat gingiva, Am. J. Anat. **123:**283, 1968.

Geisenheimer, J., and Han, S. S.: A quantitative electron microscopic study of desmosomes and hemidesmosomes in human crevicular epithelium, J. Periodontal. **42:**396, 1971.

Gottlieb, B.: Der Epithelansatz am Zähne, Dtsch. Monatsschr. Zahnheilkd. **39:**142, 1921.

Gottlieb, B.: Zur Biologie des Epithelansatzes und des Alveolarrandes, Dtsch. Zahnaerztl. Wochenschr. **25:**434, 1922.

Gottlieb, B., and Orban, B.: Biology and pathology of the tooth (translated by M. Diamond), New York, 1938, The Macmillan Co.

Grant, D. A., and Orban, B.: Leukocytes in the epithelial attachment, J. Periodontol. **31:**87, 1960.

Grant, D. A., Stern, I. B., and Everett, F. G.: Orban's periodontics, ed. 4, St. Louis, 1972, The C. V. Mosby Co.

Haim, G.: Elektronenmikroskopische Untersuchungen des normalen Epithels der Menschlichen Mundschleimhaut, Munich, 1964, Carl Hanser Verlag.

Hamilton, A. I., and Blackwood, H. J. J.: Cell renewal of oral mucosal epithelium of the rat, J. Anat. **117:**313, 1974.

Hansen, E. R.: Mitotic activity of the gingival epithelium in colchicinized rats, Odontol. T. **74:**229, 1966.

Hashimoto, K., Dibella, R. J., and Shklar, G.: Electron microscopic studies of the normal human buccal mucosa, J. Invest. Dermatol. **47:**512, 1966.

Hayward, A. F., Hamilton, A. I., and Hackemann, M. M.: Histological and ultrastructural observations on the keratinizing epithelia of the palate of the rat, Arch. Oral Biol. **18:**1041, 1973.

Hayward, A. F., and Hackemann, M. M.: Electron microscopy of membrane-coating granules and a cell surface coat in keratinized and nonkeratinized human oral epithelium, J. Ultrastruct. Res. **43:**205, 1973.

Huang, L. Y., Stern, I. B., Clagett, J. A., and Chi, E. Y.: Two polypeptide chain constituents of the major protein of the cornified layer of newborn rat epidermis, Biochemistry **14:**3573, 1975.

Ito, H., Enomoto, S., and Kobayashi, K.: Electron microscopic study of the human epithelial attachment, Bull. Tokyo Med. Dent. Univ. **14:**267, 1967.

Karring, T., and Löe, H.: The three dimensional concept of the epithelium-connective tissue boundary of gingiva, Acta Odontol. Scand. **28:**917, 1970.

Korman, M., Rubinstein, A., and Gargiulo, A.: Preservation of palatal mucosa: I. Ultrastructural changes and freezing technique, J. Periodontol. **44:**464, 1973.

Kurahashi, Y., and Takuma, S.: Electron microscopy of human gingival epithelium, Bull. Tokyo Dent. Col. 3:29, 1962.

Lange, D., and Schroeder, H. E.: Cytochemistry and ultrastructure of gingival sulcus cells, Helv. Odontol. Acta 15:65, 1971.

Listgarten, M. A.: The ultrastructure of human gingival epithelium, Am. J. Anat. 114: 49, 1964.

Listgarten, M. A.: Phase contrast and electron microscopic study of the junction between reduced enamel epithelium and enamel in unerupted human teeth, Arch. Oral Biol. 11:999, 1966.

Listgarten, M. A.: Electron microscopic study of the gingivo-dental junction of man, Am. J. Anat. 119:147, 1966.

Listgarten, M. A.: Changing concepts about the dento-epithelial junction, J. Can. Dent. Assoc. 36:70, 1970.

Löe, H., Karring, T., and Hara, K.: The site of mitotic activity in rat and human oral epithelium. Scand. J. Dent. Res. 80:111, 1972.

Luzardo-Baptista, M.: Intraepithelial nerve fibers in the human oral mucosa, Oral Surg. 35:372, 1973.

McDougall, W. A.: Pathways of penetration and effects of horseradish peroxidase in rat molar gingiva, Arch. Oral Biol. 15:621, 1970.

McHugh, W. D.: Keratinization of gingival epithelium in laboratory animals, J. Periodontol. 35:338, 1964.

McMillan, M. D.: A scanning electron study of keratinized epithelium of the hard palate of the rat, Arch. Oral Biol. 19:225, 1974.

Mahrle, G., and Orfanos, C. E.: Merkel cells as human cutaneous neuroreceptor cells. Their presence in dermal neural corpuscles and in the external hair root sheath of human adult skin, Arch. Derm. Forsch. 251: 19, 1974.

Mattern, C. F. T., Daniel, W. A., and Henkin, R. I.: The ultrastructure of the human circumvallate papilla. I. Cilia of the papillary crypt, Anat. Rec. 167:175, 1970.

Melcher, A. H.: Gingival reticulin: Identification and role in histogenesis of collagen fibers, J. Dent. Res. 45:426, 1966.

Melcher, A., and Bowen, W. H.: Biology of the periodontium, London, 1969, Academic Press Inc.

Meyer, J., and Gerson, S. J.: A comparison of human palatal and buccal mucosa, Periodontics 2:284, 1964.

Mignon, M. L.: Ultrastructure of the gingival epithelium in the new born cat—some characteristics of the intercellular junctions, J. Dent. Res. 53:1484, 1974.

Murray, R. G., Murray, A., and Fujimoto, S.: Fine structure of gustatory cells in rabbit taste buds, J. Ultrastruct. Res. 27:444, 1969.

Nuki, K., and Hock, J.: The organisation of the gingival vasculature, J. Periodont. Res. 9:305, 1974.

Odland, G. F.: Tonofilaments and keratohyalin. In Montagna, W., and Lobitz, W. C., Jr., editors: The epidermis, New York, 1964, Academic Press Inc., pp. 237-249.

Orban, B.: Zahnfleischtasche und Epithelansatz, Z. Stomatol. 22:353, 1924.

Orban, B., and Mueller, E.: The gingival crevice, J. Am. Dent. Assoc. 16:1206, 1929.

Orban, B.: Hornification of the gums, J. Am. Dent. Assoc. 17:1977, 1930.

Orban, B., and Sicher, H.: The oral mucosa, J. Dent. Educ. 10:94, 163, 1946.

Orban, B.: Clinical and histologic study of the surface characteristics of the gingiva, Oral Surg. 1:827, 1948.

Orban, B., Bhattia, H., et al.: Epithelial attachment (the attached gingival cuff). J. Periodontol. 27:167, 1956.

Palade, G. E., and Farquhar, M. G.: A special fibril of the dermis, J. Cell Biol. 27: 215, 1965.

Petitet, N. F., and Stern, I. B.: Ultrastructure de l'épithélium gingival humain. In Favard, P., editor: Microscopie électronique, Paris, 1970, Société Française de Microscopie Électronique, vol. 3, p. 223.

Rhodin, J. A. G., and Reith, E. J.: Ultrastructure of keratin in oral mucosa, skin, esophagus, claw, and hair. In Butcher, E. O., and Sognnaes, R. F., editors: Fundamentals of keratinization, Washington, D.C., 1962, American Association for the Advancement of Science.

Schroeder, H. E., and J. Theilade: Electron microscopy of normal human gingival epithelium, J. Periodont. Res. 1:95, 1966.

Schroeder, H. E.: Melanin-containing organelles in cells of the human gingiva. 1. Epithelial melanocytes, J. Periodont. Res. 4: 1, 1969.

Schroeder, H. E.: Ultrastructure of the junctional epithelium of the human gingiva, Helv. Odontol. Acta 13:65, 1969.

Schroeder, H. E., and Listgarten, M. A.: Fine structure of the developing epithelial attachment of human teeth (Monographs in developmental biology, vol. 2), Basel, 1971, S. Karger AG.

Schroeder, H. E., and Munzel-Pedrazzoli, S.: Correlated morphometric and biochemical analysis of gingival tissue, J. Microscopy **99**:301, 1973.

Skillen, W. G.: The morphology of the gingiva of the rat molar, J. Am. Dent. Assoc. **17**:645, 1930.

Skougaard, M. R.: Cell renewal, with special reference to the gingival epithelium, Adv. Oral Biol. **4**:261, 1970.

Smith, C. J.: Gingival epithelium. In Melcher, A. H., and Bowen, W. H., editors: Biology of the periodontium, New York, 1969, Academic Press Inc.

Squier, C. A.: The permeability of keratinized and nonkeratinized oral epithelium to horseradish peroxidase, J. Ultrastruct. Res. **43**:160, 1973.

Squier, C. A., and Waterhouse, L. P.: The ultrastructure of the melanocyte in human gingival epithelium, J. Dent. Res. **46**:112, 1967.

Squier, C. A., and Meyer, J.: Current concepts of the histology of oral mucosa, Springfield, Ill., 1971, Charles C Thomas, Publisher.

Stern, I. B.: Electron microscopic observations of oral epithelium. 1. Basal cells and the basement membrane, Periodontics **3**:224, 1965.

Stern, I. B.: The fine structure of the ameloblast—Enamel junction in rat incisors, epithelial attachment and cuticular membrane, 5th International Congress for Electron Microscopy, New York, 1966, Academic Press Inc., vol. B, p. 6.

Stern, I. B.: Further electron microscopic observations of the epithelial attachment, Int. Assoc. Dent. Res. Abstr., no. 325, 45th general meeting, 1967, p. 118.

Stern, I. B., and Sekeri-Pataryas, K. H.: The uptake of $^{14}$C-leucine and $^{14}$C-histidine by cell suspension of isolated strata of neonatal rat epidermis, J. Invest. Dermatol. **59**:251, 1972.

Stern, I. B., Dayton, L., and Duecy, J.: The uptake of tritiated thymidine by the dorsal epidermis of the fetal and newborn rat, Anat. Rec. **170**:225, 1971.

Susi, F. R., Belt, W. D., and Kelly, J. W.: Fine structure of fibrillar complexes associated with the basement membrane in human oral mucosa, J. Cell Biol. **34**:686, 1967.

Susi, F. R.: Histochemical, autoradiographic and electron microscopic studies of keratinization in oral mucosa, Ph.D. thesis, Tufts University, October 1967.

Susi, F. R.: Studies of cellular renewal and protein synthesis in mouse oral mucosa utilizing H$^3$-thymidine and H$^3$-cystine, J. Invest. Dermatol. **51**:403, 1968.

Susi, F. R.: Anchoring fibrils in the attachment of epithelium to connective tissue in oral mucous membranes, J. Dent. Res. **48**: 144, 1969.

Svejda, J., and Janota, M.: Scanning electron microscopy of the papillae foliatae of the human tongue, Oral Surg. **37**:208, 1974.

Thilander, H., and Bloom, G. D.: Cell contacts in oral epithelia, J. Periodont. Res. **3**: 96, 1968.

Toto, P. D., and Sicher, H.: The epithelial attachment, Periodontics **2**:154, 1964.

Toto, P. D., and Grundel, E. R.: Acid mucopolysaccharides in the oral epithelium, J. Dent. Res. **45**:211, 1966.

Turesky, S., Glickman, I., and Litvin, T.: Histochemical evaluation of normal and inflamed human gingiva, J. Dent. Res. **30**: 792, 1951.

Weinmann, J. P.: The keratinization of the human oral mucosa, J. Dent. Res. **19**:57, 1940.

Weinmann, J. P., and Meyer, J.: Types of keratinization in the human gingiva, J. Invest. Dermatol. **32**:9, February 1959.

Weinstock, M., and Wilgram, G. F.: Fine-structural observations on the formation and enzymatic activity of keratinosomes in mouse tongue filiform papilla, J. Ultrastruct. Res. **30**:262, 1970.

Wentz, F. M., Maier, A. W., and Orban, B.: Age changes and sex differences in the clinically "normal" gingiva, J. Periodontol. **23**:13, 1952.

Zelickson, A. S.: Electron microscopy of skin and mucous membrane, Springfield, Ill., 1963, Charles C Thomas, Publisher.

# 10 Salivary glands

The salivary glands are exocrine glands whose secretions flow into the oral cavity. There are three pairs of large glands, located extraorally, known as the major salivary glands (Plate 3), and numerous small glands widely distributed in the mucosa and submucosa of the oral cavity, known as the minor salivary glands. Both the major and minor glands are composed of parenchymal elements invested in and supported by connective tissue. The parenchymal elements are derived from the oral epithelium and consist of terminal secretory units leading into ducts that eventually open into the oral cavity. The connective tissue forms a capsule around the gland and extends into it, dividing groups of secretory units and ducts into lobes and lobules. The blood and lymph vessels and nerves that supply the gland are contained within the connective tissue. The most important function of the salivary glands is the production of saliva, which contains various organic and inorganic substances and assists in the mastication, deglutition, and digestion of food.

## STRUCTURE AND FUNCTION OF SALIVARY GLAND CELLS

The terminal secretory units are composed of serous, mucous, and myoepithelial cells arranged into acini or secretory tubules. The secretions of these units are collected by the intercalated ducts, which empty into the striated ducts. The structure and function of each of these components will be considered in detail, followed by a description of the connective tissue elements and nerves.

### Serous cells

Serous cells are specialized for the synthesis, storage, and secretion of proteins. The typical serous cell is pyramidal in shape, with its broad base resting

**328**

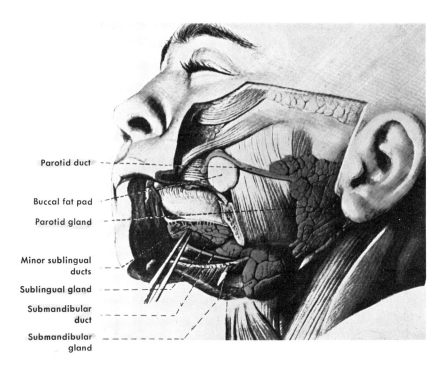

Parotid duct

Buccal fat pad

Parotid gland

Minor sublingual
ducts

Sublingual gland

Submandibular
duct

Submandibular
gland

**Plate** 3. Salivary glands of major secretion. Part of the mandible and mylohyoid muscle removed. (From Sicher, H., and Tandler, J.: Anatomie für Zahnärtze [Anatomy for dentists], Berlin, 1928, Julius Springer Verlag.)

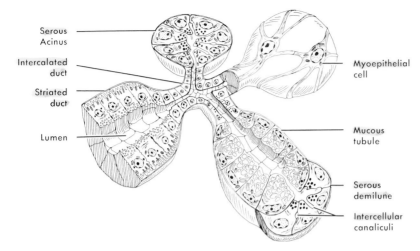

Serous
Acinus

Intercalated
duct

Striated
duct

Lumen

Myoepithelial
cell

Mucous
tubule

Serous
demilune

Intercellular
canaliculi

**Fig. 10-1.** Drawing of main features of parenchymal cells of salivary glands and their arrangement to form ducts and terminal secretory units.

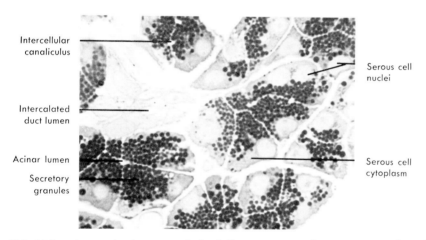

Intercellular
canaliculus

Intercalated
duct lumen

Acinar lumen

Secretory
granules

Serous cell
nuclei

Serous cell
cytoplasm

**Fig. 10-2.** Light micrograph of rat parotid gland illustrating general arrangement and cytologic features of serous cells. Gland was incubated in a cytochemical medium to demonstrate the secretory enzyme peroxidase, resulting in unstained nuclei, lightly stained cytoplasm, and heavily stained secretory granules. Cells of intercalated duct are unreactive. (One-micron section of plastic-embedded tissue; ×1240.)

on a thin basal lamina and its narrow apex bordering on the lumen (Figs. 10-1 and 10-2). The spherical nucleus is located in the basal region of the cell; occasionally binucleated cells are observed.

The most prominent feature of the serous cell is the accumulation of secretory granules in the apical cytoplasm (Fig. 10-2). These granules are about 1 micron in diameter, and by electron microscopy are observed to have a distinct limiting membrane and a dense homogeneous content (Fig. 10-3). In some salivary

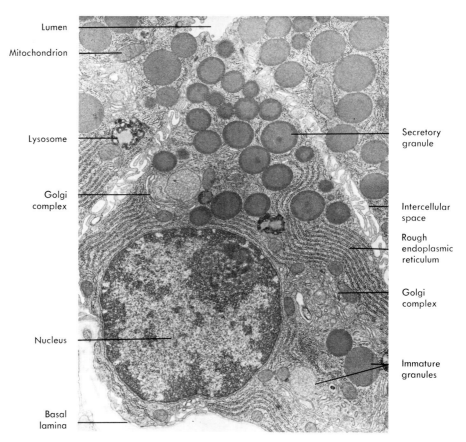

Lumen

Mitochondrion

Lysosome

Golgi complex

Nucleus

Basal lamina

Secretory granule

Intercellular space

Rough endoplasmic reticulum

Golgi complex

Immature granules

**Fig. 10-3.** Electron micrograph of typical serous cell. Round nucleus and flattened RER cisternae are located in basal half of cell. Golgi complex and immature granules are located apical and lateral to nucleus, and dense secretory granules are located in cell apex. Folds of cell membranes interdigitate in intercellular spaces. Note faint basal lamina. Rat parotid gland. (×15,700.) (From Hand, A. R.: Am. J. Anat. **135**:71, 1972; reprinted by permission of the Wistar Institute Press.)

glands, including those of the human, the serous granules may contain a dense core within a lighter matrix, or a dense, twisted skeinlike structure. The granules may be very closely apposed to one another, the plasma membrane, or other organelles, but under ordinary unstimulated conditions they retain their individual nature and do not fuse with other structures. In routine histologic preparations, the serous granules are usually not well resolved, because of section thickness and the conditions of fixation, and the apical portion of the cell may appear as an acidophilic mass. However, in semithin (1 micron) sections of plastic-embedded tissue, stained with toluidine blue or by specific cytochemical techniques (Fig. 10-2), the secretory granules are clearly seen.

The basal portion of the cytoplasm is filled with ribosome-studded (rough) endoplasmic reticulum (RER), a closed system of membranous sacs or cisternae

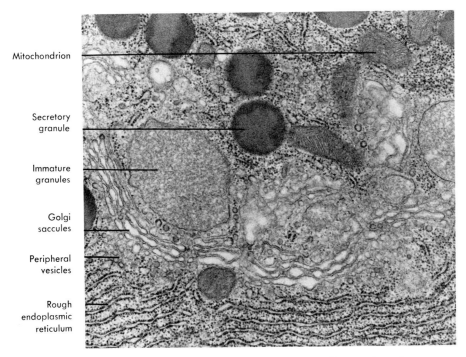

Mitochondrion

Secretory
granule

Immature
granules

Golgi
saccules

Peripheral
vesicles

Rough
endoplasmic
reticulum

**Fig. 10-4.** Electron micrograph of Golgi complex of serous cell. Saccules of outer convex surface of Golgi complex are wider than saccules of inner concave surface. Immature granules are located at inner surface; their irregular membranes suggest fusion with small vesicles. Note peripheral vesicles between RER and outer Golgi saccules. Rat parotid gland. (×25,400.)

(Fig. 10-3). The ribosomes, consisting of ribonucleic acid (RNA) and proteins, are the basic units of protein synthesis. Acting under the direction of messenger RNA from the nucleus, the ribosomes translate the encoded message, coupling the appropriate amino acids to their proper positions in the protein being synthesized. The growing polypeptide chain is transferred across the RER membrane into the cisternal space. In cells that produce large amounts of protein for secretion, the RER is characteristically well developed and arranged in parallel stacks, usually basal and lateral to the nucleus.

A second system of membranous cisternae, the Golgi complex, is located apical or lateral to the nucleus (Figs. 10-3 and 10-4). The Golgi complex consists of 4 to 6 smooth-surfaced saccules that are slightly curved or cup-shaped, with the concave portion usually oriented toward the secretory surface of the cell. The Golgi complex is functionally interconnected with the RER through vesicles budding from the ends of the RER cisternae, which approach the periphery or convex portion of the Golgi (Fig. 10-4). The newly synthesized secretory proteins within the RER are transported to the Golgi complex via these small vesicles. The vesicles may fuse either with the peripheral Golgi saccule, contributing their content to it, or directly with vacuoles of various sizes at the concave or inner face of the Golgi complex (Figs. 10-3 and 10-4). These vacuoles are the forming secretory granules and are called immature granules, prosecretory granules, or condensing vacuoles. When the proteins are transported through the Golgi saccules, the content of the saccules usually increases in density from the convex to the concave surface, and direct connections exist between the inner saccule and the immature granules. The smaller immature granules have a light flocculent content; as they increase in size, their content increases in density until it is near that of the mature granules. The increase in density of the secretory material suggests that as it is being transported and packaged for storage in granules, it is also being concentrated by the Golgi complex.

The Golgi complex is also an important site of addition of carbohydrate residues to the secretory proteins. With the notable exception of a majority of the amylase molecules, most secretory proteins are actually glycoproteins. They have a variable number of oligosaccharide chains attached to the amino acids serine, threonine, and asparagine in the protein core. The carbohydrates of secretory glycoproteins include galactose, mannose, fucose, glucosamine, galactosamine, and sialic acid. Addition of the carbohydrate residues begins in the RER, but it is completed in the Golgi complex.

The completed glycoproteins are stored in the secretory granules in the cell apex. Secretion or discharge of the granule content occurs by a process called exocytosis. This involves fusion of the granule membrane with the plasma membrane at the lumen or intercellular canaliculus, followed by the opening of the fused portion (Fig. 10-5). In this manner, the granule membrane becomes continuous with the plasma membrane, and the granule content is exteriorized without loss of cytoplasm. During rapid secretion, such as that occurring after

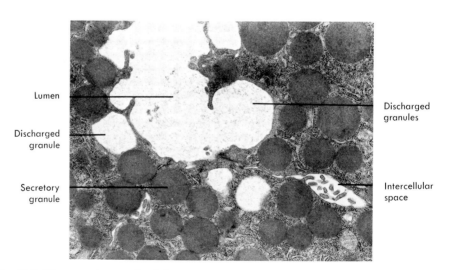

**Fig. 10-5.** Electron micrograph of three serous cells illustrating exocytosis of secretory granules induced by isoproterenol. Flask-shaped invaginations of the lumen into cell apices mark sites of granule discharge. Rat lingual serous gland (×17,600.)

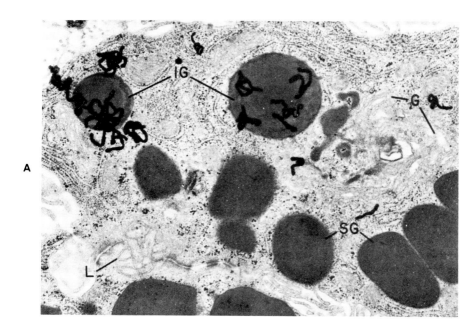

A

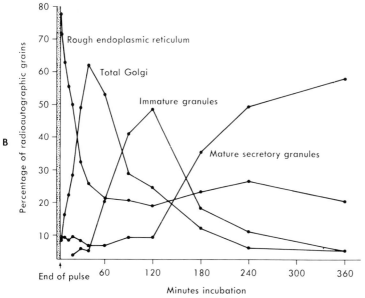

B

Fig. 10-6. **A,** Electron microscope radioautograph of serous cell of rabbit parotid gland, pulse-labeled with [3]H-leucine for 4 minutes and incubated in vitro for 116 minutes. Radio-autographic grains, indicating presence of radioactive leucine incorporated into newly synthesized proteins, are concentrated over the immature granules, *IG.* A few grains are present over RER and Golgi complex, *G,* but none are localized over mature secretory granules, *SG.* Lumen, *L.* **B,** Radioautographic grain counts of rabbit parotid serous cells after pulse-labeling with [3]H-leucine and in vitro incubation. Newly synthesized proteins move in wavelike fashion from RER, through Golgi complex, and into immature and finally mature secretory granules. About 20% of the label remains with the RER as nonsecretory proteins. (**A,** ×19,000.) (**A** and **B** from Castle, J. D., Jamieson, J. D., and Palade, G. E.: J. Cell Biol. **53:**290, 1972; reprinted by permission of the Rockefeller University Press.)

stimulation by various pharmacologic agents, a second granule may fuse with the membrane of a previously discharged granule; continuation of this process can lead to a long string of interconnected granule profiles extending into the cytoplasm. The addition of granule membranes results in a great enlargement of the plasma membrane at the secretory surface; during recovery the cell removes this excess membrane, but it is not yet clear how this is accomplished.

In summary, then, secretory proteins are synthesized by membrane-bound ribosomes and migrate to the Golgi complex, where carbohydrate addition is completed and they are packaged into secretory granules. After a variable period of storage in the cell apex, they are discharged by exocytosis at the secretory surface of the cell. The incorporation of amino acids into the secretory proteins and the movement of the proteins through the various compartments of the cell has been studied by electron microscope radioautography (Fig. 10-6, *A*). Counts of the radioautographic grains at various times after administration of radioactive amino acids reveal the sequential flow of proteins from the RER to the Golgi complex, their accumulation in immature granules, and finally storage in the mature secretory granules (Fig. 10-6, *B*). Similar studies with radioactive sugars have shown a rapid initial accumulation in the Golgi complex, followed by a more gradual movement into the forming and then mature secretory granules.

The serous cell contains several other cytoplasmic organelles, which are also found in most other salivary gland cells. Free or unattached ribosomes are located in the cytoplasm throughout the cell; they are concerned with the synthesis of nonsecretory cellular proteins. Mitochondria are also found throughout the cell, most frequently between the RER cisternae, around the Golgi complex, and along the lateral and basal plasma membranes. The mitochondria contain the enzymes of the citric acid cycle, electron transport, and oxidative phosphorylation; hence they are the major source of high-energy compounds necessary for the numerous synthetic and transport processes that occur in the cell. Lysosomes, organelles that contain potent hydrolytic enzymes, are also occasionally seen. They function to destroy foreign materials taken up by the cells, as well as portions of the cells themselves, such as worn-out mitochondria or other membranous organelles. Their typical heterogeneous content of granular and membranous debris and lipidlike droplets probably reflects the role of lysosomes in this latter process. A few peroxisomes (microbodies), small organelles containing the enzyme catalase and possibly other oxidative enzymes, can be demonstrated in the serous cells by cytochemical techniques; their function is currently unknown. Bundles of tonofilaments, associated with desmosomes, and microfilaments may be seen in the cytoplasm, as well as an occasional microtubule.

### Mucous cells

The mucous cell, like the serous cell, is specialized for the synthesis, storage, and secretion of a secretory product. However, its structure differs from that of

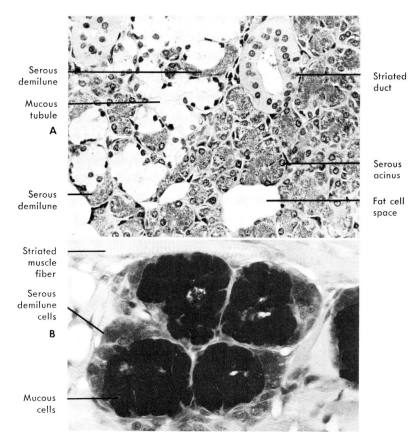

Serous demilune

Mucous tubule

A

Serous demilune

Striated muscle fiber

Serous demilune cells

B

Mucous cells

Striated duct

Serous acinus

Fat cell space

**Fig. 10-7. A,** Light micrograph of human submandibular gland illustrating the different appearance of mucous and serous cells. Mucous tubules are capped by serous demilunes. Two striated ducts are cut in cross section. **B,** Light micrograph of posterior lingual mucous gland of rat, stained with alcian blue and periodic acid–Schiff (PAS). The mucous secretory glycoprotein stains with both alcian blue and PAS, indicating acidic carbohydrate residues. Granules of serous demilune cells stain only with PAS, indicating a neutral glycoprotein. (**A,** ×295; **B,** ×470.)

the serous cell. In routine histologic preparations, the apex of the cell appears empty except for thin strands of cytoplasm forming a trabecular network (Fig. 10-7, *A*). The nucleus and a thin rim of cytoplasm are compressed against the base of the cell.

In the electron microscope, the mucous cell is seen to be filled with pale, electron-lucent secretory droplets containing scattered flocculent material (Fig. 10-8). These droplets are usually larger than serous granules and may be irregular or compressed in shape. The tenuous cytoplasmic partitions between the droplets are often disrupted; so several droplets are fused into a larger mass. Whether this occurs in vivo or strictly as a result of processing the tissue for microscopy is unknown. The secretory products of most mucous cells differ from those of

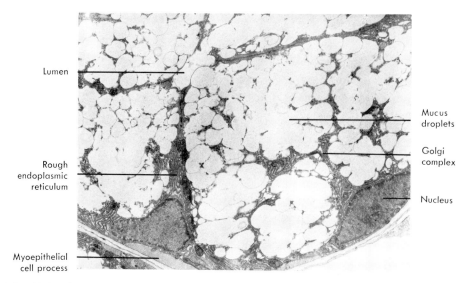

**Fig. 10-8.** Electron micrograph of portions of several mucous cells, packed with irregular, pale mucus droplets, which bulge into lumen and compress nucleus and other organelles against base of cell. Mucus droplets tend to coalesce into larger masses. Notice absence of wide intercellular spaces as seen in rat parotid gland (Figs. 10-2 and 10-3). Rat sublingual gland. (×5600.)

serous cells in two important respects: (1) they have little or no enzymatic activity and probably serve mainly for lubrication and protection of the oral tissues, and (2) the ratio of carbohydrate to protein is greater, and larger amounts of sialic acid and occasionally sulfated sugar residues are present. The differences in the carbohydrate content of the secretory material of mucous and serous cells can be demonstrated by histochemical staining techniques (Fig. 10-7, *B*).

The nucleus of the mucous cell is oval or flattened in shape and located just above the basal membrane (Fig. 10-8). The RER is limited to a narrow band of cytoplasm along the base and lateral borders of the cell and to an occasional patch of cytoplasm between the mucous droplets. The mitochondria and other organelles are also primarily limited to this band of basal and lateral cytoplasm. The Golgi complex is large, consisting of several stacks of 10 to 12 saccules sandwiched between the basal RER and mucous droplets forming from the concave surface. The Golgi complex plays an important role in these cells because of the large amount of carbohydrate that it adds to the secretory products.

The secretion of mucous droplets occurs by a somewhat different mechanism than the exocytotic process seen in the serous cells. When a single droplet is discharged, its limiting membrane fuses with the apical plasma membrane, resulting in a single membrane separating the droplet from the lumen. This separating membrane may then fragment, being lost with the discharge of mucus,

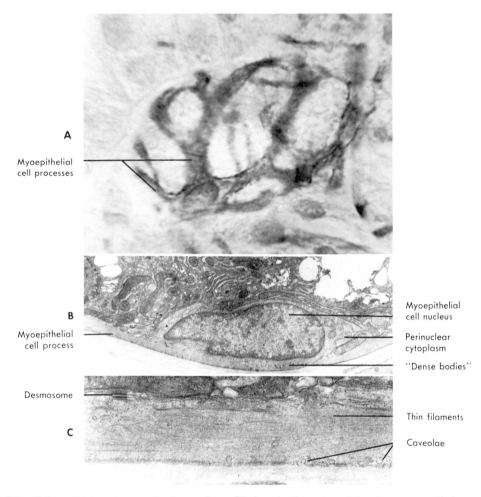

Myoepithelial
cell processes

Myoepithelial
cell nucleus

Myoepithelial
cell process

Perinuclear
cytoplasm

"Dense bodies"

Desmosome

Thin filaments

Caveolae

Fig. 10-9. **A,** Light micrograph of rat submandibular gland incubated for the enzyme alkaline phosphatase. Activity is present in branching processes of myoepithelial cells, which embrace an acinus. **B,** Electron micrograph of myoepithelial cell body showing concentration of organelles in the perinuclear cytoplasm and processes filled with fine filaments. The "dense bodies" are characteristic of myoepithelium and smooth muscle. Rat sublingual gland. **C,** Higher magnification of myoepithelial cell process filled with longitudinally arranged thin filaments. Several caveolae are located along the basal surface of cell, and a desmosome attaches the process to mucous cell. Rat sublingual gland. (**A** to **C,** ×1500, ×8500, ×28,500.) (**A,** From Leeson, C. R.: Nature **178:**858, 1956; reprinted by permission of Macmillan Journals, Ltd.)

or the droplet may be discharged with the membrane intact, surrounding it. During rapid droplet discharge, the apical cytoplasm may not seal itself off, and the entire mass of mucus may be spilled into the lumen.

### Myoepithelial cells

Myoepithelial cells are closely related to the secretory and intercalated duct cells, lying between the basal lamina and the basal membranes of the parenchymal cells (Figs. 10-1 and 10-9). The body of the cell is small, filled mostly with a flattened nucleus, and numerous branching cytoplasmic processes radiate out to embrace the parenchymal cells. Myoepithelial cells are difficult to identify in routine histologic preparations, but they are usually strongly reactive for alkaline phosphatase, and their typical stellate shape can be observed in sections incubated for this enzyme (Fig. 10-9, A). Their appearance is reminiscent of a basket cradling the secretory unit; hence the name "basket cell" in the older literature.

The usual appearance of myoepithelial cells in electron micrographs is a section through one of their processes lying in a groove on the surface of a secretory or duct cell (Figs. 10-8 and 10-10, B). The processes are filled with longitudinally oriented fine filaments about 50 Å thick (Fig. 10-9, C); the filaments frequently appear to aggregate, forming "dense bodies" in the processes. The usual cytoplasmic organelles are largely restricted to the perinuclear cytoplasm. The body of the cell, containing the nucleus, often lies in the space where the basal regions of two or three parenchymal cells come together (Fig. 10-9, B). The plasma membrane of the myoepithelial cell closely parallels the basal membrane of the parenchymal cell, and the two are joined by occasional desmosomes. Numerous micropinocytotic vesicles or caveolae are located on the plasma membranes of the myoepithelial cells.

Myoepithelial cells are considered to have a contractile function, helping to expel secretions from the lumina of the secretory units and ducts. Although direct evidence is lacking for the salivary glands, the following indirect observations suggest that this may be the case: (1) the structure of myoepithelium is similar to that of smooth muscle; (2) immunofluorescent studies suggest the presence of actin in myoepithelial cells; (3) measurements of ductal pressure after appropriate stimulation suggest a contractile process; and (4) cinemicrography of individual secretory units stimulated to secrete in vitro reveals a regular pulsatile movement of the entire unit. Studies of sweat and mammary glands, where myoepithelial cells are abundant, also support a contractile function.

### Arrangement of cells in the terminal secretory units

The structure of the terminal secretory units is different for different glands. When the gland consists entirely of serous secretory units, such as the human parotid, the serous cells are clustered in a roughly spherical fashion around a central lumen, forming an acinus (Fig. 10-1). At the apical ends of adjoining cells, the lumen is sealed off from the lateral intercellular spaces by junctional complexes, consisting of a tight junction (zonula occludens), an intermediate junction (zonula adherens), and one or more desmosomes (macula adherens). These junctions serve to hold the cells together as well as prevent leakage of the luminal contents into the intercellular spaces. Branches of the lumen, called intercellular canaliculi, extend between adjacent cells almost to their base; they increase the area of the secretory surface and are sealed by junctional complexes along their length. The remainder of the apposed lateral surfaces are joined by frequent desmosomes and an occasional gap junction (nexus).

In glands composed entirely of mucous secretory units, the arrangement of the secretory cells is similar. Rather than a spherical acinus, however, a tubular secretory end piece may be formed (Fig. 10-1). The central lumen is usually larger than in serous acini, and intercellular canaliculi are not usually present, although they have recently been observed between the mucous cells of the human labial glands.

In mixed glands, the proportion of serous and mucous cells may vary from predominantly serous, as in the human submandibular gland, to predominantly mucous, as in the human sublingual gland. Separate serous and mucous units may exist, in addition to secretory units composed of both cell types. In the latter arrangement, the mucous cells form a typical tubular portion that is capped at the blind end by crescents of several serous cells, known as demilunes (Figs. 10-1 and 10-7). The secretion of the serous demilune cells reaches the lumen through the intercellular canaliculi.

The disposition of the myoepithelium in relation to the parenchymal cells has already been described. In some glands, the cell bodies may be restricted to the intercalated ducts with only the branching processes reaching the acini. Myoepithelial cells are not usually present along the striated ducts.

### Ducts

The duct system of the salivary glands is formed by the confluence of small ducts into ones of progressively larger caliber. Within a lobule, the smallest ducts are the intercalated ducts (Fig. 10-1); they are thin branching tubes of variable length that connect the terminal secretory units to the next larger ducts, the striated ducts. In the interlobular connective tissue, the ducts continue to join one another, increasing in size until the main excretory duct is formed.

*Intercalated ducts.* The intercalated ducts (Figs. 10-1, 10-2, and 10-10, *A*) are lined by a single layer of low cuboid cells with relatively empty-appearing cytoplasm. They are often difficult to identify in the light microscope as they are compressed between secretory units. In electron micrographs, the intercalated duct cells share several characteristics of serous cells (Fig. 10-10, *B*). A small amount of RER is located in the basal cytoplasm, and a Golgi complex of moderate size is found apically. In proximally located cells (near the secretory

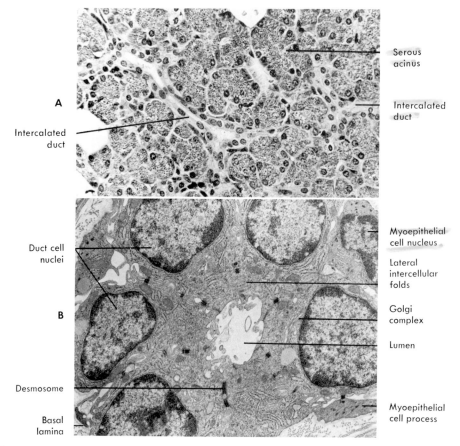

Serous
acinus

Intercalated
duct

A

Intercalated
duct

Myoepithelial
cell nucleus

Duct cell
nuclei

Lateral
intercellular
folds

Golgi
complex

B

Lumen

Desmosome

Myoepithelial
cell process

Basal
lamina

**Fig. 10-10.** **A,** Light micrograph of human parotid gland showing long branching intercalated ducts between the serous acini. **B,** Electron micrograph of intercalated duct cut in cross section. Duct cells contain a moderate amount of RER and a prominent Golgi complex, but few or no secretory granules. Prominent desmosomes and interlocking folds are present between adjacent cells. Myoepithelial cell processes extend longitudinally along the duct, inside the basal lamina. Rat parotid gland. (**A,** ×295; **B,** ×13,100.)

units) a few small secretory granules may be found. The lateral membranes of adjacent cells are joined apically by junctional complexes and several desmosomes. One or two areas of prominent interlocking folds of the lateral surface are located further basally. At the periphery of the duct, processes of myoepithelial cells may be found, attached by desmosomes to the duct cells.

**Striated ducts.** The striated ducts are lined by a layer of tall columnar epithelial cells with large, spherical, centrally placed nuclei (Figs. 10-1, 10-7, A, and 10-11). The cytoplasm is abundant and eosinophilic and shows prominent striations at the basal ends of the cells, perpendicular to the basal surface. An occasional basally located cell can be identified by the position of its nucleus, below the level of those of the other cells (Fig. 10-7, A).

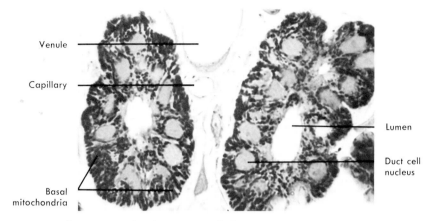

Venule

Capillary

Lumen

Duct cell
nucleus

Basal
mitochondria

**Fig. 10-11.** Light micrograph of two striated ducts cut in cross section. Large, primarily radially oriented mitochondria, stained for cytochrome oxidase activity, fill basal regions of duct cells. Unstained nuclei are centrally located, and smaller mitochondria are found in apical cytoplasm. One-micron section of plastic-embedded rat parotid gland. (×1240.)

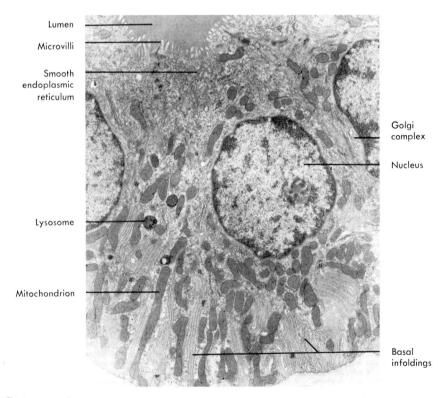

Lumen

Microvilli

Smooth
endoplasmic
reticulum

Golgi
complex

Nucleus

Lysosome

Mitochondrion

Basal
infoldings

**Fig. 10-12.** Electron micrograph of striated duct cells of rat parotid gland. Numerous mitochondria are located between the infoldings of basal plasma membrane. A few lysosomes and small Golgi complexes are located in perinuclear region, and smooth ER is found in cell apices. Short microvilli project into lumen. (×11,100.)

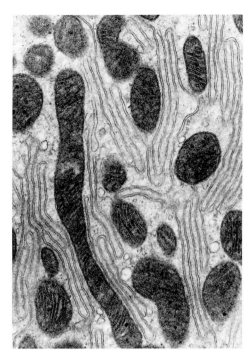

**Fig. 10-13.** Higher magnification of basal region of striated duct of rat sublingual gland (×23,900.)

In electron micrographs the basal cytoplasm of the striated duct cells is partitioned by deep infoldings of the plasma membrane, producing numerous sheet-like folds that extend beyond the lateral boundaries of the cell and interdigitate with similar folds of adjacent cells (Figs. 10-12 and 10-13). Abundant large mitochondria, usually radially oriented, are located in portions of the cytoplasm between the membrane infoldings (Figs. 10-11 to 10-13). The combination of infoldings and mitochondria accounts for the striations seen in the light microscope. A few short RER cisternae and small Golgi complexes are found in the perinuclear cytoplasm. Apically the cytoplasm may contain a variable amount of branching, tubular, smooth endoplasmic reticulum, a few small granules of moderate density, or small, empty-appearing vesicles. Several lysosomes, numerous small peroxisomes, bundles of cytoplasmic filaments, free ribosomes, and a moderate amount of glycogen are also usually present. Numerous short microvilli on the apical surfaces project into the lumen, and adjacent cells are joined by apical junctional complexes and several desmosomes along their lateral surfaces.

In larger ducts the epithelium becomes pseudostratified, with increasing numbers of smaller basal cells between the tall columnar cells. The characteristics of the striated cells are maintained to a variable degree, becoming less pronounced as the duct increases in size. In the largest ducts occasional mucous goblet cells may be found, and the epithelium of the main duct gradually becomes stratified as it merges with the epithelium of the oral cavity.

*Functions of salivary ducts.* The microscopic observations suggest that the intercalated ducts serve mainly as passive conduits between the terminal secretory units and striated ducts. However, the presence of some cells with apparent secretory granules indicates a possible minor contribution to the primary secretion of the serous and mucous cells. In contrast, the structure of the striated ducts suggest that they are actively involved in modification of the primary secretion. The basal infoldings and concentration of mitochondria in these cells are typical of tissues involved in water and electrolyte transport, such as the kidney tubules and the choroid plexus. The accumulation of granules and vesicles in the apices of the cells suggests secretion or reabsorption by pinocytosis, although these have not yet been documented.

Important contributions to the knowledge of salivary duct function have come from studies of electrolyte concentrations of saliva of experimental animals under various conditions of secretion. Analysis of the primary secretion, obtained by micropuncture techniques from the lumen of an intercalated duct draining several secretory units, reveals that it is isotonic or slightly hypertonic to plasma, with $Na^+$ and $Cl^-$ concentrations approximately equal to those in plasma. $K^+$ concentration is low compared to that of $Na^+$, but it is significantly higher than the $K^+$ concentration of plasma. Analysis of fluid collected from the excretory ducts reveals that it is hypotonic, with low $Na^+$ and $Cl^-$ and high $K^+$ concentrations. Furthermore, the concentration of these electrolytes varies with the flow rate of the saliva: with increasing flow, $Na^+$ and $Cl^-$ increase, while $K^+$ decreases. Apparently, the striated ducts actively reabsorb $Na^+$ from the primary secretion and secrete $K^+$; $Cl^-$ tends to follow the electrochemical gradient established by $Na^+$ reabsorption. At increased flow rates $Na^+$ reabsorption becomes less efficient and the secretion is in contact with the ductal epithelium for a shorter time; hence $Na^+$ concentrations of the saliva tend to increase. Microperfusion studies of the main excretory duct have shown that it too is able to reabsorb $Na^+$ and secrete $K^+$. In addition, the main excretory duct is highly impermeable to water; therefore $Na^+$ and $Cl^-$ are reabsorbed in excess of water, leaving a hypotonic luminal fluid. Since active transport of water does not occur, the ducts cannot secrete water against the osmotic gradient to produce the hypotonic saliva.[*]

## Connective tissue elements

The cells found in the connective tissue of the salivary glands are the same as those in other connective tissues of the body and include fibroblasts, macrophages, mast cells, occasional leukocytes, fat cells, and plasma cells. The cells, along with collagen and reticular fibers, are embedded in a ground substance composed of proteoglycans and glycoproteins. The vascular supply to the glands is also embedded within the connective tissue, entering the glands along the

---

[*]Electrolyte secretion and transport by the salivary glands is a complex process and not yet completely understood. For a more extensive discussion, please refer to the publications by Schneyer, Young, and Schneyer (1972) and Young and Martin (1972).

excretory ducts and branching to follow them into the individual lobules. The ducts, to the level of the intralobular striated ducts, are supplied with a dense capillary network; the capillary loops to the intercalated ducts and terminal secretory units are less extensive. A system of arteriovenous anastomoses has also been described around the larger interlobular ducts.

*Nerves.* The main branches of the nerves supplying the glands follow the course of the vessels, breaking up into terminal plexuses in the connective tissue adjacent to the terminal portions of the parenchyma. Nerve bundles, consisting of unmyelinated axons embedded within Schwann cell cytoplasm, are distributed to the smooth muscle of the arterioles, the secretory cells and myoepithelium, and possibly the intercalated and striated ducts.

The secretory cells receive their innervation by one of two patterns. In the intraepithelial type, the axons split off from the nerve bundle and penetrate the basal lamina, lying adjacent to or between the secretory cells (Fig. 10-14, *A*). As the axons pass through the basal lamina, the Schwann cell covering is usually lost; occasionally it may be continued into the parenchyma and lie between the axon and the secretory cell. The site of innervation (neuroeffector site) is considered to be at varicosities of the axon, which contain small vesicles and mitochondria. The vesicles are believed to contain the chemical neurotransmitters norepinephrine and acetylcholine and presumably release them by an exocytosis-like process. The membranes of the axon and secretory cell are separated by a space of only 100 to 200 Å, but no specializations of the membranes have been detected at these sites. A single axon may have several varicosities along its length, making contact with the same cell or with two or more cells.

The second type of innervation is subepithelial. Instead of penetrating the basal lamina, the axons remain associated with the nerve bundle in the connective tissue (Fig. 10-14, *B*). Where the nerve bundles approach the secretory cells, some of the axonal varicosities, which contain the small neurotransmitter vesicles, lose their covering of Schwann cell cytoplasm. Presumably, these bared axonal varicosities are the sites of transmitter release. The axons remain separated from the secretory cells by 1000 to 2000 Å, and the transmitters must diffuse across this space, which includes the basal laminae of the secretory cells and the nerve bundle.

The pattern of innervation varies between glands in the same animal and between the same gland in different species. The parotid serous cells and the sublingual mucous cells of the rat receive an intraepithelial type of innervation, as do the mucous cells of human labial glands. In contrast, the innervation of the secretory cells of the rat submandibular and the serous cells of the human parotid and submandibular glands is of the subepithelial type.

Both divisions of the autonomic nervous system may participate in the innervation of the secretory cells. In some glands both sympathetic (adrenergic) (Fig. 10-14, *C*) and parasympathetic (cholinergic) terminals (distinguished by special fixation and cytochemical techniques) have been observed in proximity

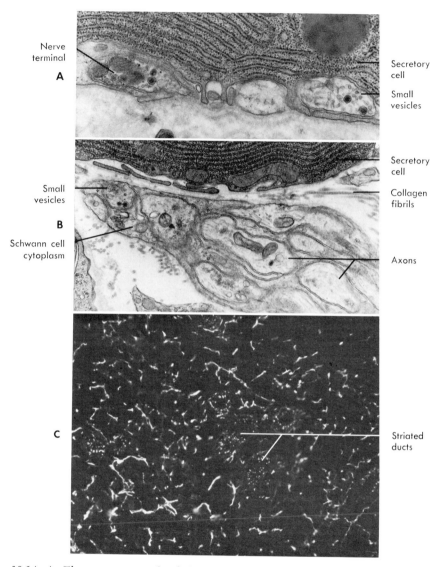

**Fig. 10-14. A,** Electron micrograph of three nerves of the intraepithelial type at base of a secretory cell. Axons are on epithelial side of basal lamina, in close contact with secretory cell. Nerve terminals contain mitochondria, small vesicles, a few larger dense-cored vesicles, and neurotubules. Rat parotid gland. **B,** Electron micrograph of nerve bundle of the subepithelial type in rat submandibular gland. Several axons are enclosed by a Schwann cell; innervation of the secretory cell presumably occurs where the axonal varicosities are bared of covering Schwann cell cytoplasm. **C,** Light micrograph of human parotid gland treated with formaldehyde vapor, which causes fluorescence of adrenergic nerves. Fluorescent structures seen here are nerve bundles, such as that in Fig. 10-14, *B,* located in the connective tissue around the parenchymal cells. The extensive nature of the sympathetic innervation of the human parotid is evident. Fluorescence of the striated ducts is caused by lysosomes. (**A,** ×28,500; **B,** ×20,800; **C,** courtesy Prof. J. R. Garrett, London, England.)

to the secretory cells. Similarly, physiologic studies indicate that the cells of some glands respond to both sympathetic and parasympathetic stimulation by changes in their membrane potential. However, the extent of participation by each division varies between glands and animals, and the composition of the saliva secreted in response to stimulation of each division is distinctly different. In general, a copious flow of watery saliva is secreted in response to parasympathetic stimulation, whereas that produced by sympathetic stimulation is thicker, higher in organic content, and comparatively less in quantity.

The innervation of duct cells is not clear. Intraepithelial terminals in ducts have been observed only rarely, but histochemical studies suggest that cholinergic and adrenergic nerves are found in the connective tissue around the ducts. Physiologic studies indicate that the ductal system is responsive to autonomic stimulation or administration of autonomic drugs: membrane potential changes in duct cells have been recorded, as well as changes in the transductal ion flux.

## CLASSIFICATION AND STRUCTURE OF HUMAN SALIVARY GLANDS

The salivary glands have been classified in a variety of ways by different histologists; the two most commonly used groupings are based on (1) the size and location and (2) the histochemical nature of the secretory products. In this chapter the former classification will be used, although the latter is not without considerable merit. To a large extent, the nature of the secretion produced by a gland depends on its cellular makeup in terms of serous and mucous cells. However, all serous cells are not alike; they may differ considerably in the type and amount of enzymes they produce and in the amount and nature of the carbohydrates attached to the secretory proteins. Mucous cells show a similar variability in the nature of their carbohydrate component. Furthermore, in salivary glands of some animals, the secretory cells may have a structure that cannot be readily classified as serous or mucous; histochemical characterization of their secretory products is useful for comparisons with other glands.

### Major salivary glands

The largest of the glands are the three bilaterally paired major salivary glands (Plate 3). They are all located extraorally and their secretions reach the mouth by variably long ducts.

*Parotid gland.* The parotid gland is enclosed within a well-formed connective tissue capsule, with its superficial portion lying in front of the external ear and its deeper part filling the retromandibular fossa. The main excretory duct (Stensen's duct) opens into the oral cavity on the buccal mucosa opposite the maxillary second molar. The opening is usually marked by a small papilla.

The parotid gland is a pure serous gland (Fig. 10-15, *A*); all the acinar cells are similar in structure to the serous cells described earlier. In the infant, however, a few mucous secretory units may be found. Electron microscopic studies indicate that the serous granules may have a dense central core. The intercalated

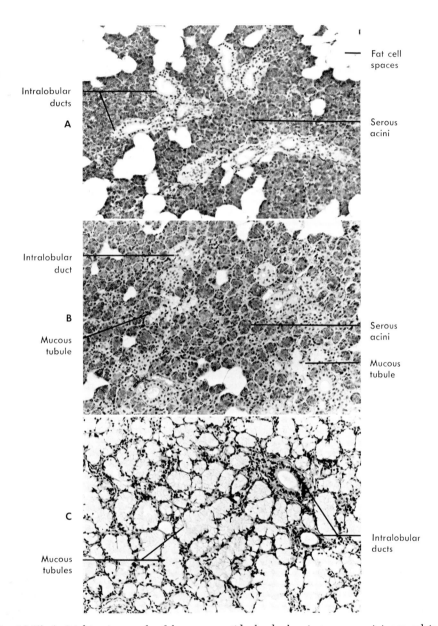

Fat cell spaces

Intralobular ducts

A

Serous acini

Intralobular duct

B

Serous acini

Mucous tubule

Mucous tubule

C

Intralobular ducts

Mucous tubules

**Fig. 10-15. A,** Light micrograph of human parotid gland, showing serous acini, several intralobular striated ducts, and numerous fat cell spaces. **B,** Light micrograph of human submandibular gland. Serous acini predominate, but a few mucous secretory units are present. Several intralobular striated ducts are cut in cross section. **C,** Light micrograph of human sublingual gland showing large mucous secretory units with typical tubular structure. Serous demilunes are difficult to distinguish at low magnification. Intralobular ducts are poorly developed. (**A** to **C,** ×115.)

ducts of the parotid are long and branching (Fig. 10-10, *A*), and the pale-staining striated ducts are numerous and stand out conspicuously against the more densely stained acini. The connective tissue septa in the parotid contain numerous fat cells, which increase in number with age and leave an empty space in histologic sections.

*Submandibular gland.* The submandibular gland is also enveloped by a well-defined capsule; it is located in the submandibular triangle behind and below the free border of the mylohyoid muscle, with a small extension lying above the mylohyoid. The main excretory duct (Wharton's duct) opens at the *caruncula sublingualis*, a small papilla at the side of the lingual frenum on the floor of the mouth. Some isolated smooth muscle cells have been reported around the duct.

The submandibular gland is a mixed gland, with both serous and mucous secretory units (Figs. 10-7, *A,* and 10-15, *B*). The serous units predominate, but the proportions may vary from one lobule to the next. The mucous terminal portions are capped by demilunes of serous cells. Although they appear similar by light microscopy, notable differences between submandibular and parotid serous cells are observed in the electron microscope (Fig. 10-16). The basal and lateral plasma membranes are thrown into numerous folds, interdigitating with similar processes from adjacent cells. The serous granules exhibit a variable substruc-

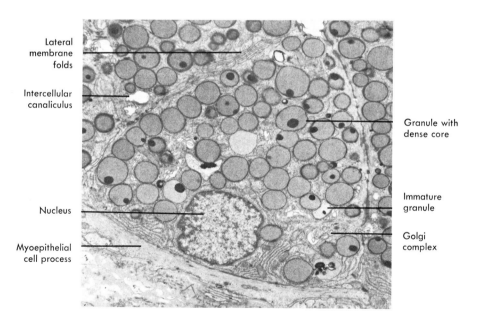

**Fig. 10-16.** Electron micrograph of serous cell of human submandibular gland, showing secretory granules with a dense core. Immature granules with similar cores are seen in the Golgi regions. Several intercellular canaliculi are cut in cross section, and extensive folding of lateral cell membranes occurs between two cells. A myoepithelial cell process is present at base of cell. (×9800.) (From Tandler, B., and Erlandson, R. A.: Am. J. Anat. **135:**419, 1972; reprinted by permission of the Wistar Institute Press.)

ture, from a granular matrix with a dense core or crescent, to an irregular skein of dense material dispersed in the matrix. The intercalated ducts tend to be somewhat shorter than those of the parotid, whereas the striated ducts are usually longer.

*Sublingual gland.* The sublingual gland lies between the floor of the mouth and the mylohyoid muscle; it is composed of one main gland and several smaller glands. The main duct (Bartholin's duct) opens with or near the submandibular duct, and several smaller ducts open independently along the sublingual fold. The capsule is poorly developed, but the connective tissue septa are particularly prominent within the gland.

The sublingual is also a mixed gland, but the mucous secretory units greatly outnumber the serous units (Fig. 10-15, *C*). The mucous cells are usually arranged in a tubular pattern; serous demilunes may be present at the blind ends of the tubules. Pure serous acini are rare or absent. The intercalated and striated ducts are poorly developed; mucous tubules may open directly into ducts lined with cuboid or columnar cells without typical basal striations.

## Minor salivary glands

The minor salivary glands are located beneath the epithelium in almost all parts of the oral cavity. These glands usually consist of several small groups of secretory units opening via short ducts directly into the mouth. They lack a distinct capsule, instead mixing with the connective tissue of the submucosa or muscle fibers of the tongue or cheek.

*Labial and buccal glands.* The glands of the lips and cheeks classically have been described as mixed, consisting of mucous tubules with serous demilunes. However, ultrastructural studies of the labial glands have revealed the presence of mucous cells only. Intercellular canaliculi have also been observed between the mucous cells. The intercalated ducts are variable in length, and the intralobular ducts possess only a few cells with basal striations. Although the buccal glands have not been examined by electron microscopy, they are usually described as a continuation of the labial glands with a similar structure.

*Glossopalatine glands.* The glossopalatine glands are pure mucous glands. They are principally localized to the region of the isthmus in the glossopalatine fold but may extend from the posterior extension of the sublingual gland to the glands of the soft palate.

*Palatine glands.* The palatine glands are also of the pure mucous variety. They consist of several hundred glandular aggregates in the lamina propria of the posterolateral region of the hard palate and in the submucosa of the soft palate and uvula. The excretory ducts may have an irregular contour with large distensions as they course through the lamina propria. The openings of the ducts on the palatal mucosa are often large and easily recognizable.

*Lingual glands.* The glands of the tongue can be divided into several groups. The anterior lingual glands (glands of Blandin and Nuhn) are located near the

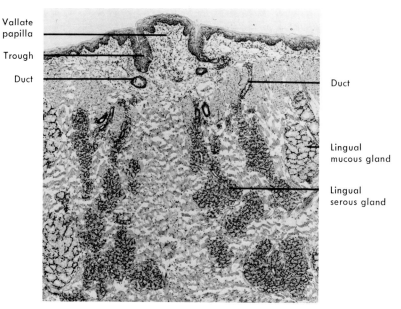

Vallate
papilla

Trough

Duct

Duct

Lingual
mucous gland

Lingual
serous gland

**Fig. 10-17.** Light micrograph of minor salivary glands of rat tongue. Lingual serous (von Ebner's) gland is located between the muscle fibers of the tongue below the vallate papilla. Its ducts empty into trough around papilla. Posterior lingual mucous glands are located lateral to the serous glands; their ducts open onto surface of tongue. (×40.) (From Hand, A. R.: J. Cell Biol. 44:340, 1970; reprinted by permission of the Rockefeller University Press.)

apex of the tongue. The anterior regions of the glands are chiefly mucous in character, while the posterior portions are mixed. The ducts open on the ventral surface of the tongue near the lingual frenum. The posterior lingual mucous glands (Fig. 10-17) are located lateral and posterior to the vallate papillae and in association with the lingual tonsil. They are purely mucous in character, and their ducts open onto the dorsal surface of the tongue. The posterior lingual serous glands (von Ebner's glands) are an extensive group of purely serous glands located between the muscle fibers of the tongue, below the vallate papillae (Fig. 10-17). Their ducts open into the trough of the vallate papillae, and at the rudimentary foliate papillae on the sides of the tongue.

Of all of the minor salivary glands, the posterior lingual serous glands have been the most thoroughly investigated. Classically, their secretions have been described as serving to wash out the trough of the papillae and ready the taste receptors (located in the epithelium of the trough) for a new stimulus. Although this may be a part of their function, recent studies suggest that these glands play an important role in the protective and digestive functions of the oral cavity. Histochemical studies have localized the enzyme peroxidase to the granules of the serous cells in man, and amylase activity has been demonstrated in these glands in the rat. Most importantly, the lingual serous glands of the rat synthesize a secretory enzyme with lipolytic activity; this lingual lipase has an acid pH optimum, so that it is capable of hydrolyzing triglycerides in the stomach. In the newborn, when fat intake is high and levels of pancreatic lipase are low, lingual lipase may play a significant role in lipid digestion. In man, a lipase with similar properties is present in aspirates from the esophagus and stomach, and preliminary investigations have revealed its presence in the lingual serous glands.*

## SPECIES VARIATION

From the preceding sections it is obvious that a number of differences exist between the individual salivary glands of man. Numerous differences in the structure and biochemical makeup of the salivary glands also exist between various mammalian species. Although many of them are relatively minor, such as variations in the proportion of serous to mucous cells or the extent of innervation by each division of the autonomic nervous system, others are important because they represent variations in the structure and biochemistry of the parenchymal cells, they may be a reflection of the particular diet of the animal, or they occur in animals that are widely used for research purposes.

The parotid gland of ruminants is specialized for the production of large amounts of fluid, up to 60 liters per day. The structure of the secretory cells reflects this function; they have little RER and few secretory granules, but extensive lateral membrane folds and numerous apical microvilli are present. The submandibular gland of rodents is one of the most interesting and widely studied of the salivary glands. In the rat and mouse, the acinar cells are intermediate in structure and carbohydrate content between serous and mucous cells; they are usually termed "seromucous." The rodent submandibular gland, at the time of sexual maturity, also undergoes a specialization of the proximal portion of the intralobular striated ducts (adjacent to the intercalated ducts) to form a granular tubule segment. The cells of the granular tubule are large, with basally situated nuclei and remnants of basal infoldings and a large number of electron-dense granules of various size in the apical cytoplasm. The granular tubules are very sensitive to hormonal influences. They are generally smaller in the female than in the male, but administration of testosterone to females results in development of a malelike structure; conversely, castration of males results in femalelike glands. Interrelationships between the pituitary, thyroid, and submandibular gland have also been shown. The male mouse shows the greatest development of the granular tubules, and several proteins with unique biologic activities are found in large amounts in this gland. Most of these have similar molecular weights and exhibit trypsinlike esteroprotease activity; however, their effects on tissues and animals are quite different. Nerve growth factor (NGF) stimulates the growth of neurites from embryonic dorsal root ganglia and sympathetic ganglia in culture; injection of antibodies to NGF into mice destroys their sym-

---

*Hamosh, M., and Burns, W. A.: Personal communication, 1974.

pathetic neurons. Epidermal growth factor (EGF) causes premature opening of the eyelids and eruption of the incisors and increases keratinization when injected into newborn mice. Renin and kallikrein, proteolytic enzymes that act on plasma proteins to liberate vasoactive peptides, can be isolated from the rodent submandibular gland; kallikrein has also been found in lesser amounts in the salivary glands of other species. The significance of these biologically active substances in the salivary glands remains obscure.

## DEVELOPMENT AND GROWTH

During fetal life each salivary gland is formed at a specific location in the oral cavity through the growth of a bud of oral epithelium into the underlying mesenchyme. The primordia of the parotid and submandibular glands of man appear during the sixth week, whereas the primordium of the sublingual gland appears after 7 to 8 weeks of fetal life. The minor salivary glands begin their development during the third month. The epithelial bud grows into an extensively branched system of cords of cells that are first solid but gradually develop a lumen and become ducts. The secretory portions develop later than the duct system and form by repeated branching and budding of the finer cell cords and ducts.

Studies of embryonic salivary glands in vitro have provided considerable information on the mechanism of glandular morphogenesis. The mesenchyme into which the glandular rudiment grows produces a factor or factors that stimulate the growth of the gland. If the mesenchyme and epithelium are separated and cultured on opposite sides of a filter, the growth of the epithelium proceeds normally; in the absence of the mesenchyme, the epithelium fails to grow. In the mouse, the submandibular gland exhibits a specific requirement for submandibular mesenchyme; however, in the rat, parotid mesenchyme, and to a lesser extent lung mesenchyme, can support morphogenesis of the submandibular epithelium. The rat parotid and sublingual rudiments appear to be somewhat less specific in their mesenchymal requirements. The process of branching morphogenesis, i.e., the formation of hollow, tubular glands from an initially flat epithelial surface, appears to be related to the presence of microfilaments. Microfilaments, about 50 to 70 Å thick, form a network beneath the cell membrane of almost all cells; they are believed to be actin, one of the contractile proteins of muscle. In developing salivary epithelium they are particularly prominent at the apical and basal ends of the cells; differential contraction could cause a group of cells to pucker outward, or clefts to form, in a solid cord or sheet of cells, sort of like pulling a purse string. Addition of the drug cytochalasin B, which disrupts the structure and function of microfilaments, to salivary gland rudiments growing in vitro prevents branching and cleft formation and causes newly formed clefts to disappear. Older clefts are unaffected, probably because they have been stabilized by the presence of mesenchymal cells and extracellular materials.

The presence of a functional innervation is also essential to proper growth and maintenance of salivary gland structure. Parasympathetic denervation of adult animals results in a 30% loss in glandular weight within 2 to 3 weeks. Sympathetic denervation causes variable responses, from atrophy of some glands to hypertrophy of others. Parasympathectomy of the developing rat parotid prevents attainment of adult gland size, cell number and size, and DNA and RNA content; sympathectomy has a moderate effect on cell and gland size only. Normal physiologic activity is also important for the proper growth of developing glands, as well as maintenance of adult structure and enzyme content. Feeding of a liquid diet to rats greatly diminishes the reflexly mediated secretory activity; the parotid rapidly decreases in weight and amylase content, and the normal diurnal pattern of synthesis and secretion is eliminated.

Conversely, chronically increased stimulation can cause an increase in glandular size. For example, increasing the bulk content of the food, which necessitates increased masticatory activity, results in hypertrophy of the rat parotid. Repeated amputation of the incisors, apparently acting reflexly through the superior cervical ganglion, also causes enlargement of the salivary glands. Treatment of mice and rats with isoproterenol, a $\beta$-adrenergic drug, causes several interesting changes in the salivary glands. A single injection results in the rapid and complete discharge of the stored secretory products and stimulation of protein synthesis; 20 to 30 hours after injection an increase in DNA synthesis and a wave of mitoses occurs. Daily injections of isoproterenol cause cellular hypertrophy and hyperplasia, resulting in glandular enlargement up to five times that of untreated animals. The effects on the salivary glands of isoproterenol and related adrenergic drugs have found wide application in experimental studies of cellular secretion and protein and nucleic acid synthesis.

## CONTROL OF SECRETION

The physiologic control of salivary glands secretion is mediated through the activity of the autonomic nervous system. The release of neurotransmitters from their storage sites (vesicles) in the nerve terminals adjacent to parenchymal cells stimulates them to discharge their secretory granules and secrete water and electrolytes. The molecular events that occur during this process, called stimulus-secretion coupling, have only recently begun to be elucidated. Although a number of conflicting observations have been reported, the following series of events is consistent with most of the experimental data. (1) Interaction of norepinephrine (or other $\beta$-adrenergic agents) with a specific receptor complex on the cell surface activates the enzyme adenyl cyclase, located in the plasma membrane. (2) Concomitantly, $Ca^{++}$ is mobilized from the plasma membrane and membrane permeability is increased, allowing influx of $Na^+$ and $Ca^{++}$, while efflux of $K^+$ occurs. This probably accounts for the observed hyperpolarization of the membrane potential. (3) Adenyl cyclase converts adenosine triphosphate (ATP) to cyclic adenosine $3',5'$-monophosphate (cyclic AMP), increasing its intracellular concentration ten- to twentyfold. (4) Cyclic AMP activates a protein kinase, an enzyme that in the presence of ATP phosphorylates additional proteins in the reaction chain leading to granule secretion. (5) The increase in intracellular $Ca^{++}$ may activate the phosphorylated proteins, and may also regulate adenyl cyclase activity. The concentration of $Ca^{++}$ is regulated by a specific $Ca^{++}$ "pump" located in the plasma membrane and an intracellular storage organelle, probably the mitochondria. (6) The secretory granules are translocated to the luminal surface, and their membranes fuse with it. (7) Cyclic AMP is hydrolyzed to inactive 5'-adenosine monophosphate by the enzyme phosphodiesterase.

There is some evidence that the phosphorylated proteins may be, or may interact with, microtubules or microfilaments, which would serve as a cytoskeletal framework or contractile mechanism for granule movement. Colchicine, a drug that disrupts microtubules, and cytochalasin B both inhibit amylase release from rat parotid gland in vitro. However, in other secretory cells, colchicine has no effect on secretion, and cytochalasin B may cause enhanced secretion. Furthermore, definite associations of microtubules and microfilaments with secretory granules have been observed only rarely in the electron microscope. Conclusions regarding the involvement of a microtubular-microfilament system in salivary secretion cannot be made at present.

Cholinergic stimulation of secretion is not mediated by cyclic AMP, nor is the release of $K^+$ that occurs with stimulation of $\alpha$-adrenergic receptors. Recent experiments on the pancreas suggest that cholinergic agents may act through a system similar to that for cyclic AMP, but involving cyclic guanosine 3',5'-monophosphate (cyclic GMP). These and other processes involved in exocrine secretion are currently under investigation in a number of laboratories.

## SALIVA: COMPOSITION AND FUNCTIONS

The most important function of the salivary glands is the production and secretion of saliva. At the outset, it is important to make a distinction between pure glandular secretions, collected by special devices from the ducts, and whole saliva obtained from the mouth, usually by expectoration. In addition to the components contributed by the glands, whole saliva contains desquamated oral epithelial cells, leukocytes, microorganisms and their products, fluid from the gingival sulcus, and food remnants. The total volume of saliva secreted daily by humans is approximately 750 ml., of which 60% to 70% is produced by the submandibular glands, 25% to 35% by the parotids, and about 5% or less from the sublinguals. These proportions may change considerably with stimulation of various intensities, however. Water accounts for 99% or more of the saliva; inorganic ions, secretory glycoproteins, certain serum constituents, and other substances make up the remaining 1% or less. The major inorganic ions of saliva are $Na^+$, $K^+$, $C^-$, and $HCO_3^-$; the levels of these ions are variable, depending on the type of stimulation and rate of salivary flow (see p. 353). Other ions found in smaller amounts include $Ca^{++}$, $Mg^{++}$, $HPO_4^-$, $I^-$ and $F^-$. The pH of whole saliva varies from 6.7 to about 7.4, whereas parotid saliva may vary over a greater range, from pH 6.0 to 7.8.

Secretory glycoproteins represent the main category of organic substances in the saliva. The enzymes found in the glandular secretions include amylase, ribonuclease, deoxyribonuclease, lysozyme, peroxidase, and acid phosphatase. At least four isoenzymes of amylase have been identified in man; two of these, representing 25% to 30% of the total amylase protein, have small amounts of bound carbohydrate. In contrast, the glycoproteins, or mucins, produced by the mucous cells of the submandibular and sublingual glands, may have up to 800 oligosaccharide groups attached to the protein core. Blood group substances, also glycoproteins, and blood clotting factors are found in saliva, as are serum albumin and certain immunoglobulins. Small organic molecules are present in saliva and include amino acids, urea, uric acid, various lipids, and corticosteroids.

Saliva participates in digestion by providing a fluid environment for solubilization of food and taste substances and through the action of its digestive enzymes, principally amylase. The action of amylase on ingested carbohydrates to produce glucose and maltose begins in the mouth and may continue for up to 30 minutes in the stomach, before the amylase is inactivated by the acid pH and proteolysis. The recent discovery of a lipolytic enzyme, produced by the lingual serous glands and capable of hydrolyzing triglycerides to diglycerides and fatty acids in the stomach, suggests that the digestion of dietary lipids may be initiated by the saliva.

Saliva also has several protective functions. It keeps the oral tissues moist, and the glycoproteins provide lubrication for the movement of tissues against each other. Saliva also helps to protect the teeth from dental caries. In disease states or conditions when the flow of saliva is reduced or absent, the incidence of caries increases. At least four proteins that are capable of inhibiting the growth of microorganisms and possibly preventing infection are found in saliva; however, the specific contribution of these substances to the protection of the oral cavity has not been determined. The secretion of peroxidase by the acinar cells and the concentration and secretion of iodide by the duct system establish a bactericidal system in saliva. In the presence of hydrogen peroxide, peroxidase can iodinate the tyrosine residues of bacterial proteins. Another antibacterial protein present in saliva is lysozyme, an enzyme that hydrolyzes the polysaccharide of bacterial cell membranes. Immunofluorescent staining suggests that lysozyme may be produced by the basally located cells of the intralobular striated ducts. The third group of defensive substances in saliva are the immunoglobulins. The predominant salivary immunoglobulin is IgA. It is produced in the glands by plasma cells located in the connective tissue stroma. Salivary IgA differs from serum IgA in that it is a dimer of two IgA molecules plus an additional glycoprotein called secretory component, which is apparently produced by the parenchymal cells. Secretory component, possibly acting as a specific receptor in the parenchymal cell membrane for dimeric IgA, may facilitate the transfer of the IgA to the lumen, either by translation in the cell membrane or by pinocytosis and secretion along with the secretory products of the parenchymal cells. Small amounts of IgG and IgM have also been detected in saliva, and occasional plasma cells in the stroma can be stained by fluorescent antibodies specific for these immunoglobulins. The fourth antibacterial substance is lactoferrin, an iron-binding protein. In the presence of specific antibody, lactoferrin that is not saturated with iron enhances the inhibitory effect of the antibody on the micro-organisms. Lactoferrin has been localized by immunofluorescent techniques to the serous cells of human parotid and submandibular glands.

The salivary glands of animals other than man have additional specialized functions, such as thermoregulation in mammals lacking sweat glands. In some reptiles and amphibians the homologous venom glands produce a variety of toxic substances. The salivary glands, as are many other tissues, are affected by secretions of the endocrine glands. The pronounced sexual dimorphism of the rodent submandibular gland has already been discussed. Thyroid and pituitary hormones have also been implicated in structural and functional changes of the salivary glands. The sodium and potassium content of saliva can be influenced by the administration of adrenocorticotropic hormone or mineralocorticoids, and alterations of salivary $Na^+ : K^+$ ratios are observed in patients with Addison's disease or Cushing's syndrome. There is also some evidence, though not yet thoroughly accepted, that the human parotid gland produces a hormone called parotin. Parotin is said to promote the growth of mesenchymal tissues; it also lowers serum calcium levels in rabbits, stimulates calcification of rat incisor dentin, and increases bone marrow temperature with an accompanying increase in circulating leukocytes. Other growth-promoting substances produced by certain salivary glands have already been considered.

## CLINICAL CONSIDERATIONS

An understanding of the anatomy, histology, and physiology of the salivary glands is essential for good dental practice. There is hardly any aspect of clinical practice in which salivary glands and saliva do not play an obvious or hidden role.

With the exception of a portion of the anterior part of hard palate, salivary glands are seen everywhere in the oral cavity. They may, by developmental coincidence, even be included within the jaws. In the mandible, this occurs in an area just posterior to the third molar teeth. In the maxilla, salivary glands may be present in the nasoplatine canal. Because of these features, lesions of salivary glands, including tumors, can occur almost anywhere within the mouth. In a differential diagnosis of oral lesions, therefore, a salivary gland origin must always be kept in mind.

The salivary glands in general, but the major glands in particular, undergo a striking change with age. This consists of a gradual replacement of parenchyma with fatty tissue and is most prominent in the parotid. Since the parotid is the major source of serous saliva, with advancing age, patients often complain of dryness and an increase in the viscosity of saliva. These changes in salivary flow may also contribute to the pain and atrophy of the oral mucosa.

The quality and quantity of saliva is believed to have a relationship to the incidence of dental caries. In diseases associated with reduction of flow the incidence of decay increases. Fluorides in the saliva are known to be taken up by the enamel surface. The enzymes as well as the antibacterial factors in the saliva have been investigated extensively, but their precise role in caries and gingival disease is as yet unknown.

The major salivary glands, specifically the parotid, are often associated with lymph nodes. This association is brought about by a common area of development of the cervical lymph nodes and the major salivary glands. Because of this association, pathologic conditions of the lymph nodes that are within these glands are often mistaken for salivary gland diseases. Cat-scratch disease and Mikulicz's disease are classic examples of this phenomenon.

The major salivary glands, but especially the parotid, may become enlarged in a variety of metabolic states such as starvation, protein deficiency, alcoholism, pregnancy, and liver disease. In such cases the treatment must consist of the removal of the cause rather than local therapy.

One of the most common surface lesions of the oral mucosa is a vesicular elevation called mucocele. This is produced from the severance of the duct of a minor salivary gland and pooling of the saliva in the tissues.

A blockage of the duct of a minor or major salivary gland occurs after the formation of a mucus or calcified plug within a duct. If this occurs in minor glands, it usually causes no symptoms, but in major glands such obstruction can be very painful and may require surgical treatment.

## REFERENCES

Amsterdam, A., Ohad, I., and Schramm, M.: Dynamic changes in the ultrastructure of the acinar cell of the rat parotid gland during the secretory cycle, J. Cell Biol. **41:** 753, 1969.

Archer, F. L., and Kao, V. C. Y.: Immunohistochemical identification of actomyosin in myoepithelium of human tissues, Lab. Invest. **18:**669, 1968.

Ball, W. D.: Development of the rat salivary glands. III. Mesenchymal specificity in the morphogenesis of the embryonic submaxillary and sublingual glands of the rat, J. Exp. Zool. **188:**277, 1974.

Batzri, S., Selinger, Z., Schramm, M., and Robinovitch, M. R.: Potassium release mediated by the epinephrine α-receptor in rat parotid slices. Properties and relation to enzyme secretion, J. Biol. Chem. **248:** 361, 1973.

Bdolah, A., and Schramm, M.: The function of 3'5'-cyclic AMP in enzyme secretion, Biochem. Biophys. Res. Commun. **18:**452, 1965.

Beaudoin, A. R., Marois, C., Dunnigan, J., and Morisset, J.: Biochemical reactions involved in pancreatic enzyme secretion. I. Activation of the adenylate cyclase complex, Can. J. Physiol. Pharmacol. **52:**174, 1974.

Bhaskar, S. N.: Synopsis of oral pathology, ed. 4, St. Louis, 1974, The C. V. Mosby Co.

Bhaskar, S. N.: Radiographic interpretation for the dentist, ed. 2, St. Louis, 1975, The C. V. Mosby Co.

Bienenstock, J., Tourville, D., and Tomasi, T. B., Jr.: The secretion of immunoglobulins by the human salivary glands. In Botelho, S. Y., Brooks, F. P., and Shelley, W. B., editors: The exocrine glands, Philadelphia, 1969, University of Pennsylvania Press, pp. 187-194.

Blair-West, J. R., Coghlan, J. P., Denton, D. A., and Wright, R. D.: Effect of endocrines on salivary glands. In Code, C. F., editor: Handbook of physiology, Section 6, vol. 2, Washington, D.C., 1967, American Physiological Society, pp. 633-664.

Brandtzaeg, P.: Mucosal and glandular distribution of immunoglobulin components: Differential localization of free and bound SC in secretory epithelial cells, J. Immunol. 112:1553, 1974.

Bullen, J. J., Rogers, H. J., and Griffiths, E.: Iron binding proteins and infection, Br. J. Haematol. 23:389, 1972.

Burgen, A. S. V., and Emmelin, N. G.: Physiology of the salivary glands, Baltimore, 1961, The Williams & Wilkins Co.

Case, R. M.: Cellular mechanisms controlling pancreatic exocrine secretion, Acta Hepato-Gastroenterol. 20:435, 1973.

Castle, J. D., Jamieson, J. D., and Palade, G. E.: Radioautographic analysis of the secretory process in the parotid acinar cell of the rabbit, J. Cell Biol. 53:290, 1972.

Chiang, T. S., Erdös, E. G., Miwa, I., Tague, L. L., and Coalson, J. J.: Isolation from a salivary gland of granules containing renin and kallikrein, Circ. Res. 23:507, 1968.

Ekfors, T. O., and Hopsu-Havu, V. K.: Immunofluorescent localization of trypsin-like esteropeptidases in the mouse submandibular gland, Histochem. J. 3:415, 1971.

Ekfors, T. O., Malmiharju, T., and Hopsu-Havu, V. K.: Isolation of six trypsin-like esteropeptidases from the mouse submandibular gland, Enzymologia 43:151, 1972.

Ellison, S. A.: Proteins and glycoproteins of saliva. In Code, C. F., editor: Handbook of physiology, Section 6, vol. 2, Washington, D.C., 1967, American Physiological Society, pp. 531-559.

Emmelin, N.: Nervous control of salivary glands. In Code, C. F., editor: Handbook of physiology, Section 6, vol. 2, Washington, D.C., 1967, American Physiological Society, pp. 595-632.

Feinstein, H., and Schramm, M.: Energy production in rat parotid gland. Relation to enzyme secretion and effects of calcium, Eur. J. Biochem. 13:158, 1970.

Franks, D. J., Perrin, L. S., and Malamud, D.: Calcium ion: A modulator of parotid adenylate acylase activity, FEBS Letters 42:267, 1974.

Garrett, J. R.: The innervation of normal human submandibular and parotid salivary glands. Demonstrated by cholinesterase histochemistry, catecholamine fluorescence and electron microscopy, Arch. Oral Biol. 12:1417, 1967.

Garrett, J. R.: Neuro-effector sites in salivary glands. In Emmelin, N., and Zotterman, Y., editors: Oral physiology, Oxford, 1972, Pergamon Press, pp. 83-97.

Grobstein, C.: Epithelio-mesenchymal specificity in the morphogenesis of mouse submandibular rudiments in vitro, J. Exp. Zool. 124:383, 1953.

Hall, H. D., and Schneyer, C. A.: Salivary gland atrophy in rat induced by liquid diet, Proc. Soc. Exp. Biol. Med. 117:789, 1964.

Hamosh, M., Klaeveman, H. L., Wolf, R. O., and Scow, R. O.: Pharyngeal lipase and digestion of dietary triglyceride in man, J. Clin. Invest. 55:908, 1975.

Hamosh, M., and Scow, R. O.: Lingual lipase and its role in the digestion of dietary fat, J. Clin. Invest. 52:88, 1973.

Hand, A. R.: The fine structure of von Ebner's gland of the rat, J. Cell Biol. 44:340, 1970.

Hand, A. R.: Morphology and cytochemistry of the Golgi apparatus of rat salivary gland acinar cells, Am. J. Anat. 130:141, 1971.

Hand, A. R.: Adrenergic and cholinergic nerve terminals in the rat parotid gland. Electron microscopic observations on permanganate-fixed glands, Anat. Rec. 173:131, 1972.

Hand, A. R.: Morphologic and cytochemical identification of peroxisomes in the rat parotid and other exocrine glands, J. Histochem. Cytochem. 21:131, 1973.

Ito, Y.: Parotin: A salivary gland hormone, Ann. New York Acad. Sci. 85:228, 1960.

Jamieson, J. D., and Palade, G. E.: Intracellular transport of secretory proteins in the pancreatic exocrine cell. I. Role of the peripheral elements of the Golgi complex, J. Cell Biol. 34:577, 1967.

Jamieson, J. D., and Palade, G. E.: Intracellular transport of secretory proteins in the pancreatic exocrine cell. II. Transport to condensing vacuoles and zymogen granules, J. Cell Biol. 34:597, 1967.

Jamieson, J. D., and Palade, G. E.: Intracellular transport of secretory proteins in the pancreatic exocrine cell. III. Dissociation of intracellular transport from protein synthesis, J. Cell Biol. **39**:580, 1968.

Jamieson, J. D., and Palade, G. E.: Intracellular transport of secretory proteins in the pancreatic exocrine cell. IV. Metabolic requirements, J. Cell Biol. **39**:589, 1968.

Jamieson, J. D., and Palade, G. E.: Condensing vacuole conversion and zymogen granule discharge in pancreatic exocrine cells: Metabolic studies, J. Cell Biol. **48**:503, 1971.

Johnson, D. A., and Sreebny, L. M.: Effect of food consistency and starvation on the diurnal cycle of the rat parotid gland, Arch. Oral Biol. **16**:177, 1971.

Johnson, D. A., and Sreebny, L. M.: Effect of increased mastication on the secretory process of the rat parotid gland, Arch. Oral Biol. **18**:1555, 1973.

Kauffman, D. L., Zager, N. I., Cohen, E., and Keller, P. J.: The isoenzymes of human parotid amylase, Arch. Biochem. Biophys. **137**:325, 1970.

Kim, S. K., Nasjleti, C. E., and Han, S. S.: The secretion processes in mucous and serous secretory cells of the rats sublingual gland, J. Ultrastruct. Res. **38**:371, 1972.

Klebanoff, S. J.: Iodination of bacteria: A bactericidal mechanism, J. Exp. Med. **126**:1063, 1967.

Klebanoff, S. J., and Luebke, R. G.: The antilactobacillus system of saliva. Role of salivary peroxidase, Proc. Soc. Exp. Biol. Med. **118**:483, 1965.

Kraus, F. W., and Mestecky, J.: Immunohistochemical localization of amylase, lysozyme and immunoglobulins in the human parotid gland, Arch. Oral Biol. **16**:781, 1971.

Kurtz, S. M.: The salivary glands. In Kurtz, S. M., editor: Electron microscopic anatomy, New York, 1964, Academic Press Inc., pp. 97-122.

Lawson, K. A.: The role of mesenchyme in the morphogenesis and functional differentiation of rat salivary epithelium, J. Embryol. Exp. Morphol. **27**:497, 1972.

Leeson, C. R.: Localization of alkaline phosphatase in the submaxillary gland of the rat, Nature **178**:858, 1956.

Leeson, C. R.: Structure of salivary glands. In Code, C. F., editor: Handbook of physiology, Section 6, vol. 2, Washington, D.C., 1967, American Physiological Society, pp. 463-495.

Levi-Montalcini, R., and Angeletti, P. U.: Nerve growth factor, Physiol. Rev. **48**:534, 1968.

Masson, P. L., Heremans, J. L., and Dive, C.: An iron-binding protein common to many external secretions, Clin. Chim. Acta **14**:735, 1966.

Mayo, J. W., and Carlson, D. M.: Protein composition of human submandibular secretions, Arch. Biochem. Biophys. **161**:134, 1974.

Mayo, J. W., and Carlson, D. M.: Isolation and properties of four α-amylase isozymes from human submandibular saliva, Arch. Biochem. Biophys. **163**:498, 1974.

Monnard, P., and Schorderet, M.: Cyclic adenosine 3',5'-monophosphate concentration in rabbit parotid slices following stimulation by secretagogues, Eur. J. Pharmacol. **23**:306, 1973.

Myant, N. B.: Iodine metabolism of salivary glands, Ann. New York Acad. Sci. **85**:208, 1960.

Neutra, M., and Leblond, C. P.: Synthesis of the carbohydrate of mucus in the Golgi complex shown by electron microscope radioautography of goblet cells from rats injected with glucose-$H^3$, J. Cell Biol. **30**:119, 1966.

Parks, H. F.: On the fine structure of the parotid gland of mouse and rat, Am. J. Anat. **108**:303, 1961.

Pedersen, G. L., and Petersen, O. H.: Membrane potential measurement in parotid acinar cells, J. Physiol. **234**:217, 1973.

Rasmussen, H.: Cell communication, calcium ion, and cyclic adenosine monophosphate, Science **170**:404, 1970.

Riva, A., Motta, G., and Riva-Testa, F.: Ultrastructural diversity in secretory granules of human major salivary glands, Am. J. Anat. **139**:293, 1974.

Riva, A., and Riva-Testa, F.: Fine structure of acinar cells of human parotid gland, Anat. Rec. **176**:149, 1973.

Robberecht, P., Deschodt-Lanckman, M., De Neef, P., Borgeat, P., and Christophe, J.: In vivo effects of pancreozymin, secretin, vasoactive intestinal polypeptide and pilocarpine on the levels of cyclic AMP and cyclic GMP in the rat pancreas, FEBS Letters **43**:139, 1974.

Rutberg, U.: Ultrastructure and secretory mechanisms of the parotid gland, Acta Odontol. **19**:suppl. 30, 1961.

Schneyer, C. A., and Hall, H. D.: Autonomic regulation of postnatal changes in cell number and size of rat parotid gland, Am. J. Physiol. **219**:1268, 1970.

Schneyer, L. H., and Schneyer, C. A.: Inorganic composition of saliva. In Code, C. F., editor: Handbook of physiology, section 6, vol. 2, Washington, D.C., 1967, American Physiological Society, pp. 497-530.

Schneyer, L. H., Young, J. A., and Schneyer, C. A.: Salivary secretion of electrolytes, Physiol. Rev. **52**:720, 1972.

Schramm, M.: Secretion of enzymes and other macromolecules, Annu. Rev. Biochem. **36**:307, 1967.

Schramm, M., and Naim, E.: Adenyl cyclase of rat parotid gland. Activation by fluoride and norepinephrine, J. Biol. Chem. **245**:3225, 1970.

Scott, B. L., and Pease, D. C.: Electron microscopy of the salivary and lacrimal glands of the rat, Am. J. Anat. **104**:115, 1959.

Selye, H., Veilleux, R., and Cantin, M.: Excessive stimulation of salivary gland growth by isoproterenol, Science **133**:44, 1961.

Shackleford, J. M., and Klapper, C. E.: Structure and carbohydrate histochemistry of mammalian salivary glands, Am. J. Anat. **111**:25, 1962.

Shackleford, J. M., and Schneyer, L. H.: Ultrastructural aspects of the main excretory duct of rat submandibular gland, Anat. Rec. **169**:679, 1971.

Shackleford, J. M., and Wilborn, W. H.: Ultrastructure of bovine parotid glands, J. Morphol. **127**:453, 1969.

Spooner, B. S., and Wessells, N. K.: An analysis of salivary gland morphogenesis: Role of cytoplasmic microfilaments and microtubules, Dev. Biol. **27**:38, 1972.

Sreebny, L. M., Johnson, D. A., and Robinovitch, M. R.: Functional regulation of protein synthesis in the rat parotid gland, J. Biol. Chem. **246**:3879, 1971.

Suddick, R. P., and Dowd, F. J.: The microvascular architecture of the rat submaxillary gland: Possible relationship to secretory mechanisms, Arch. Oral Biol. **14**:567, 1969.

Tamarin, A., Pickering, R., Johnson, D., and Robinovitch, M.: Correlative studies of biochemical and kinematic aspects of acinar secretion in dissociated rat parotid glands. In Han, S. S., Sreebny, L., and Suddick, R., editors: Symposium on the mechanism of exocrine secretion, Ann Arbor, 1973, University of Michigan Press, pp. 1-9.

Tamarin, A., and Sreebny, L. M.: The rat submaxillary salivary gland. A correlative study by light and electron microscopy, J. Morphol. **117**:295, 1965.

Tandler, B.: Ultrastructure of the human submaxillary gland. I. Architecture and histological relationships of the secretory cells, Am. J. Anat. **111**:287, 1962.

Tandler, B.: Ultrastructure of the human submaxillary gland. III. Myoepithelium, Z. Zellforsch. **68**:852, 1965.

Tandler, B., Denning, C. R., Mandel, I. D., and Kutscher, A. H.: Ultrastructure of human labial salivary glands. I. Acinar secretory cells, J. Morph. **127**:383, 1969.

Tandler, B., Denning, C. R., Mandel, I. D., and Kutscher, A. H.: Ultrastructure of human labial salivary glands. III. Myoepithelium and ducts, J. Morphol. **130**:227, 1970.

Tandler, B., and Erlandson, R. A.: Ultrastructure of the human submaxillary gland. IV. Serous granules, Am. J. Anat. **135**:419, 1972.

Taubman, M. A., and Smith, D. J.: Secretory immunoglobulins and dental disease. In Han, S. S., Sreebny, L., and Suddick, R., editors: Symposium on the mechanism of exocrine secretion, Ann Arbor, 1973, University of Michigan Press, pp. 152-172.

Taylor, T., and Erlandsen, S. L.: Peroxidase localization in von Ebner's gland of man, J. Dent. Res. **52**:635, 1973.

Tomasi, T. B., Jr., Tan, E. M., Solomon, A., and Prendergast, R. A.: Characteristics of an immune system common to certain external secretions, J. Exp. Med. **121**:101, 1965.

Wells, H.: Functional and pharmacological studies on the regulation of salivary gland growth. In Schneyer, L. H., and Schneyer, C. A., editors: Secretory mechanisms of salivary glands, New York, 1967, Academic Press Inc., pp. 178-190.

Young, J. A., and Martin, C. J.: Electrolyte transport in the excurrent duct system of the submaxillary gland. I. Studies on the intact gland. In Emmelin, N., and Zotterman, Y., editors: Oral physiology, Oxford, 1972, Pergamon Press, pp. 99-113.

# 11 Tooth eruption

## DEFINITION

Although the word eruption properly refers to the cutting of the tooth through the gum (from the Latin *erumpere,* meaning 'to break out') it is generally understood to mean the axial or occlusal movement of the tooth from its developmental position within the jaw to its functional position in the occlusal plane. However, eruption is only part of the total pattern of physiologic tooth movement, as teeth also undergo complex movements related to maintaining their position in the growing jaws and compensating for masticatory wear.

## PATTERN OF TOOTH MOVEMENT

*Preeruptive tooth movement.* When deciduous tooth germs first differentiate, there is a good deal of space between them. However, because of their rapid growth, this available space is utilized and the developing teeth become crowded together, especially in the incisor and canine region. This crowding is relieved by growth in the length of the infant jaws, which provides room for the second deciduous molars to drift backward and the anterior teeth to drift forward. At the same time the tooth germs also move outward as the jaws increase in width, and upward (downward in the upper jaw) as the jaws increase in height.

Permanent teeth with deciduous predecessors also undergo complex movements before they reach the position from which they will erupt (Chapter 12). For example, the permanent incisors and canines first develop lingual to the deciduous tooth germs at the level of their occlusal surfaces and in the same bony crypt. As their deciduous predecessors erupt, they move to a more apical position and occupy their own bony crypts (Fig. 11-1). Permanent premolars begin their development lingual to their predecessors at the level of their occlusal surfaces and in the same bony crypt. They also shift so that they are eventually situated in their own crypts beneath the divergent roots of the deciduous molars (Fig. 11-2).

The permanent molars, which have no deciduous predecessors, also move considerably from the site of their initial differentiation. For example, the upper permanent molars, which develop in the tuberosity of the maxilla, at first have their occlusal surfaces facing distally (Fig. 11-3) and swing round only when the maxilla has grown sufficiently to provide the necessary space. Similarly, mandibu-

**361**

lar molars develop with their occlusal surfaces inclined mesially and only become upright as room becomes available. All these movements are linked to jaw growth and may be considered as movements positioning the tooth and its crypt within the jaws preparatory to tooth eruption.

*Eruptive tooth movement.* During this phase the tooth moves from its position within the bone of the jaw to its functional position in occlusion and the principal direction of movement is occlusal or axial. However, it is important to recognize that because jaw growth continues during the replacement of the deciduous dentition by the permanent dentition, movements in planes other than axial are superimposed on eruptive movement.

*Posteruptive tooth movement.* Posteruptive tooth movements are those that (1) maintain the position of the erupted tooth while the jaw continues to grow and (2) compensate for occlusal and proximal wear. The former movement, like eruptive movement, occurs principally in an axial direction so as to keep pace with the increase in height of the jaws. It involves both the tooth and its socket and ceases when jaw growth is completed. The movements compensating

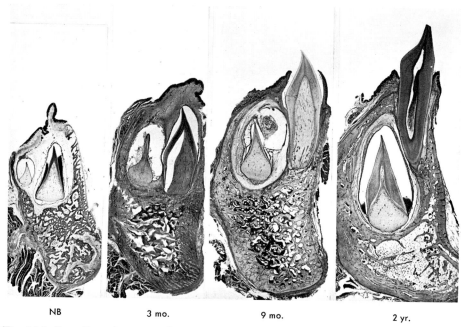

|   NB   |   3 mo.   |   9 mo.   |   2 yr.   |

**Fig. 11-1.** Buccolingual sections through central incisor region of mandible at representative stages of development from birth to 9 years of age. At birth both the deciduous and permanent tooth germs occupy the same bony crypt. Notice how, by excentric growth and eruption of the deciduous tooth, the permanent tooth germ comes to occupy its own bony crypt apical to erupted incisor. At 4½ years, resorption of deciduous incisor has begun. At 6 years, the deciduous incisor has been shed and its successor is erupting. Notice active deposition of new bone at base of socket at this time.

for occlusal and proximal wear continue throughout life and consist of axial and mesial migration respectively.

## HISTOLOGY OF TOOTH MOVEMENT

*Preeruptive phase.* During this phase, movement of the developing tooth germ is achieved in two ways. First there is a total bodily movement of the germ and second there is its excentric growth. Excentric growth means that one part of the developing tooth germ remains stationary while the remainder continues to grow leading to a shift in its center. This type of movement explains, for example, how the deciduous incisors maintain their superficial position as the jaws grow in height (Fig. 11-1). Histologically preeruptive tooth movement is reflected in the pattern of bony remodeling of the crypt wall. Thus during bodily movement of the tooth, osteoclastic bone resorption occurs on the surface of the crypt wall in advance of the moving tooth while bone deposition occurs on the

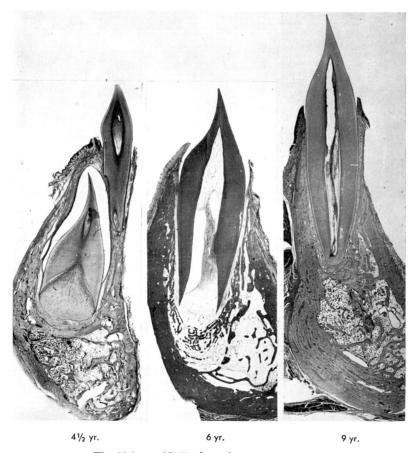

4½ yr.　　　　　　6 yr.　　　　　　9 yr.

**Fig. 11-1, cont'd.** For legend see opposite page.

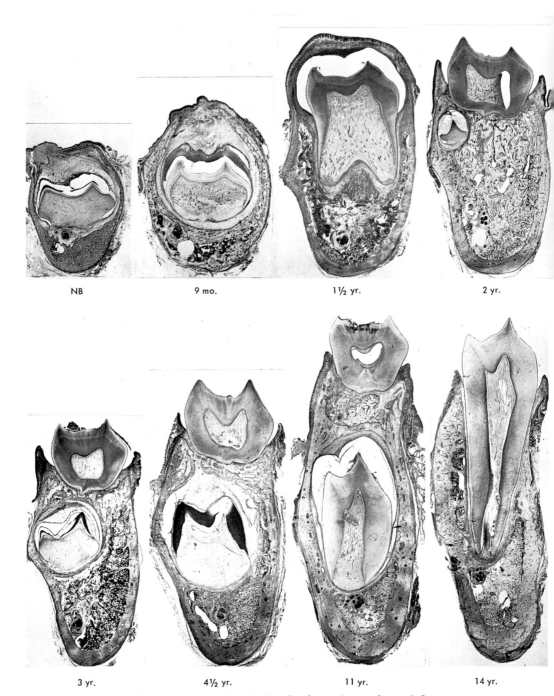

NB   9 mo.   1½ yr.   2 yr.

3 yr.   4½ yr.   11 yr.   14 yr.

**Fig. 11-2.** Buccolingual sections through the deciduous first molar and first permanent pre-molar of the mandible at representative stages of development from birth to 14 years. Notice how permanent tooth germ shifts its position. In the section of the 4½ year mandible, gubernacular canal is clearly visible. Lack of roots in the 2, 3, 4½, and 11 year sections is not the result of resorption but of the section's being cut in midline of tooth with widely divergent roots.

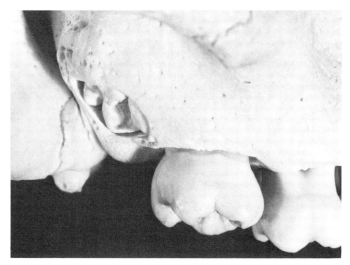

**Fig. 11-3.** Region of maxillary tuberosity of dried skull of 4-year-old child. At this stage of development the first permanent molar is still within its bony crypt. Notice how occlusal surface faces backward. With further growth of maxilla the molar swings down so that it eventually erupts into the occlusal plane.

crypt wall behind it. During excentric movement bone resorption is seen on the surface of the crypt that faces the growing tooth germ.

*Eruptive phase.* During this phase significant developmental changes occur and they include the formation of the roots, periodontal ligament and dentogingival junction of the tooth.

Root formation is initiated by proliferation of Hertwig's epithelial root sheath (Chapter 2). The forming root first grows toward the floor of the bony crypt and, as a result, there is resorption of bone in this location to provide room for the advancing root tip. However, with the onset of eruptive tooth movement (probably coincident with periodontal ligament formation) space is created for the forming root, and resorption no longer occurs on the floor of the crypt. Indeed, in some instances, the distance moved by the tooth outstrips the rate of root formation and bone deposition occurs on the crypt floor (Fig. 11-4).

As the roots form, important changes that are associated with the development of the supporting apparatus of the tooth occur in the dental follicle. There is bone deposition on the crypt wall, cement deposition on the newly formed root surface, and organization of a periodontal ligament from the dental follicle (Chapter 7). These changes lag behind root formation.

Significant changes occur within the tissues that cover the erupting tooth. There is a loss of the intervening connective tissue between the reduced enamel epithelium covering the crown of the tooth and the overlying oral epithelium. Because of this loss the two epithelia proliferate and form a solid plug of cells in advance of the erupting tooth. The central cells of this epithelial mass degenerate

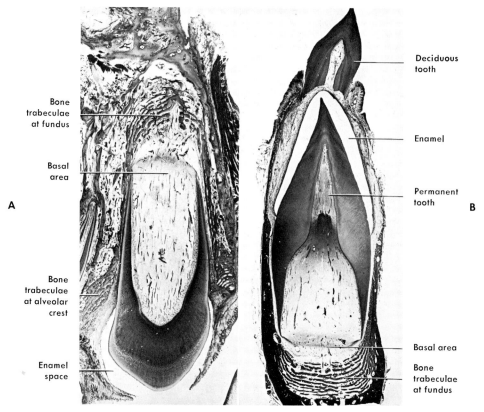

Bone
trabeculae
at fundus

Basal
area

A

Bone
trabeculae
at alveolar
crest

Enamel
space

Deciduous
tooth

Enamel

Permanent
tooth

B

Basal area

Bone
trabeculae
at fundus

**Fig. 11-4.** Erupting upper deciduous canine, **A**, and lower permanent canine, **B**. Note formation of numerous parallel bone trabeculae at alveolar fundus. Formation of bone trabeculae at alveolar crest of deciduous canine, **A**, is a sign of rapid growth of maxilla in height. (From Kronfeld, R.: Dent. Cosmos **74**:103, 1932.)

and form an epithelium-lined canal through which the tooth erupts without any hemorrhage. This epithelial cell mass is also involved in the generation of the dentogingival junction (Chapter 9).

Once the tooth has broken through the oral mucosa, it continues to erupt at the same rate until it reaches the occlusal plane and meets its antagonist. Immediate and rapid eruptive movements then cease. Root formation, however, is not yet complete, and because further occlusal movement is restricted, additional root growth is accommodated by removal of bone on the socket floor.

The above description generally applies to all teeth. Successional teeth, however, possess an additional anatomic feature, the *gubernacular canal* and its contents the *gubernacular cord*, which may have an influence on eruptive tooth movement. When the successional tooth germ first develops within the same crypt as its deciduous predecessor, bone surrounds both tooth germs but does not completely close over them. As the deciduous tooth erupts, the permanent tooth germ becomes situated apically and entirely enclosed by bone (Figs. 11-1 and

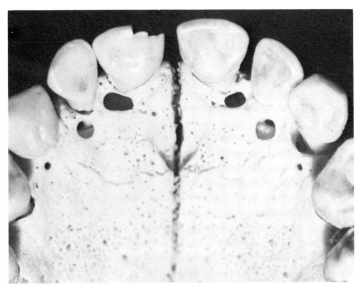

**Fig. 11-5.** Incisor region of dried mandible of 4-year-old child. Notice the foramina lingual to deciduous teeth. These are the gubernacular canals.

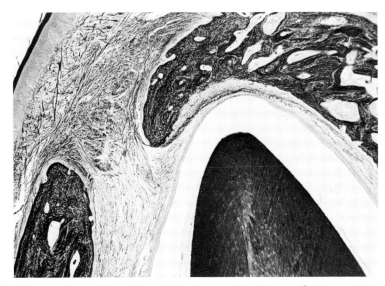

**Fig. 11-6.** Gubernacular cord consists mainly of connective tissue and often contains a central strand of epithelium surrounded by connective tissue.

11-2) except for a small canal which contains remnants of dental lamina and connective tissue. Together, these structures are termed the *gubernacular cord* (Figs. 11-5 and 11-6). This cord may have a function in guiding the permanent tooth as it erupts.

A problem associated with tooth eruption is to explain how the collagen fiber bundles of the periodontal ligament readjust to permit movement between tooth and alveolar bone. It has been suggested that there is an intermediate plexus within the periodontal ligament in which remodeling of the ligament fiber bun-

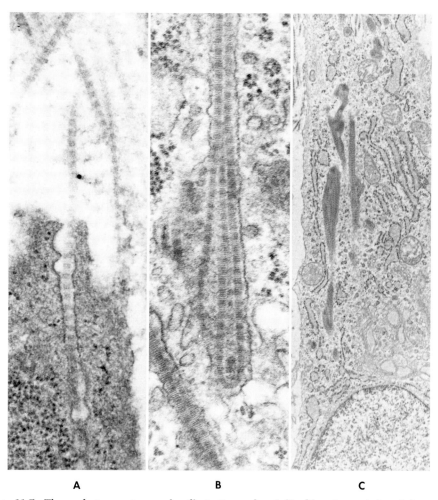

**A**                    **B**                    **C**

**Fig. 11-7.** Three electron micrographs illustrating role of fibroblast in periodontal ligament remodeling and turnover. **A,** Phagocytosis (ingestion) of collagen fibril. Once within the fibroblast, lysosomes containing catabolic enzymes fuse with the vesicle containing the collagen, **B,** and degradation continues in phagolysosomes, **C.** (From Ten Cate, A. R.: Anat. Rec. **182:**1, 1975.)

dles occurs without any necessity to continually reembed their terminal ends in cement and bone. However, it is doubtful whether such a plexus exists, as no evidence for it can be detected in the periodontal ligament of the actively erupting tooth using the high magnifications provided by the electron microscope (Chapter 7). This instrument has been able to show, however, that many of the fibroblasts of the ligament are actively ingesting and degrading old collagen fibrils while, at the same time, forming new collagen fibrils (Fig. 11-7). Fibroblasts with such characteristics are found across the entire width of the periodontal ligament, and there is no evidence for their concentration in an intermediate zone. Also studies using tritiated proline as a marker have shown that there is a high rate of collagen remodeling across the entire width of the ligament. Thus it is through the remodeling of the fibrils in the fiber bundle of the periodontal ligament by the fibroblasts that the ligament adjusts to the eruption of the tooth. This activity occurs throughout the periodontal ligament rather than being an isolated area, which was once called the intermediate plexus.

*Posteruptive phase.* Those movements the tooth makes after eruption to accommodate for further jaw growth represent a total movement of the tooth and its socket. The principal movement is in an axial direction to keep pace with the increase in height of the jaws and is brought about by the active deposition of new bone at the alveolar crest and at the base of the socket.

Then there are those movements made to compensate for occlusal and proximal wear of the tooth. It is generally assumed that the continuous deposition of cement around the apices of the roots of teeth is sufficient to compensate for occlusal wear. However, there is no evidence that this deposition of cement actually moves the tooth. It is more likely that the forces causing tooth eruption, discussed later in this chapter, are still available to bring about sufficient axial movement of the tooth to compensate for occlusal wear. The cement deposition that occurs is probably an infilling phenomenon.

Wear also takes place at the contact points between teeth, and to maintain tooth contact, mesial or proximal drift takes place. Histologically this is seen as a selective deposition and resorption of bone on the socket walls. The ligament of the functioning tooth, like that of the erupting tooth, has a high rate of remodeling and also possesses fibroblasts, which are simultaneously synthesizing and degrading collagen. There is thus no reason to suppose that ligament remodeling to accommodate for mesial drift differs in any way from the ligament remodeling that occurs during eruption.

## MECHANISM OF TOOTH MOVEMENT

The mechanism or mechanisms that determine and bring about tooth movement are not properly understood. How preeruptive tooth movements are determined is unknown and the facile explanation is to attribute a genetic basis to them.

A good deal more is known about the possible mechanisms responsible for eruptive tooth movement. Although many theories have been proposed, only four merit serious consideration. They are (1) root growth, (2) vascular pressure, (3) bone growth, and (4) ligament traction. Briefly stated, the theory of root growth supposes that the proliferating root impinges upon a fixed base thus converting an apically directed force into occlusal movement; the vascular pressure theory supposes that a local increase in tissue fluid pressure in the periapical region is sufficient to move the tooth; bony remodeling supposes that selective deposition and resorption of bone brings about eruption; finally, the ligament traction theory proposes that the cells and fibers of the ligament pull the tooth into occlusion.

As a result of elegant and careful studies with bone markers, it now seems certain that selective bone deposition and resorption around the roots of moving teeth is the result of, not the cause of, tooth movement and therefore need not be discussed further.

Root formation is also unlikely to be the cause of tooth eruption although at first glance this may seem to be an obvious mechanism. It has long been recognized that some teeth move a greater distance than the length of their fully formed roots. If root formation is responsible for eruption, it would be expected that the onset of root formation and eruptive movement would coincide, but, as has already been stated, the onset of root formation is not synchronous with the onset of axial tooth movement. Indeed initial root formation results in bone resorption at the base of the socket. This is a very important observation, for it illustrates a fundamental point of bone biology, which is that when pressure is applied to bone it is removed by osteoclastic action. Thus, for root formation to result in an eruptive force, the apical growth of the root needs to be translated into occlusal movement and requires the presence of a fixed base. No such fixed base exists. The bone at the base of the socket cannot act as a fixed base for, as we have seen, pressure on bone results in its resorption. Advocates seeking in root growth the mechanism for tooth eruption postulated the existence of a ligament, the cushioned-hammock ligament, straddling the base of the socket from one bony wall to the other like a sling. Its function was to provide a fixed base for the growing root to react against. Unfortunately the structure described as the cushioned-hammock ligament is the pulp-delineating membrane that runs across the apex of the tooth and has no bony insertion. It cannot act as a fixed base.

Experiments also indicate the improbability of root growth providing the force for tooth eruption. Before the discussion of these experiments a slight note of caution is warranted, as most of them have been carried out on the continuously erupting rodent incisor (Fig. 11-8). Although eruption is a basic mammalian phenomenon and although there is no reason to suspect any species difference, one must recognize that these experimental findings are being extrapolated to human tooth eruption.

If the incisor is prevented from erupting, root growth still continues and is

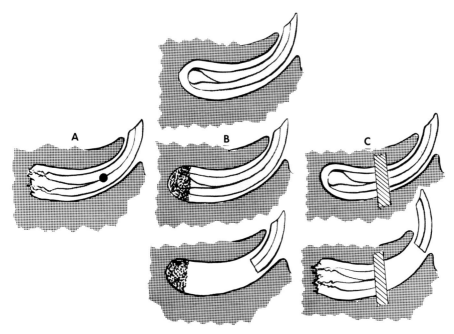

**Fig. 11-8.** Diagram summarizing some of the experimental work undertaken on continuously erupting rodent incisor. As this tooth erupts continuously, dental tissues are also continually being generated at base of tooth. If tooth is pinned, **A**, eruptive movement is prevented and the continual generation of new dental tissue results in a buckling of the root and a resorption of bone at base of socket. If, on the other hand, the basal generative tissues are removed surgically, **B**, the distal fragment of the tooth continues to erupt and undergoes eventual exfoliation. **C**, Combination of both experiments. Here, incisor is cut in half and an artificial rigid barrier is inserted between the two halves. The distal fragment continues to erupt and is eventually shed. The proximal fragment can no longer erupt, and as a result the growing end buckles and also retreats.

accommodated by reabsorption of bone at the base of the socket and some buckling of the newly formed dental tissues (Fig. 11-8, *A*). This situation is very much akin to the start of root formation in teeth of limited growth such as those of man where, with the onset of root formation and the absence of occlusal movement, bone resorption occurs in the socket floor. It is also similar to impaction of developing human third molars. When this occurs, the roots grow into bone and become deformed. This experiment tells us that root formation does indeed generate a force. However, if the periapical tissues of the incisor i.e., Hertwig's epithelial root sheath, proliferating papilla cells, and the apical portion of the periodontal ligament, are removed surgically, eruption of the distal portion of the tooth continues, with eventual exfoliation even though no further root formation takes place (Fig. 11-8, *B*). This result tells us that root formation is not responsible for eruptive movement. A variation of this experiment is to transect the incisor and place a barrier (plaster of paris gauze) between the two halves of the tooth. This has the effect of isolating the active cellular elements of the tooth from the distal fragment. The distal fragments erupt (Fig. 11-8, *C*). This experiment indicates that the force of eruption most likely is generated within the periodontal ligament, as this is the only tissue remaining in association with the distal fragment. The last two experiments would also seem to suggest that tissue fluid pressure is not responsible for tooth movement, as the periapical vasculature has either been eliminated or isolated. However, there is the slight possibility that an accumulation of tissue fluid, as a result of the surgical inter-ference, might occur and be sufficient to cause tooth movement. Tissue fluid pressure as an eruptive force must always be considered, as direct measurements have been made of the pressures below and above erupting, but as yet unerupted, teeth in the dog. A pressure differential, which could be sufficient to cause tooth movement, exists between the two.

There is further evidence to indicate the periodontal ligament as the prime mover of teeth in an axial direction. The fact that the collagen of the periodontal ligament has a high rate of turnover has already been referred to. It is possible to interfere specifically with ligament turnover by halting collagen synthesis and in turn distort the normal architecture of the ligament. When this is done, eruptive movements are retarded, with consequent buckling of the growing roots and resorption of the socket floor—a result similar to pinning of the incisor. The result of all these experiments indicate that eruption takes place so long as liga-ment tissue is present and its architecture is undisturbed. Although the ligament is indicated as the prime mover of teeth, it is still not known how a tractile force is generated within this tissue. Two possibilities have been suggested. First, in some way the synthesis of collagen involves contraction, and second, the fibroblasts provide the contractile force. The latter suggestion is biologically the most feasible as isolated fibroblasts have been shown to have contractile proper-ties and also to be responsible for the contraction that occurs during wound repair.

With respect to posteruptive movements of the tooth, the mechanisms for moving the tooth axially during eruption are most likely utilized to compensate for occlusal wear.

The mechanism of mesial or proximal drift is understood. The forces bringing about this movement are the forces of mastication resolved in a mesial direction by the inclined planes of the tooth cusps. They are controlled by the transseptal ligaments, which connect adjacent teeth.

## CLINICAL CONSIDERATIONS

From all that has been written so far in this chapter it should be evident that the principal supporting tissues of the tooth, the periodontal ligament and the bone of the jaw, possess a remarkable "plasticity" that enables the tooth to react either favorably or unfavorably to its immediate environment. This "plasticity" of the supporting tissues is utilized by the orthodontist to achieve a favorable clinical response. By applying forces to the tooth and by relying on the biologic

**Table 5.** Chronology of human dentition*

| Tooth | | Formation of enamel matrix and dentin begins | Amount of enamel matrix formed at birth | Enamel completed | Emergence into oral cavity | Root completed |
|---|---|---|---|---|---|---|
| **Primary dentition** | | | | | | |
| Maxillary | Central incisor | 4 mo. in utero | Five-sixths | 1½ mo. | 7½ mo. | 1½ yr. |
| | Lateral incisor | 4½ mo. in utero | Two-thirds | 2½ mo. | 9 mo. | 2 yr. |
| | Canine | 5 mo. in utero | One-third | 9 mo. | 18 mo. | 3¼ yr. |
| | First molar | 5 mo. in utero | Cusps united | 6 mo. | 14 mo. | 2½ yr. |
| | Second molar | 6 mo. in utero | Cusp tips still isolated | 11 mo. | 24 mo. | 3 yr. |
| Mandibular | Central incisor | 4½ mo. in utero | Three-fifths | 2½ mo. | 6 mo. | 1½ yr. |
| | Lateral incisor | 4½ mo. in utero | Three-fifths | 3 mo. | 7 mo. | 1½ yr. |
| | Canine | 5 mo. in utero | One-third | 9 mo. | 16 mo. | 3¼ yr. |
| | First molar | 5 mo. in utero | Cusps united | 5½ mo. | 12 mo. | 2¼ yr. |
| | Second molar | 6 mo. in utero | Cusp tips still isolated | 10 mo. | 20 mo. | 3 yr. |
| **Permanent dentition** | | | | | | |
| Maxillary | Central incisor | 3-4 mo. | | 4-5 yr. | 7-8 yr. | 10 yr. |
| | Lateral incisor | 10-12 mo. | | 4-5 yr. | 8-9 yr. | 11 yr. |
| | Canine | 4-5 mo. | | 6-7 yr. | 11-12 yr. | 13-15 yr. |
| | First premolar | 1½-1¾ yr. | | 5-6 yr. | 10-11 yr. | 12-13 yr. |
| | Second premolar | 2-2¼ yr. | | 6-7 yr. | 10-12 yr. | 12-14 yr. |
| | First molar | At birth | Sometimes a trace | 2½-3 yr. | 6-7 yr. | 9-10 yr. |
| | Second molar | 2½-3 yr. | | 7-8 yr. | 12-13 yr. | 14-16 yr. |
| | Third molar | 7-9 yr. | | 12-16 yr. | 17-21 yr. | 18-25 yr. |
| Mandibular | Central incisor | 3-4 mo. | | 4-5 yr. | 6-7 yr. | 9 yr. |
| | Lateral incisor | 3-4 mo. | | 4-5 yr. | 7-8 yr. | 10 yr. |
| | Canine | 4-5 mo. | | 6-7 yr. | 9-10 yr. | 12-14 yr. |
| | First premolar | 1¾-2 yr. | | 5-6 yr. | 10-12 yr. | 12-13 yr. |
| | Second premolar | 2¼-2½ yr. | | 6-7 yr. | 11-12 yr. | 13-14 yr. |
| | First molar | At birth | Sometimes a trace | 2½-3 yr. | 6-7 yr. | 9-10 yr. |
| | Second molar | 2½-3 yr. | | 7-8 yr. | 11-13 yr. | 14-15 yr. |
| | Third molar | 8-10 yr. | | 12-16 yr. | 17-21 yr. | 18-25 yr. |

*From Logan, W. H. G., and Kronfeld, R.: J. Am. Dent. Assoc. **20:**379, 1933; slightly modified by McCall and Schour.

responses of bone and periodontal ligament, malalignment of teeth can often be corrected.

Table 5 gives the time of tooth emergence, and one should note that there is considerable variation in these times. However, only teeth emerging significantly outside these ranges should be considered as abnormal and indicative of some fault in eruptive movement. By far the greatest number of aberrations in eruption times are delayed eruptive movements. Premature eruption of teeth occurs infrequently. Sometimes infants are born with "erupted" lower central incisors, but this is an example of gross maldevelopment. Such teeth need to be extracted as soon as possible because they prevent suckling. Premature loss of a deciduous tooth without closure of the gap may lead to early eruption of its successor. Far more common, however, is the occurrence of delayed or retarded eruption. This may be caused by either local or systemic factors. Systemic factors are those such as nutritional, genetic, or endocrine deficiencies. Local factors may be a loss of a deciduous tooth and drifting of opposing teeth to block the eruptive pathway. Severe trauma may eliminate the dental follicle, and hence periodontal ligament formation is prevented. When this happens, the bone of the jaw fuses with tooth, a condition known as ankylosis and eruption is not possible.

The Caucasian exhibits an evolutionary trend to a diminution in the size of the jaws. This trend has not been accompanied by a corresponding decrease in the size of the teeth, and as a result crowding is a common occurrence. The third molars are the last teeth to erupt and frequently all the available space has been utilized. As a result these teeth become impacted. Canines are also often impacted because of their late eruption time. Finally, it has been shown that the moment a tooth breaks through the oral epithelium an acute inflammatory response occurs in the connective tissue adjacent to the tooth. This is seen even in the germ-free animals and is seen in varying degrees around all teeth throughout life. Clinically, as teeth break through the oral mucosa, there is often some pain, slight fever, and general malaise, all signs of an inflammatory process. In infants these symptoms are popularly called "teething." Whether the inflammatory response associated with eruption is responsible for these symptoms has not been established. It has been suggested that these symptoms represent primary infections with the herpes simplex virus.

## REFERENCES

Berkovitz, B. K. B., and Thomas, N. R.: Unimpeded eruption in the root resected lower incisor of the rat with a preliminary note on root transection, Arch. Oral Biol. **14:**771, 1969.

Berkovitz, B. K. B.: The effect of root transection and partial root resection on the unimpeded eruption rate of the rat incisor, Arch. Oral Biol. **16:**1033, 1971.

Berkovitz, B. K. B.: The healing process in the incisor tooth socket of the rat following root resection and exfoliation, Arch. Oral Biol. **16:**1045, 1971.

Berkovitz, B. K. B.: The effect of preventing eruption on the proliferative basal tissues of the rat lower incisor, Arch. Oral Biol. **17:**1279, 1972.

Brash, J. C.: The growth of the alveolar bone and its relation to the movements of the teeth, including eruption, Int. J. Orthod. Oral Surg. Radiogr. **14:**196, 283, 398, 487, 494, 1928.

Brodie, A. G.: The growth of alveolar bone

and the eruption of the teeth, Oral Surg. **1**:342, 1948.

Bryer, L. W.: An experimental evaluation of physiology of tooth eruption, Int. Dent. J. **7**:432, 1957.

Cahill, D. R.: The histology and rate of tooth eruption with and without temporary impaction in the dog, Anat. Rec. **166**:225, 1970.

Cahill, D. R.: Histological changes in the bony crypt and gubernacular canal of erupting permanent premolars during deciduous premolar exfoliation in beagles, J. Dent. Res. **53**:786, 1974.

Carollo, D. A., Hoffman, R. L., and Brodie, A. G.: Histology and function of the dental gubernacular cord, Angle Orthod. **41**:300, 1971.

Herzberg, F., and Schour, I.: Effects of the removal of pulp and Hertwig's sheath on the eruption of incisors in the albino rat, J. Dent. Res. **20**:264, 1941.

Jenkins, G. N.: The physiology of the mouth, ed. 3, Oxford, 1966, Blackwell Scientific Publications Ltd.

Logan, W. H. G., and Kronfeld, R.: Development of the human jaws and surrounding structures from birth to the age of fifteen years, J. Am. Dent. Assoc. **20**:379, 1933.

Magnusson, B.: Tissue changes during molar tooth eruption, Trans. R. Sch. Dent. Stockholm **13**:1, 1968.

Main, J. H. P.: A histological survey of the hammock ligament, Arch. Oral Biol. **10**:343, 1965.

Main, J. H. P., and Adams, D.: Experiments on the rat incisor into the cellular proliferation and blood pressure theories of tooth eruption, Arch. Oral Biol. **11**:163, 1966.

Manson, J. D.: Bone changes associated with tooth eruption. In The mechanisms of tooth support, a symposium, Oxford, 6-8 July, 1965, Bristol, 1967, John Wright & Sons, Ltd.

Moss, J. P., and Picton, D. C. A.: Mesial drift of teeth in adult monkeys *(Macaca irus)* when forces from the cheeks and tongue had been eliminated, Arch. Oral Biol. **15**:979, 1970.

Orban, B.: Growth and movement of the tooth germs and teeth, J. Am. Dent. Assoc. **15**:1004, 1928.

Sicher, H.: Tooth eruption: The axial movement of continuously growing teeth, J. Dent. Res. **21**:201, 1942.

Sicher, H.: Tooth eruption: The axial movement of teeth with limited growth, J. Dent. Res. **21**:395, 1942.

Sicher, H., and Weinmann, J. P.: Bone growth and physiological tooth movement, Am. J. Orthod. **30**:109, 1944.

Taylor, A. C., and Butcher, E. O.: The regulation of eruption rate in the incisor teeth of the white rat, J. Exp. Zool. **117**:165, 1951.

Ten Cate, A. R.: The mechanism of tooth eruption. In Melcher, A. H., and Bowen, W. H., editors: The biology of the periodontium, New York, 1969, Academic Press Inc.

Ten Cate, A. R.: Physiological resorption of connective tissue associated with tooth eruption. An electron microscope study, J. Periodont. Res. **6**:168, 1971.

Ten Cate, A. R.: Morphological studies of fibrocytes in connective tissue undergoing rapid remodelling, J. Anat. **112**:401, 1972.

Thomas, N. R.: The properties of collagen in the periodontium of an erupting tooth. In The mechanisms of tooth support, a symposium, Oxford, 6-8 July, 1965, Bristol, 1967, John Wright & Sons, Ltd.

Thomas, N. R.: The effect of inhibition of collagen maturation on eruption in rats, J. Dent. Res. **44**:1159, 1969.

Weinmann, J. P.: Bone changes related to eruption of the teeth, Angle Orthod. **11**:83, 1941.

# 12 Shedding of deciduous teeth

## DEFINITION

The human dentition, like those of most mammals, consists of two generations. The first generation is known as the deciduous (primary) dentition and the second as the permanent (secondary) dentition. The necessity for two dentitions exists because infant jaws are small and the size and number of teeth they can support is limited. Since teeth, once formed, cannot increase in size, a second dentition, consisting of larger and more teeth, is required for the larger jaws of the adult. The physiologic process resulting in the elimination of the deciduous dentition is called *shedding* or *exfoliation*.

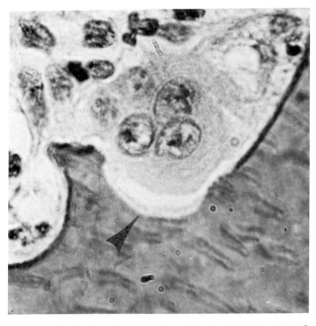

**Fig. 12-1.** Photomicrograph of odontoclast resorbing dentin. Note brush border *(arrow)* where odontoclast is in contact with dentin. (From Furseth, R.: Arch. Oral Biol. **13:**417, 1968.)

## PATTERN OF SHEDDING

The shedding of deciduous teeth is the result of a progressive resorption of the roots by specialized cells called odontoclasts (Fig. 12-1). In general, the pressure generated by the growing and erupting permanent tooth dictates the pattern of deciduous tooth resorption. At first this pressure is directed against the root surface of the deciduous tooth itself (Fig. 12-2). Because of the developmental position of the permanent incisor and canine tooth germs and their subsequent physiologic movement in an occlusal and vestibular direction, resorption of the roots of the deciduous incisors and canines begins on their lingual surfaces (Fig. 12-3). Later, these developing tooth germs occupy a position directly apical to the deciduous tooth, which permits them to erupt in the position formerly occupied by the deciduous tooth (Fig. 12-4). Frequently, however, and especially

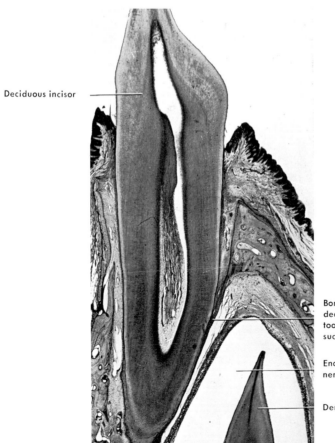

Deciduous incisor

Bone between deciduous tooth and successor

Enamel of permanent incisor

Dentin

**Fig. 12-2.** Thin lamella of bone separates a permanent tooth germ from its predecessor.

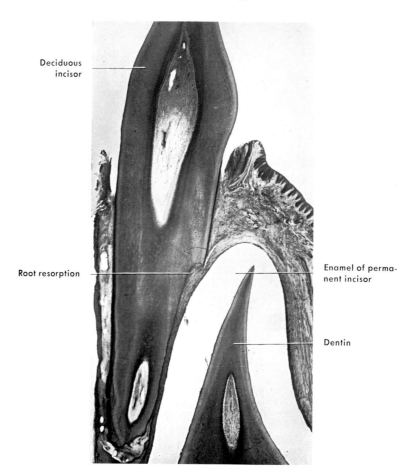

Deciduous
incisor

Root resorption

Enamel of perma-
nent incisor

Dentin

**Fig. 12-3.** Resorption of lingual aspect of root of deciduous incisor caused by pressure of erupting successor.

in the case of the permanent mandibular incisors, this apical positioning of the tooth germs does not occur and the permanent tooth erupts lingual to the still functioning deciduous tooth (Fig. 12-5).

Resorption of the roots of deciduous molars often first begins on their inner surfaces as the early developing bicuspids are found between them (Fig. 12-6). This resorption occurs long before the deciduous molars are shed and reflects the expansion of their growing permanent successors. However, as a result of the continued growth of the jaws and occlusal movement of the deciduous molars, the successional tooth germs come to lie apical to the deciduous molars (Fig. 12-7). This change in position provides the growing bicuspids with adequate space for their continued development and also relieves the pressure on the roots of the overlying deciduous molars. The areas of early resorption are repaired by the deposition of a cementum-like tissue. When the bicuspids begin

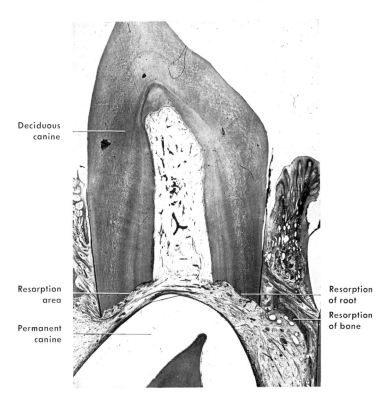

Deciduous
canine

Resorption
area

Permanent
canine

Resorption
of root

Resorption
of bone

**Fig. 12-4.** Resorption of root of deciduous canine. Note apical position of permanent successor. (From Kronfeld, R.: Dent. Cosmos **74**:103, 1932.)

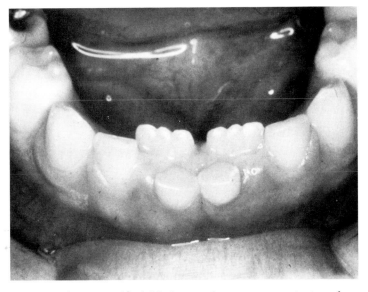

**Fig. 12-5.** Dentition of six-year-old child showing how permanent incisors frequently erupt lingually to deciduous incisors before the latter teeth are shed.

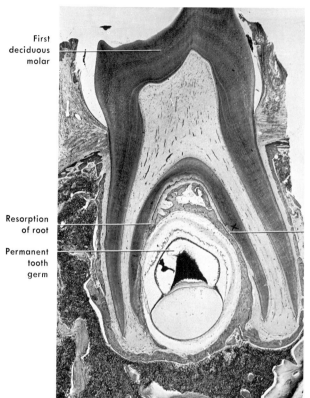

First deciduous molar

Resorption of root

Permanent tooth germ

Repaired resorption of dentin (X)

**Fig. 12-6.** Germ of lower first permanent premolar between roots of first deciduous molar. Repair of previously resorbed dentin has occurred at x. (See also Figs. 12-16 and 12-17.)

to erupt, resorption of the deciduous molars is again initiated and this time continues until the roots are completely lost and the tooth is shed (Fig. 12-8). The bicuspids thus erupt in the position of deciduous molars.

## HISTOLOGY OF SHEDDING

The cells responsible for the removal of dental hard tissue are identical to osteoclasts, the highly specialized cells responsible for the removal of bone, and are called *odontoclasts*.

Odontoclasts are readily identifiable in the light microscope as large, multinucleated cells occupying resorption bays on the surface of a dental hard tissue. Their cytoplasm is vacuolated, and the surface of the cell adjacent to the resorbing hard tissue forms a "brush" border (Fig. 12-1). Histochemically, a characteristic feature of the odontoclast is a high level of activity of the enzyme acid phosphatase. These light-microscope observations have been confirmed and extended with the electron microscope (Fig. 12-9). The brush border is resolved as a ruffled border produced by extensive folding of the cell membrane into a

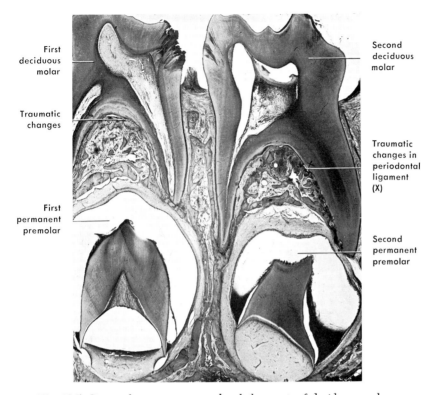

First
deciduous
molar

Traumatic
changes

First
permanent
premolar

Second
deciduous
molar

Traumatic
changes in
periodontal
ligament
(X)

Second
permanent
premolar

**Fig. 12-7.** Germs of permanent premolars below roots of deciduous molars.

series of invaginations 2 to 3 microns deep, with mineral crystallites within the depths of the invaginations. The cytoplasm of the odontoclast is characterized by an exceptionally high content of mitochondria and many vacuoles, which are especially concentrated adjacent to the ruffled border. Acid phosphatase activity occurs within these vacuoles (Fig. 12-10).

Odontoclasts are able to resorb all the dental hard tissues including, on occasions, enamel. When dentine is being resorbed, the presence of the tubules provides a pathway for the easy extension of odontoclast processes (Fig. 12-11).

The origin of odontoclasts and their distribution during tooth resorption is debatable. It is believed that odontoclasts originate from a similar source as osteoclasts do, and since neither mitotic nor amitotic division can be demonstrated with the latter cells as they differentiate, it is believed that their multinucleated appearance is the result of cell fusion. Which cells fuse, however, is entirely unknown.

Odontoclasts are most commonly found on surfaces of the roots in relation to the advancing permanent tooth. However, they have also been described in the root canals and pulp chambers of resorbing teeth lying against the predentine surface. Although their location in the pulp chamber has been disputed, most

*Text continued on p. 387.*

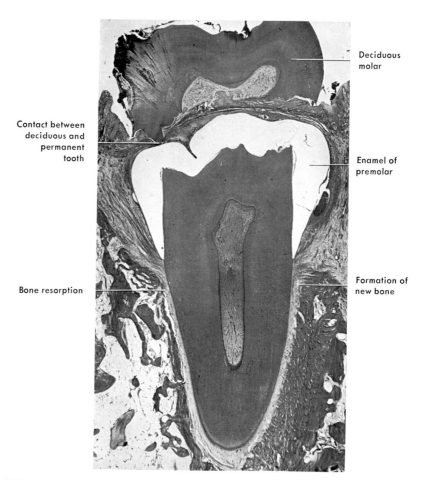

**Fig. 12-8.** Roots of primary molar completely resorbed. Dentin of primary tooth in contact with enamel of premolar. Resorption of bone on one side and formation of new bone on opposite side of premolar caused by transmitted excentric pressure to premolar. (From Grimmer, E. A.: J. Dent. Res. **18:**267, 1939.)

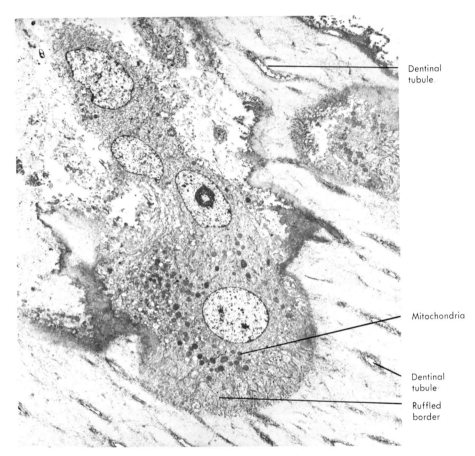

Dentinal
tubule

Mitochondria

Dentinal
tubule

Ruffled
border

**Fig. 12-9.** A multinucleated odontoclast displays a ruffled border well-adapted to resorption lacuna in root dentin. Dense mitochondria are aggregated toward "resorptive" (lower) pole of cell, and most of the cytoplasm is highly vacuolated. Dentinal tubules are visible in oblique section. (×3000.) (From Freilich, L. S.: J. Dent. Res. **50:**1047, 1971.)

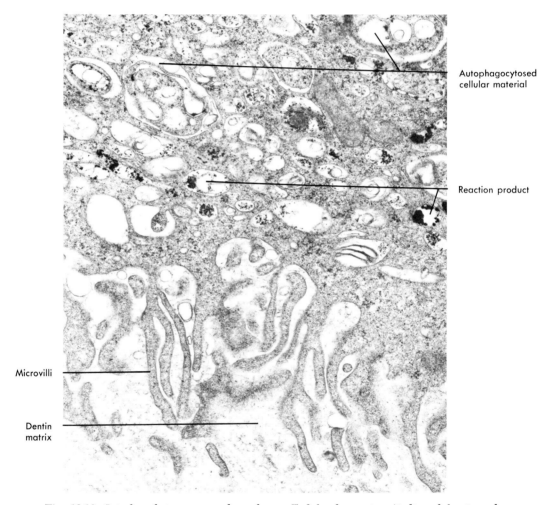

**Fig. 12-10.** Interface between an odontoclast ruffled border region (indicated by irregular microvilli) and disintegrated dentin matrix of root surface undergoing resorption. Numerous membrane-bound vacuoles in odontoclast cytoplasm show varied contents, including autophagocytosed cellular material and dense patches of reaction product, indicating acid phosphatase activity. (×40,000.) (From Freilich, L. S.: J. Dent. Res. **50:**1047, 1971.)

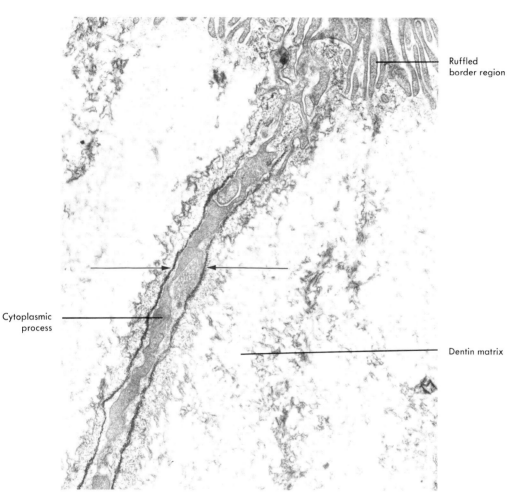

Ruffled
border region

Cytoplasmic
process

Dentin matrix

**Fig. 12-11.** Electron micrograph showing cytoplasmic process emanating from ruffled border region of an odontoclast and occupying a dentinal tubule. Dentin matrix occupies bulk of field. (×25,000.) (From Freilich, L. S.: J. Dent. Res. **50**:1047, 1971.)

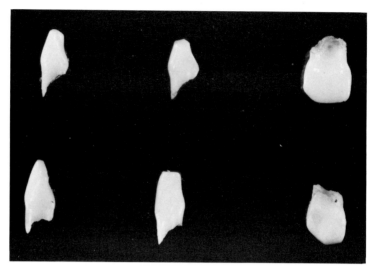

**Fig. 12-12.** Random selection of exfoliated deciduous incisor and canine teeth showing that a considerable amount of root dentin remains at time of exfoliation.

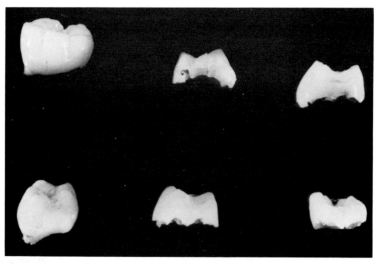

**Fig. 12-13.** Random selection of exfoliated deciduous molars showing that total loss of roots usually occurs before these teeth are shed. This photograph also shows occurrence of enamel resorption.

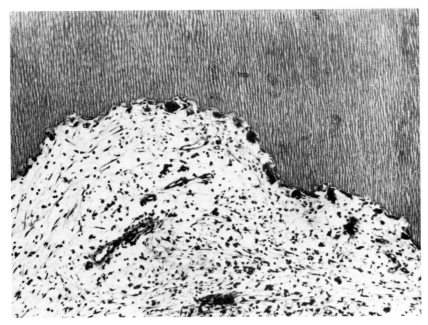

**Fig. 12-14.** Osteoclastic resorption in surface of coronal dentin of deciduous first molar tooth. Odontoblast layer is absent and numerous odontoblasts can be seen lining the pulp chamber. (From Weatherell, J. A., and Hargreaves, J. A.: Arch. Oral Biol. **11:**749, 1966.)

likely the reason is that different patterns of resorption exist for different teeth. For example, single-rooted teeth are usually shed before root resorption is complete (Fig. 12-12), and odontoclasts are not therefore found within the pulp chambers of these teeth and the odontoblast layer remains intact. In molars, however, the roots are usually completely resorbed and the crown is also partially resorbed before exfoliation. When this happens (Fig. 12-13), the odontoblast layer is replaced by odontoclasts (Fig. 12-14), which resorb both primary and secondary dentin (Fig. 12-15). Sometimes all the dentin is removed, and the vascular connective tissue is visible beneath the translucent cap of enamel.

The process of tooth resorption is not continuous, since there are periods of rest and repair; although in the long term, resorption predominates over repair. Repair is achieved by cells resembling cementoblasts that lay down a dense collagenous matrix in which spotty mineralization occurs. The final repair tissue resembles cellular cementum but is less mineralized (Figs. 12-16 and 12-17).

## MECHANISM OF RESORPTION AND SHEDDING

The mechanisms involved in bringing about tooth resorption and exfoliation are not yet fully understood. It seems clear that pressure from the erupting successional tooth plays a key role as the odontoclasts differentiate at predicted sites of pressure.

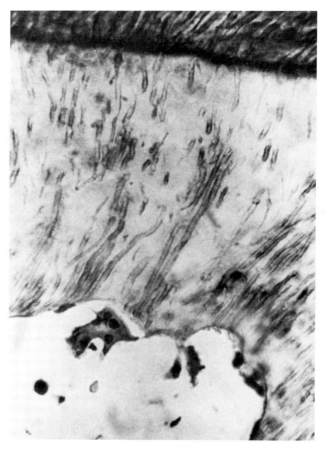

**Fig. 12-15.** Odontoclasts resorbing secondary dentin. (From Weatherell, J. A., and Hargreaves, J. A.: Arch. Oral Biol. **11**:749, 1966.)

How the odontoclast actually resorbs dental hard tissue is not known. The finding of mineral crystallites in the depths of the ruffled border and the fact that scanning electron microscopy indicates that the collagenous matrix of the dentin becomes exposed during resorption suggests that mineral is removed first. How the dissolution of the crystallites is achieved is not known. Nor is it known how the organic matrix, that is the collagen and associated ground substance, is dispersed. The acid-phosphatase content of the vesicles close to the ruffled border suggests that these structures are phagosomes in which breakdown of ingested material is taking place. The most likely sequence of events is resorption of dental hard tissue by the odontoclast is an initial removal of mineral followed by extracellular dissolution of the organic matrix (mainly collagen) to smaller molecules, which are then taken up by the odontoclast and degraded further.

Although pressure obviously has a key role in initiating tooth resorption, other factors must also be involved. It is a common clinical observation that when a

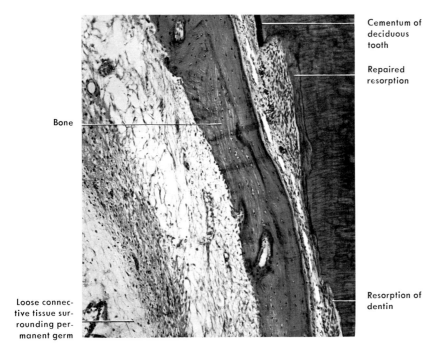

Cementum of
deciduous
tooth

Repaired
resorption

Bone

Resorption of
dentin

Loose connec-
tive tissue sur-
rounding per-
manent germ

Fig. 12-16. High magnification of repaired resorption from area X of Fig. 12-6.

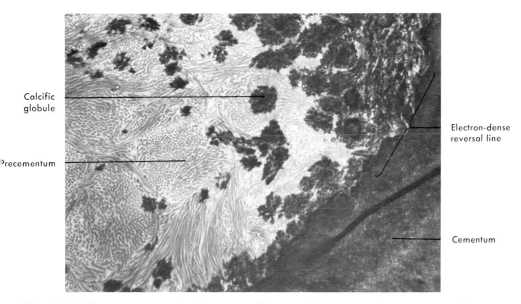

Calcific
globule

Precementum

Electron-dense
reversal line

Cementum

**Fig. 12-17.** Electron micrograph of resorption lacunae where repair of cementum is taking place. Newly deposited repair tissue is not as electron dense as underlying cementum. Note electron-dense reversal line and calcific globules in precementum. (From Furseth, R.: Arch. Oral Biol. **13:**417, 1968.)

successional tooth germ is missing, shedding of the deciduous tooth is delayed. Also, experimental removal of a permanent tooth germ delays, but does not prevent, shedding of its deciduous predecessor. It is more than likely that the forces of mastication applied to the deciduous tooth are also capable of initiating the resorption. As an individual grows, the muscles of mastication increase in size and exert forces on the deciduous tooth greater than its periodontal ligament can withstand. This leads to trauma to the ligament and the initiation of resorption. That this is so has been established experimentally by placing a splint bridge into the mouth of an experimental animal in such a way as to protect the deciduous tooth from occlusal stress. When this is done, resorption of the deciduous tooth is halted and repair takes place.

In practice a combination of both factors likely determines the rate and pattern of resorption. As resorption of the roots initiated by pressure of the underlying tooth occurs, there is a progressive loss of surface area for attachment of the periodontal ligament fiber bundles. This weakening of tooth support occurs because it has to stand increasingly greater occlusal forces generated by the growing muscles of mastication.

Finally, though the resorption of the dental hard tissues has been studied extensively, little, if anything, is known as to how the dental soft tissues are removed, especially the periodontal ligament.

## CLINICAL CONSIDERATIONS

*Remnants of deciduous teeth.* Sometimes parts of the roots of deciduous teeth are not in the path of erupting permanent teeth and may escape resorption. Such remnants, consisting of dentin and cementum, may remain embedded in the jaw

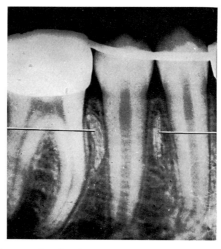

Root remnant of deciduous tooth

Root remnant of deciduous tooth

Fig. 12-18. Remnants of roots of a deciduous molar embedded in interdental septa. (Courtesy Dr. G. M. Fitzgerald, University of California.)

for a considerable time. They are most frequently found in association with the permanent premolars, especially in the region of the lower second premolars (Fig. 12-18). The reason is that the roots of the lower second deciduous molar are strongly curved or divergent. The mesiodistal diameter of the second premolars is much smaller than the greatest distance between the roots of the deciduous molar. Root remnants may later be found deep in the bone, completely surrounded by and ankylosed to the bone (Fig. 12-19). Frequently they are cased in heavy layers of cellular cementum. When the remnants are close to the surface of the jaw (Fig. 12-20), they may ultimately be exfoliated. Progressive resorption of the root remnants and replacement by bone may cause the disappearance of these remnants.

*Retained deciduous teeth.* Deciduous teeth may be retained for a long time beyond their usual shedding schedule. Such teeth are usually out of function. This occurs most frequently in the upper lateral incisor (Fig. 12-21, A), less

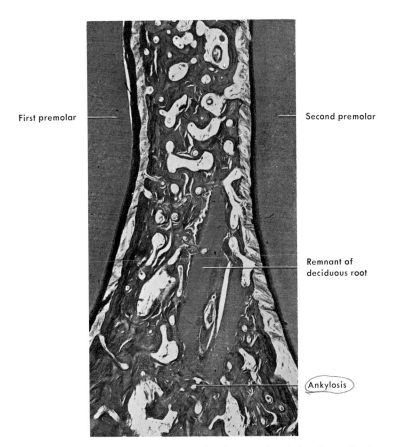

First premolar

Second premolar

Remnant of deciduous root

Ankylosis

**Fig. 12-19.** Remnant of deciduous tooth embedded in, and ankylosed to, the bone. (From Schoenbauer, F.: Z. Stomatol. **29:**892, 1931.)

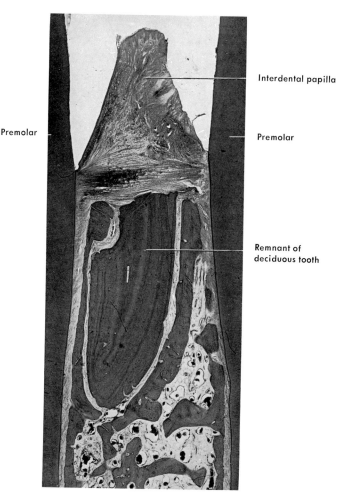

Premolar

Interdental papilla

Premolar

Remnant of
deciduous tooth

Fig. 12-20. Remnant of deciduous tooth at alveolar crest.

frequently in the second permanent premolar, especially in the mandible (Fig. 12-21, B), and rarely in the lower central incisor (Fig. 12-21, C). If a permanent tooth is embedded, its deciduous predecessor may also be retained (Fig. 12-21, D). This is most frequently seen in the deciduous and permanent canine teeth.

If the permanent lateral incisor is missing, the deciduous tooth is often resorbed under the pressure of the erupting permanent canine. This resorption may be simultaneous with that of the deciduous canine (Fig. 12-22). Sometimes the permanent canine causes resorption of the deciduous lateral incisor only and erupts in its place. In such cases the deciduous canine may be retained distally to the permanent canine. A supernumerary tooth or an odontogenic tumor may occasionally prevent the eruption of a permanent tooth or teeth. In such cases ankylosis of the deciduous tooth may occur.

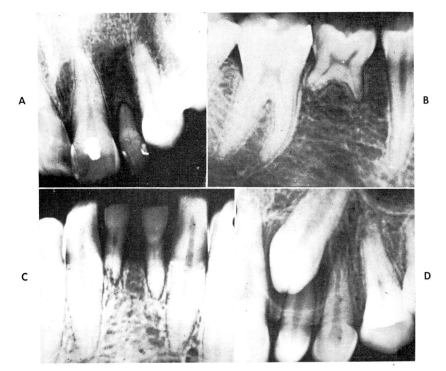

Fig. 12-21. Roentgenograms of retained deciduous teeth. **A,** Upper permanent lateral incisor missing, and deciduous tooth retained (age 56 years). **B,** Lower second premolar missing and deciduous molar retained. Roots partly resorbed. **C,** Permanent lower central incisors missing and deciduous teeth retained. **D,** Upper permanent canine embedded and deciduous canine retained. (**A** and **B,** Courtesy Dr. M. K. Hine, Indiana University. **C** and **D,** Courtesy Dr. Rowe Smith, Texarkana, Texas.)

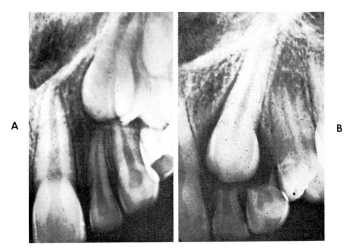

Fig. 12-22. Upper permanent lateral incisor missing. Deciduous lateral incisor and deciduous canine are resorbed because of pressure of erupting permanent canine. **A,** At age of 11 years. **B,** At age of 13 years.

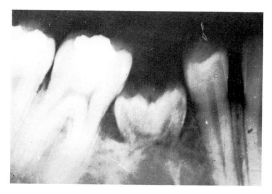

**Fig. 12-23.** Submerging deciduous lower second molar. Second premolar missing. (Courtesy Dr. M. K. Hine, Indiana University.)

**Submerged deciduous teeth.** Trauma may result in damage to either the dental follicle or the developing periodontal ligament. If this happens, the eruption of the tooth ceases and it becomes ankylosed to the bone of the jaw. Because of continued eruption of neighboring teeth and increase in the height of the alveolar bone, the ankylosed tooth may be either "shortened" (Fig. 12-23) or submerged in the alveolar bone. Submerged deciduous teeth prevent the eruption of their permanent successors or force them from their position. Submerged deciduous teeth should therefore be removed as soon as possible.

**REFERENCES**

Boyde, A., and Lester, K. S.: Electron microscopy of resorbing surfaces of dental hard tissues, Z. Zellforsch. **83**:538, 1967.

Freilich, L. S.: Ultrastructure and acid phosphatase cytochemistry of odontoclasts: Effect of parathyroid extract, J. Dent. Res. **50**:1047, 1971.

Furseth, R.: The resorption processes of human deciduous teeth studied by light microscopy, microradiography and electron microscopy, Arch. Oral Biol. **13**:417, 1968.

Kronfeld, R.: The resorption of the roots of deciduous teeth, Dent. Cosmos **74**:103, 1932.

Morita, H., Yamashiya, H., Shimizu, M., and Sasaki, S.: The collagenolytic activity during root resorption of bovine deciduous tooth, Arch. Oral Biol. **15**:503, 1970.

Weatherell, J. A., and Hargreaves, J. A.: Effect of resorption on the fluoride content of human deciduous dentine, Arch. Oral Biol. **11**:749, 1966.

Westin, G.: Über Zahndurchbruch und Zahnwechsel, Z. Mikrosk. Anat. Forsch. **51**:393, 1942.

Yaeger, J. A., and Kraucunas, E.: Fine structure of the resorptive cells in the teeth of frogs, Anat. Rec. **164**:1, 1969.

# 13 Temporomandibular joint

## ANATOMIC REMARKS

The mandibular articulation (temporomandibular or craniomandibular joint) is a bilateral diarthrosis between the articular tubercle eminences of the temporal bone and the condyles (capitula) of the mandible. A fibrous plate, the articular disc, is interposed on either side between the articular surfaces of the two bones. The temporomandibular joint is a joint that permits the mandible to move as a unit. The mandible can be depressed or elevated, protruded or retracted. The lateral movements consist of alternate protrusion and retraction of the mandible on each side. All these movements show a characteristic pattern for each individual, are controlled by interaction of muscles, and are involved in the injestion and mastication of food. The anatomy and histology of the joint are related to its functional activity.

The temporomandibular joint is a synovial joint formed by the mandibular fossa of the temporal bone above and the condyle of the mandible below. The articular disc divides the joint into upper and lower joint cavities.

The articular surface of the temporal bone is concave in its posterior part and convex in its anterior part. The articular fossa extends from the squamotympanic and petrotympanic fissures posteriorly to the convex articular tubercle anteriorly. The latter is strongly convex in a sagittal plane and slightly concave in a frontal plane. The convexity varies considerably, with the radius ranging from 5 to 15 mm. The long axes of the articular tubercles are directed medially and slightly posteriorly. The articular surfaces of the mandibular condyles are arcuate, with their axes placed in the same direction as those of the articular tubercles on the temporal bone. The articulating parts of the temporomandibular joint are covered by a fibrous or fibrocartilaginous tissue and not by hyaline cartilage, as in most other articulations of the human body. The absence of hyaline cartilage on the articulating surface was wrongly interpreted as indicating that the joint is not a stress-bearing joint. The hyaline cartilage present in the head of the condyle is the growth center of the mandible. It is comparable to the epiphyseal cartilage in a long bone but does not disappear entirely with maturity and cessation of growth.

The articular disc is an oval fibrous plate that fuses at its anterior margin

**395**

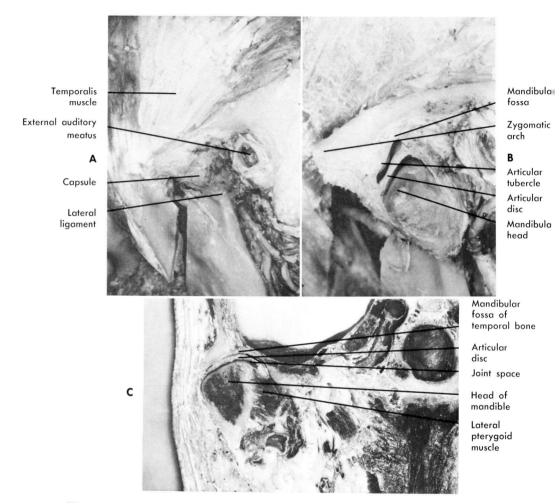

Temporalis
muscle

External auditory
meatus

**A**

Capsule

Lateral
ligament

Mandibula
fossa

Zygomatic
arch

**B**

Articular
tubercle

Articular
disc

Mandibula
head

Mandibular
fossa of
temporal bone

Articular
disc

Joint space

Head of
mandible

Lateral
pterygoid
muscle

**C**

Fig. 13-1. **A,** Lateral view of temporomandibular joint with capsule and lateral ligament in situ. **B,** Sagittal section through temporomandibular joint. **C,** Frontal section of head through condyle of mandible. (Courtesy Dr. F. R. Suarez, Georgetown University, Washington, D.C.)

with the fibrous capsule. Its posterior border is connected to the capsule by loose connective tissue, which allows its anterior movement (Fig. 13-1). Its medial and lateral corners are directly attached to the poles of the condyle. The articular space is divided into two compartments: a lower, between the condyle and the disc (condylodiscal), and an upper, between the disc and temporal bone (temporodiscal). The disc is biconcave in sagittal section, with the central part thin and the anterior and posterior borders thickened (Fig. 13-2). Some fibers of the lateral pterygoid muscle attach to the anterior border of the disc. The disc produces a movable articulation for the condyles. In the inferior portion of the joint, rotational movement about an axis through the heads of the condyles per-

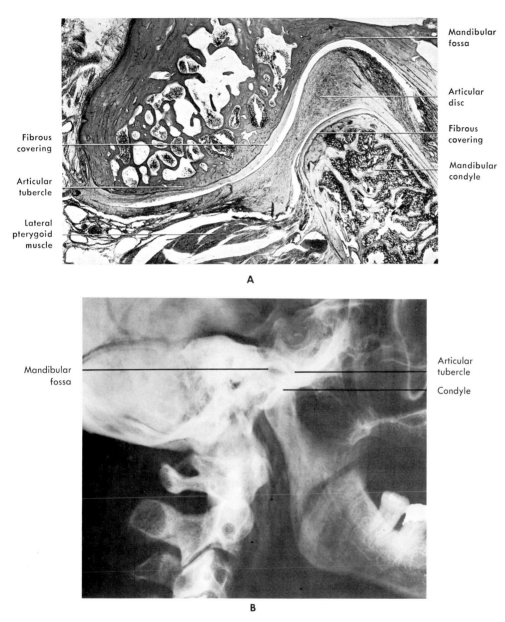

Mandibular
fossa

Articular
disc

Fibrous
covering

Mandibular
condyle

Fibrous
covering

Articular
tubercle

Lateral
pterygoid
muscle

**A**

Mandibular
fossa

Articular
tubercle

Condyle

**B**

Fig. 13-2. **A,** Sagittal section through temporomandibular joint. **B,** Radiograph of temporo-mandibular joint showing fossa, articular tubercle, and condyle in closed relation. (Courtesy Dr. F. R. Suarez, Georgetown University, Washington, D.C.)

mits opening of the jaws. This is designated as a hinge movement. The superior portion of the joint permits a translatory movement as the discs and the condyles traverse anteriorly along the inclines of the articular tubercles to provide an anterior and inferior movement of the mandible.

The articular capsule is a fibrous sac that surrounds the joint with its attachment to the mandibular fossa above and the neck of the mandible below. It is strengthened laterally by the temporomandibular ligament (lateral ligament). The inner aspect of the capsule is lined by a synovial membrane, which is especially well developed behind the disc. It lines the capsule in each of the two cavities but does not extend over the surfaces of the discs, the articular tubercle, or the condyle.

## HISTOLOGY

*Bony structures.* The condyle of the mandible is composed of cancellous bone covered by a thin layer of compact bone (Fig. 13-2, A). The trabeculae are grouped in such a way that they radiate from the neck of the mandible and reach the cortex at right angles, thus giving maximal strength to the condyle. The large marrow spaces decrease in size with progressing age by a noticeable thickening of the trabeculae. The red marrow in the condyle is of the myeloid or cellular type. In older individuals it is sometimes replaced by fatty marrow.

During the period of growth a layer of hyaline cartilage lies underneath the fibrous covering of the condyle. This cartilaginous plate grows by apposition from the deepest layers of the covering connective tissue. At the same time its deep surface is replaced by bone (Fig. 13-3). Remnants of this cartilage may persist into old age (Fig. 13-4).

The roof of the mandibular fossa (Fig. 13-2) consists of a thin compact layer of bone. The articular tubercle is composed of spongy bone covered with a thin layer of compact bone. In rare cases islands of hyaline cartilage are found in the articular tubercle.

*Articular fibrous covering.* The condyle as well as the articular tubercle is covered by a rather thick layer of fibrous tissue containing a variable number of chondrocytes. The fibrous covering of the mandibular condyle is of fairly even thickness (Fig. 13-4). Its superficial layers consist of a network of strong collagenous fibers. Chondrocytes may be present, and they have a tendency to increase in number with age. They can be recognized by their thin capsule, which stains heavily with basic dyes. The deepest layer of the fibrocartilage is rich in chondroid cells as long as growing hyaline cartilage is present in the condyle. It contains only a few thin collagenous fibers. In this zone the appositional growth of the hyaline cartilage of the condyle takes place during the period of growth.

The fibrous layer covering the articulating surface of the temporal bone (Fig. 13-5) is thin in the articular fossa and thickens rapidly on the posterior slope of the articular tubercle (Fig. 13-2, A). In this region the fibrous tissue shows a definite arrangement in two layers, with a small transitional zone between them. The

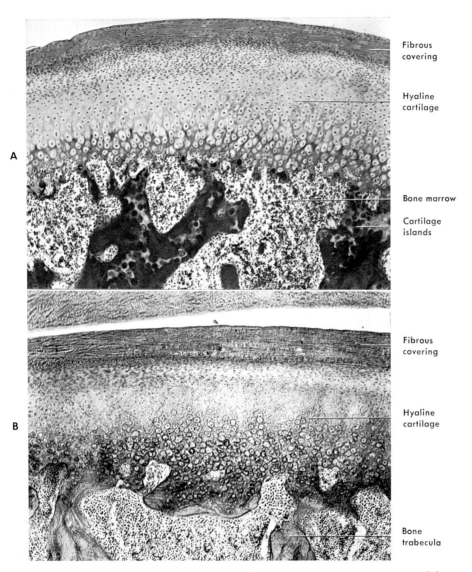

Fibrous
covering

Hyaline
cartilage

**A**

Bone marrow

Cartilage
islands

Fibrous
covering

Hyaline
**B** cartilage

Bone
trabecula

**Fig. 13-3.** Sections through the mandibular head. **A,** Newborn infant. **B,** Young adult. Note transitional zone between fibrous covering and hyaline cartilage, characteristic for appositional growth of cartilage.

two layers are characterized by the different course of the constituent fibrous bundles. In the inner zone the fibers are at right angles to the bony surface. In the outer zone they run parallel to that surface. As in the fibrous covering of the mandibular condyle, a variable number of chondrocytes are found in the tissue on the temporal surface. In adults the deepest layer shows a thin zone of calcification.

There is no continuous cellular lining on the free surface of the fibrocartilage.

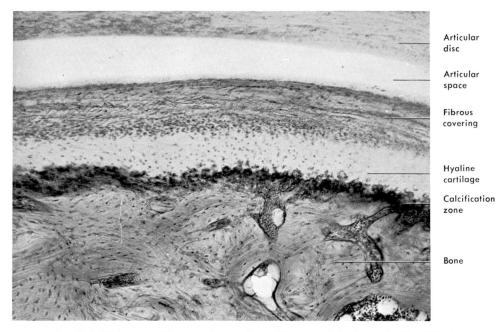

Articular
disc

Articular
space

Fibrous
covering

Hyaline
cartilage

Calcification
zone

Bone

**Fig. 13-4.** Higher magnification of part of mandibular condyle shown in Fig. 13-2, *A*.

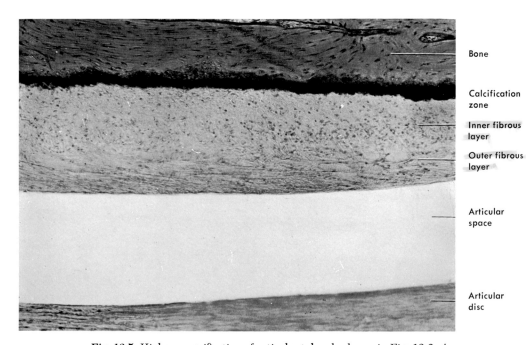

Bone

Calcification
zone

Inner fibrous
layer

Outer fibrous
layer

Articular
space

Articular
disc

**Fig. 13-5.** Higher magnification of articular tubercle shown in Fig. 13-2, *A*.

Only isolated fibroblasts are situated on the surface itself. They are characterized by the formation of long, flat cytoplasmic processes.

*Articular disc.* In young individuals the articular disc is composed of dense fibrous tissue. The interlacing fibers are straight and tightly packed (Fig. 13-6). Elastic fibers are found only in relatively small numbers. The fibroblasts in the disc are elongated and send flat cytoplasmic winglike processes into the interstices between the adjacent bundles.

With advancing age, some of the fibroblasts develop into chondroid cells, which later may differentiate into true chondrocytes. Even small islands of hyaline cartilage may be found in the discs of older persons. Chondroid cells, true cartilage cells, and hyaline ground substance develop in situ by differentiation of the fibroblasts. In the discs as well as in the fibrous tissue covering the articular surfaces this cellular change seems to be dependent on mechanical influences.

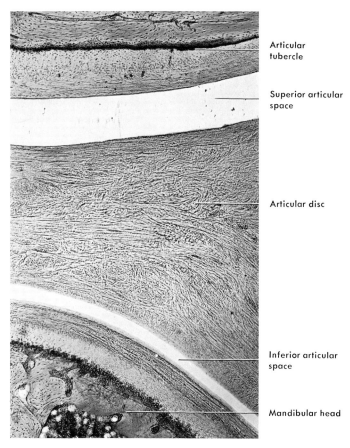

Fig. 13-6. Higher magnification of articular disc shown in Fig. 13-2, *A*.

The presence of chondrocytes may increase the resistance and resilience of the fibrous tissue.

The fibrous tissue covering the articular eminence and mandibular condyle as well as the large central area of the disc is devoid of blood vessels and nerves and has limited reparative ability.

*Articular capsule.* As in all other joints, the articular capsule consists of an outer fibrous layer that is strengthened on the lateral surface to form the temporomandibular ligament. The inner or synovial layer is a thin layer of connective tissue. It contains numerous blood vessels that form a capillary network close to its surface. From its surface, folds or fingerlike processes (synovial folds and villi) protrude into the articular cavity (Fig. 13-7). A few fibroblasts of the synovial membrane reach the surface and, with some histiocytes and lymphatic wandering cells, form an incomplete lining of the synovial membrane.

A small amount of a clear, straw-colored viscous fluid, synovial fluid, is found in the articular spaces. It is a lubricant and also a nutrient fluid for the avascular tissues covering the condyle and the articular tubercle and for the disc. It is elaborated by diffusion from the rich capillary network of the synovial membrane, augmented by mucin possibly secreted by the synovial cells.

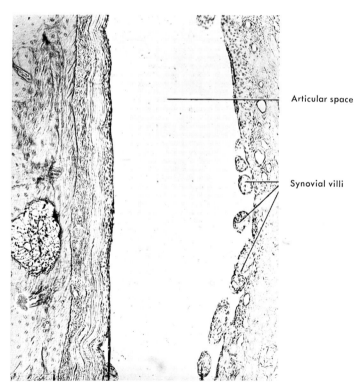

Articular space

Synovial villi

**Fig. 13-7.** Villi on synovial capsule of temporomandibular joint.

*Innervation and blood supply.* Sensations from the joint structures have usually been considered proprioceptive in nature. The auriculotemporal and masseteric nerves from the mandibular branch of the trigeminal nerve supply the joint. It has been suggested that there exist a number of free, complex, and encapsulated receptors among the synovial villi of the joint capsule. The primary source of blood supply comes from the superficial temporal and the maxillary arteries of the external carotid.

## CLINICAL CONSIDERATIONS

The thinness of the bone in the articular fossa is responsible for fractures if the mandibular head is driven into the fossa by a heavy blow. In such cases injuries of the dura mater and the brain have been reported.

The finer structure of the bone and its fibrocartilaginous covering depends on mechanical influences. A change in force or direction of stress, occurring especially after loss of posterior teeth, may cause structural changes. These are characterized by degeneration of the fibrous covering of the articulating surfaces and of the disc. Abnormal functional activity produces injury to the fibrous covering and the articular bones. Compensation and partial repair may be accomplished by the development of hyaline cartilage on the condylar surface and in the disc. In severe trauma the articular bone is destroyed, and cartilage and new bone develop in the marrow spaces and at the periphery of the condyle. Then the function of the joint is severely impaired.

There is considerable literature on the disturbances that occur in the articulation of the result of disharmony in the relation of the teeth and the temporomandibular joint. Disharmony of the factors that govern occlusion may produce extensive degenerative changes in the mandibular articulation. The clinical symptoms are pain in the region of the joint and pain radiating to the temporal, infraorbital, supraorbital, and postauricular areas, which may be of such severity as to produce trismus. A variety of noises can be observed during function, depending on the type and severity of the alterations produced.

Dislocation of the temporomandibular joint may take place without the impact of an external force. The dislocation of the jaw is usually bilateral and the displacement is anterior. When the mouth is opened unusually wide during yawning, the head of the mandible may slip forward into the infratemporal fossa causing articular dislocation of the joint.

Many explanations have been advanced for these variable symptoms: pressure on the external auditory meatus exerted by the mandibular condyle, which is driven deeply into the articular fossa; compression of the auriculotemporal nerve; compression of the chorda tympani; compression of the auditory tube; and impaired function of the tensor palati muscle. Anatomic findings do not substantiate any one of these explanations. Hypersensitivity and spasm of the muscles of mastication account for many of the symptoms.

## REFERENCES

Bauer, W.: Anatomische und mikroskopische Untersuchungen über das Kiefergelenk [Anatomical and microscopic investigations on the temporo-mandibular joint], Z. Stomatol. **30**:1136, 1932.

Bauer, W. H.: Osteo-arthritis deformans of the temporo-mandibular joint, Am. J. Pathol. **17**:129, 1941.

Bernick, S.: The vascular and nerve supply to the temporomandibular joint of the rat, Oral Surg. **15**:488, 1962.

Breitner, C.: Bone changes resulting from experimental orthodontic treatment, Am. J. Orthod. **26**:521, 1940.

Cabrini, R., and Erausquin, J.: La articulación temporomaxilar de la rata [Temporomandibular joint of the rat], Rev. Odont. Buenos Aires, 1941.

Choukas, N. C., and Sicher, H.: The structure of the temporo-mandibular joint, Oral Surg. **13**:1263, 1960.

Cohen, D. W.: The vascularity of the articular disc of the temporo-mandibular joint, Alpha Omegan, Sept. 1955.

Cowdry, E. V.: Special cytology, ed. 2, New York, 1932, Paul B. Hoeber, Inc., pp. 981-989, 1055-1075.

Kawamura, Y.: Recent concepts of physiology of mastication, Adv. Oral Biol. **1**:102, 1964.

Ramfjord, S. P., and Ash, M. M.: Occlusion, Philadelphia, 1966, W. B. Saunders Co.

Sarnat, B. G.: The temporomandibular joint, ed. 2, Springfield, Ill., 1964, Charles C Thomas, Publisher.

Schaffer, J.: Die Stützgewebe [Supporting tissues]. In von Möllendorff, W., editor: Handbuch der mikroskopischen Anatomie des Menschen, Berlin, 1930, Julius Springer Verlag, vol. 2, pt. 2.

Shapiro, H. H., and Truex, R. C.: The temporo-mandibular joint and the auditory function, J. Am. Dent. Assoc. **30**:1147, 1943.

Sicher, H.: Temporomandibular articulation in mandibular overclosure, J. Am. Dent. Assoc. **36**:131, 1948.

Sicher, H.: Some aspects of the anatomy and pathology of the temporomandibular articulation, New York State Dent. J. **14**:451, 1948.

Sicher, H.: Positions and movements of the mandible, J. Am. Dent. Assoc. **48**:620, 1954.

Sicher, H.: Structural and functional basis for disorders of the temporomandibular articulation, J. Oral Surg. **13**:275, 1955.

Steinhardt, G.: Die Beanspruchung der Gelenkflächen bei verschiedenen Bissarten [Investigations on the stresses in the mandibular articulation and their structural consequences], Deutsch. Zahnheilk. Vortr. **91**:1, 1934.

# 14 Maxillary sinus

## DEFINITION

The maxillary sinus is the pneumatic space that is lodged inside the body of the maxilla and that communicates with the environment by way of the middle nasal meatus and the nasal vestibule.

## HISTORICAL REVIEW

A recent publication entitled *Eighteen Hundred Years of Controversy: The Paranasal Sinuses* (Blanton and Biggs, 1969) reflects quite accurately the present confused state of knowledge about the pneumatic cavities. The maxillary sinus, more than any other of these cavities, has been subjected to peculiar interpretations throughout history. As early as the second century, Galen (A.D. 130-201) made the first known descriptive remarks about the adult maxillary sinus. In the following centuries many prominent scientists (Leonardo da Vinci, 1452-1519; Berengar, 1507-1527; Massa, 1542; Vesalius, 1542; Fallopius, 1600; Veslingius, 1637; Spigelius, 1645; Highmore, 1651; Schneider, 1655; Bartholinus, 1658; Morgagni, 1723; Boerhaave, 1735; and Haller, 1763—cited by Blanton and Biggs) contributed to the ever-increasing knowledge of the structure and function of the paranasal cavities.

Despite historical uncertainty as to the specific contribution of each of these researchers, it is well accepted that Highmore was the first to describe in detail the morphology of the maxillary sinus and to advance the idea of pneumatization by the sinuses. In the later centuries the interest of investigators focused on the mechanism of pneumatizing processes and the functional significance of the paranasal sinuses as a whole, in addition to the structural, dimensional, sexual, racial, environmental, and developmental diversity among the sinuses.

## DEVELOPMENTAL ASPECTS

The initial development of the maxillary sinus follows a number of morphogenic events in the differentiation of the nasal cavity in early gestation (about 32 mm. crown-rump length [CRL] in an embryo). First, the horizontal shift of palatal shelves and subsequent fusion of the shelves with one another and with the nasal septum separate the secondary oral cavity from two secondary nasal chambers (Chapter 1). This modification presumably influences further

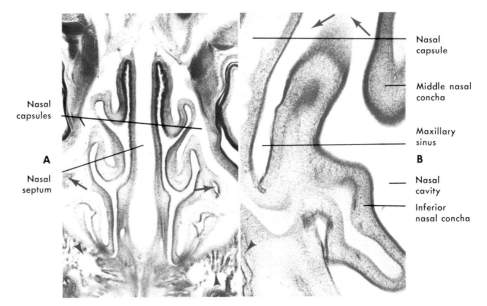

**Fig. 14-1. A,** This coronal section of a human fetal head (60 mm. CRL) demonstrates both nasal cavities bordered by the nasal septum medially, three conchae and subjacent meatuses laterally, and the palate, which shows already extensive centers of ossification inferiorly (*arrowheads at bottom*). Lateral to the conchae and continuous with their cartilaginous skeletons is the nasal capsule. Developing maxillary sinuses on both sides of the midline are indicated by *arrows*. (Hematoxylin and eosin stain; ×27.) **B,** This coronal section demonstrates the nasal cavity, the maxillary sinus, and the inferior and middle nasal conchae in a 69 mm. CRL fetus. The sinus grows into the maxilla in an inferior direction parallel to the plane of cartilaginous nasal capsule. The skeleton of both conchae is cartilaginous, while in the maxilla several centers of ossification (*arrowhead*) are present. The communication between the middle nasal meatus and the maxillary sinus is indicated by *arrows*. (Hematoxylin and eosin stain; ×67.5.) (**A,** No. 1183; **B,** No. 4291; courtesy Dr. Ronan O'Rahilly, Carnegie Laboratories of Embryology, Davis, Calif.)

expansion of the lateral nasal wall in that the wall begins to fold; thus three nasal conchae and three subjacent meatuses arise. The inferior and superior meatuses remain as shallow depressions along the lateral nasal wall for approximately the first half of the intrauterine life; the middle meatus expands immediately into the lateral nasal wall. Because the cartilaginous skeleton of the lateral nasal capsule is already established, expansion of the middle meatus proceeds primarily in an inferior direction, occupying progressively more of the future maxillary body (Fig. 14-1).

The maxillary sinus thus established in the embryo of about 32 mm. CRL expands vertically into the primordium of the maxillary body and reaches a diameter of 1 mm. in the 50 mm. fetus (at this time the first glandular primordia from the maxillary sinus epithelium are apparent), 3.5 mm. in the 160 mm. fetus, and 7.5 mm. in the 250 mm. CRL fetus (Vidić). In the perinatal period the human maxillary sinus measures about 7 to 16 mm. (standard deviation

[SD] 2.64) in the anteroposterior direction, 2 to 13 mm. (SD 1.52) in the superoinferior direction, and 1 to 7 mm. (SD 1.18) in the mediolateral direction (Cullen and Vidić). According to Shaeffer these diameters increase to 15, 6, and 5.5 mm. respectively at the age of 1 year, to 31.5, 19, and 19.5 mm. at the age of 15 years, and to 34, 33, and 23 mm. in the adult. Although the exact time at which the maxillary sinus attains the definite size is not ascertained for man, the sinus appears to modify in form and expands until the time of eruption of all permanent teeth.

## DEVELOPMENTAL ANOMALIES

Agenesis (complete absence), aplasia, and hypoplasia (altered development or underdevelopment) of the maxillary sinus occurs either alone or in association with other anomalies, e.g., choanal atresia, cleft palate, high palate, septal deformity, absence of a concha, mandibulofacial dysostosis, malformation of the external nose, and the pathologic conditions of the nasal cavity as a whole (Gouzy et al., Rosenberger, Schürch, Blair, Mocellin, Fatin, Eckel et al., and Blumenstein). The supernumerary maxillary sinus, on the other hand, is the occurrence of two completely separated sinuses on the same side. This condition is most likely initiated by outpocketing of the nasal mucosa into the primordium of the maxillary body from two points either in the middle nasal meatus or in the middle and superior or middle and inferior nasal meatuses, respectively. Consequently, the result is two permanently separated ostia of the sinus.

## STRUCTURE AND VARIATIONS

The maxillary sinus is subject to a great extent of variations in shape, size, and mode of developmental pattern. It is inconceivable, therefore, to propose any structural description that would satisfy the majority of human maxillary sinuses. Usually, however, the sinus is described as a four-sided pyramid the base of which is facing medially toward the nasal cavity and the apex of which is pointed laterally toward the body of the zygomatic bone (Fig. 14-2). The four sides are related to the surface of the maxilla in the following manner: (1) anterior to the facial surface of the body; (2) inferior, to the alveolar and zygomatic processes; (3) superior, to the orbital surface; and (4) posterior, to the infratemporal surface. The four sides of the sinus, which are usually distant from one another medially, converge laterally and meet at an obtuse angle. The identity of each of the four sides is somewhat difficult to discern and the transition of the surface from one side to the other is usually poorly defined. Thus it is apparent that the comparison of the sinus space to a geometrically well-defined body is of pedagogic value only.

The base of the sinus, which is the thinnest of all the walls, presents a perforation, the ostium, at the level of the middle nasal meatus (Fig. 14-3). In some individuals, in addition to the main ostium, two or many more accessory ostia connect the sinus with the middle nasal meatus. In 5.5% of instances the main

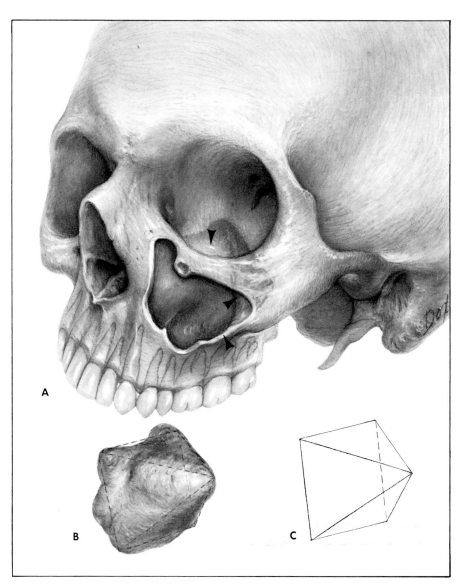

Fig. 14-2. **A,** Left semiprofile of the skull showing maxillary sinus opened through anterior wall. The outline of the superior, posterior, and inferior walls of the sinus are respectively indicated in relation to the floor of the orbit *(upper arrowhead),* infratemporal surface of the maxilla *(middle arrowhead),* and the alveolar and zygomatic processes of the maxilla *(lower arrowhead).* The basal wall separates the space of the sinus from the nasal cavity. **B** and **C,** Polysulfate rubber cast of the maxillary sinus about 10 ml. in volume and an idealized geometric form of the sinus, respectively. For the convenience of visualizing the presumed pyramidal form of the sinus the orientation is the same for the sinus in situ, **A;** the cast of the sinus, **B;** and for the closest geometric form to the sinus, **C.** (Courtesy Mr. and Mrs. B. F. Melloni, Department of Medical-Dental Communications, Georgetown University, Washington, D.C.)

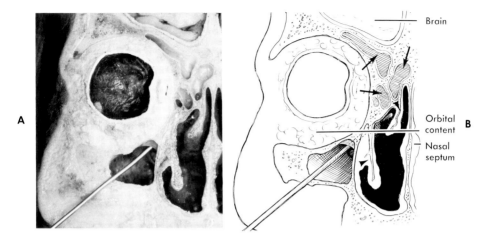

**Fig. 14-3. A,** Coronal section of adult female face was made approximately 7 mm. anterior to ostium of maxillary sinus. **B,** Drawing made from **A** (proportion, 1:1). Probe indicates ostium, or the communication between upper part of sinus lumen and middle nasal meatus. Several ethmoidal air cells *(arrows)*, middle and inferior conchae *(two arrowheads)*, orbital content, nasal septum, and frontal lobe of brain are also indicated. (**A,** Frontal section courtesy Dr. F. R. Suarez, Georgetown University, Washington, D.C. **B,** Courtesy Mr. and Mrs. B. F. Melloni, Department of Medical-Dental Communications, Georgetown University, Washington, D.C.)

ostium is located within the anterior third of the uncibullar groove (hiatus semilunaris), in 11% within the middle third, in 71.7% within the posterior third, and in 11.3% the ostium is found outside and in a posterior position to the groove. The accessory ostia are found in 23% of these instances in the middle nasal meatus (Van Alyea) and occur rarely in the inferior nasal meatus (Delaney et al.).

In the course of development the maxillary sinus quite often pneumatizes the maxilla beyond the boundaries of the maxillary body. Some of the processes of the maxilla consequently become invaded by the air space. These expansions, referred to as the *recesses*, are found in the alveolar process (50% of all instances), zygomatic process (41.5% of all instances), frontal process (40.5% of all instances), and the palatine process (1.75% of all instances) of the maxilla (Hajniš). The occurrence of the zygomatic recess usually brings the superior alveolar neurovascular bundles into proximity with the space of the sinus. The frontal recess invades and sometimes surrounds the content of the infraorbital canal, whereas the alveolopalatine recesses reduce the amount of the bone between the dental apices and the sinus space. The latter development most often pneumatizes the floor of the sinus adjacent to the roots of the first molar (Fig. 14-4) and less often to the roots of the second premolar, first premolar, and second molar, in that order of frequency (Osmont). The fully developed alveolar recess is characterized by three depressions separated by two incomplete bony

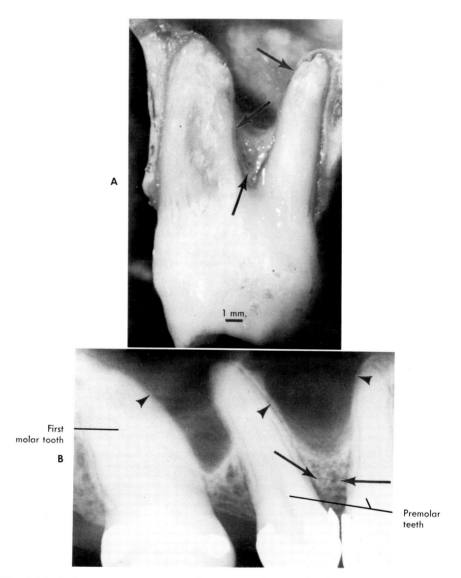

**Fig. 14-4. A** demonstrates in a coronal section made immediately mesial to the upper first molar tooth the gross relationships of the vestibular (left) and palatine (right) roots with the floor of the maxillary sinus. The amount of bone *(arrows)* interposed between the roots and the space of the sinus is reduced at certain levels to a thin lamina. **B,** Lateral radiograph of both right upper premolar and first molar teeth. Maxillary sinus expands, in this instance, deep into the alveolar process *(arrows)* between each two of the indicated teeth. Bony lamina separating the dental roots from the sinus *(arrowheads)* is extremely thin at certain levels. (**B,** Courtesy Dr. Donald Reynolds, Georgetown University, Washington, D.C.)

septa. The anterior depression, or fossa, corresponds to the original site of premolar buds, the middle to the molar buds, and the posterior to the third molar bud (Perović).

## MICROSCOPIC FEATURES

Three microscopically distinct layers surround the space of the maxillary sinus: the epithelial layer, the basal lamina, and the subepithelial layer, including the periostium (Figs. 14-5 and 14-6). The epithelium, pseudostratified columnar ciliated, is derived from the olfactory epithelium of the middle nasal meatus and therefore undergoes the same pattern of differentiation as does the respiratory segment of the nasal epithelium proper. The most numerous cellular type in the maxillary sinus epithelium is the columnar ciliated cell. In addition, there are basal cells, columnar nonciliated cells, and mucus-producing, secretory

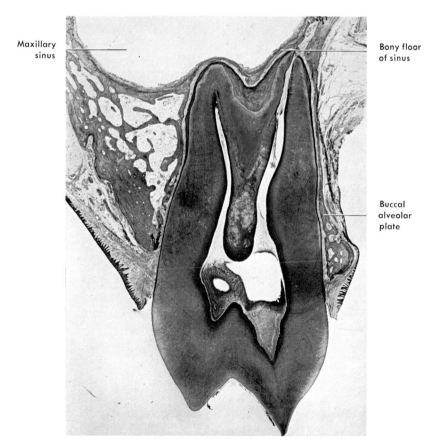

**Fig. 14-5.** Buccolingual section through first upper premolar. Apex is separated from sinus by a thin plate of bone.

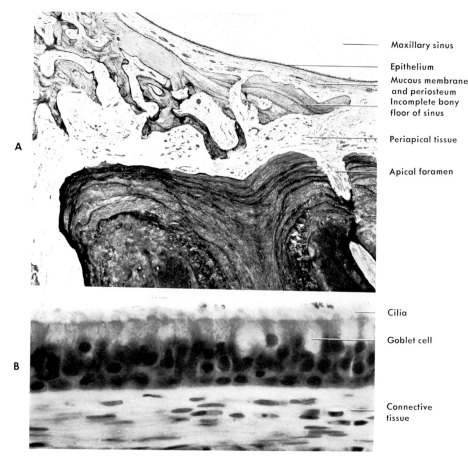

Maxillary sinus

Epithelium
Mucous membrane
and periosteum
Incomplete bony
floor of sinus

Periapical tissue

Apical foramen

Cilia

Goblet cell

Connective
tissue

A

B

**Fig. 14-6.** Mucous membrane and epithelium of maxillary sinus. **A,** Apical region of a second premolar. Lining of sinus is continuous with periapical tissue through openings in bony floor of sinus. **B,** High magnification of epithelium of maxillary sinus. (From Bauer, W. H.: Am. J. Orthodont. **29:**133, 1943.)

goblet cells (Figs. 14-6 and 14-7). A ciliated cell encloses the nucleus and an electron-lucent cytoplasm with numerous mitochondria and enzyme-containing organelles. The basal bodies, which serve as the attachment of the ciliary microtubules to the cell, are characteristic of the apical segment of the cell. The cilia are typically composed of $9+1$ pairs of microtubules, and they provide the motile apparatus to the sinus epithelium (Satir). By way of ciliary beating the mucous blanket lining the epithelial surface moves generally from the sinus interior toward the nasal cavity.

The goblet cell displays all of the characteristic features of a secretory cell. In its basal segment the cell is occupied by, in addition to the nucleus, the cytocavitary network consisting of the rough and smooth endoplasmic reticulum and the Golgi apparatus, all of which are involved in the synthesis of the secretory

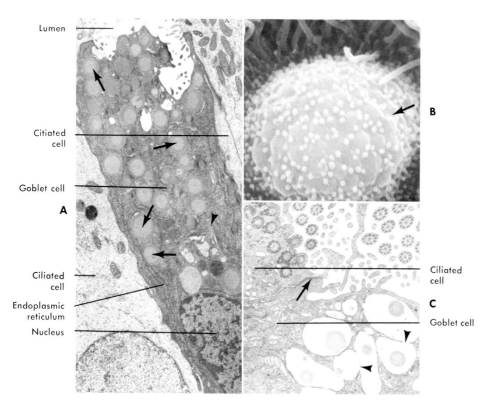

Lumen

Citiated
cell

Goblet cell

**A**

Ciliated
cell

Endoplasmic
reticulum

Nucleus

**B**

Ciliated
cell

**C**

Goblet cell

**Fig. 14-7. A,** Electron micrograph of thin section (about 350 Å) taken from rat trachea. Goblet cell is surrounded by two ciliated cells. From the nucleus toward the lumen the globlet cell is occupied by the endoplasmic reticulum, Golgi apparatus *(arrowhead)* and numerous secretory granules *(arrows)*. Luminal surface of goblet cell is covered by short microvilli. **B,** Scanning electron micrograph taken from rat trachea demonstrates surface view of a goblet cell *(arrow)* bordered above by numerous cilia from the neighboring cells. In addition to the microvilli, the surface of the goblet cell appears rough because of the projection of the apically situated secretory granules. **C,** Electron micrograph of thin section taken from human maxillary sinus demonstrates apical portions and surfaces of ciliated cell and goblet cell. Several secretory granules in the goblet cell are demonstrated as either individual organelles or coalescing with one another *(arrowheads)*. A junctional complex between the two cells is indicated by *arrow.* (**A,** Uranyl acetate and lead citrate stain; ×10,400. **B,** Fixed in aldehyde, dried by critical-point technique, and coated with a layer of gold-palladium about 200 Å thick; ×14,000. **C,** Uranyl acetate and lead citrate stain; ×22,400.)

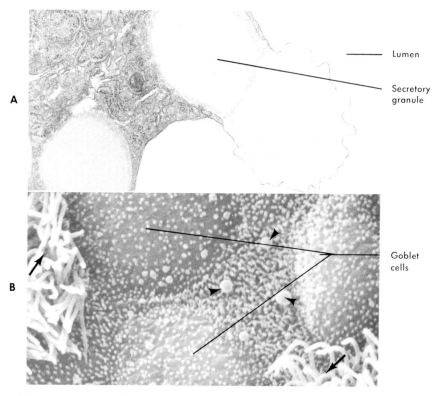

**Fig. 14-8.** Secretory material from goblet cell is released into lumen by exocytosis. **A,** Electron micrograph of thin section taken from rat trachea shows a secretory granule in the process of extrusion from cell into lumen. **B,** Scanning electron micrograph taken from rat trachea shows several goblet cells and parts of two ciliated cells *(arrows)*. *Arrowheads* indicate the surface projection of secretory granules in the process of extrusion from cell into lumen. (**A,** Uranyl acetate and lead citrate stain; ×48,000. **B,** Fixed in aldehydes, dried by critical-point technique, and coated with a layer of gold-palladium about 200 Å thick; ×11,600.)

mucosubstances. From the Golgi apparatus the zymogenic granules transport the mucopolysaccharides toward the cellular apex and finally release this material onto the epithelial surface by exocytosis (Fig. 14-8). In addition to the epithelial secretion, the surface of the sinus is provided with a mixed secretory product (serous secretion consisting primarily of water with small amounts of neutral nonspecific lipids, proteins and carbohydrates, and mucous secretion consisting of compound glycoproteins or mucopolysaccharides or both) from the subepithelial glands (Fig. 14-9). These are located in the subepithelial layer of the sinus and reach the sinus lumen by way of excretory ducts (Fig. 14-10), after the ducts have pierced the basal lamina.

On the basis of histochemical differentiation and fine structural characteristics (Vidić and Tandler) it is evident that the acini of subepithelial glands contain in varying proportions two types of secretory cells, the serous and the mucous.

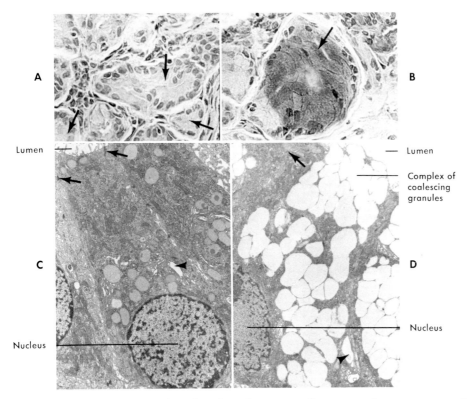

**Fig. 14-9. A** and **B,** Micrographs taken from human maxillary sinus demonstrate several serous acini (see *arrows* in **A**) and a mucous acinus (see *arrow* in **B**). Note the positive reaction of the secretory material with alcian blue in the mucous acinus and no reaction in the serous gland. **C** and **D,** Electron micrographs illustrate respectively a thin section of several serous and mucous secretory cells taken from human submucosal maxillary gland. In both representative cells, from the nucleus toward the acinar lumen the cytoplasm is occupied by the endoplasmic reticulum, mitochondria, secretory granules, and the Golgi apparatus *(arrowheads)*. Note the difference in the electron opacity between the two types of secretory granules. Serous granules are separated from one another by respective membranes, while the mucous granules frequently coalesce among them. (Note the complex of coalescing granules). Junctional complexes between cells in both illustrations are indicated by *arrows*. (**A,** Alcian blue and fast red procedure; ×1900 for serous acini and ×2000 for mucous acinus. **B,** Uranyl acetate and lead citrate stain; ×7200 for serous gland and ×6750 for mucous gland.)

The serous cell is stained with ninhydrin-Schiff and sudan black B procedures and encloses an electron-dense, homogeneous secretory material. The mucous cell reacts positive with the alcian blue 8GX procedure for acid sialomucin or sulfomucin or both and produces an electron-lucent, heterogeneous secretory material. The myoepithelial cells (Fig. 14-11) surround the acini composed of either both secretory cells or a pure population of cells of either secretory type.

The secretion from these glands, like that of the other exocrine glands, is controlled by both divisions of the autonomic nervous system (Fig. 14-11). The

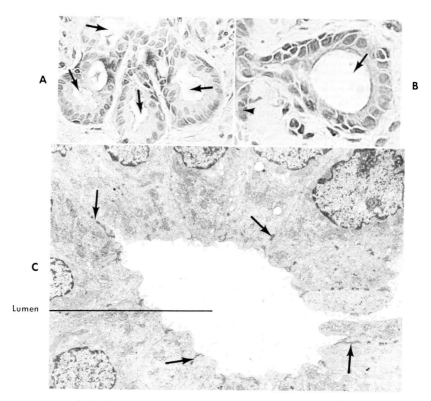

**Fig. 14-10. A** and **B,** Micrographs represent excretory ducts of maxillary gland taken from human maxillary sinus. Ductal cells, from cuboid to columnar in shape, surround lumen *(arrows),* which measures in these instances up to 12.5 microns in radius. **B,** Duct is demonstrated in a close apposition to epithelium of sinus *(arrowhead).* **C,** Thin section of several cells lining lumen of excretory duct from human maxillary gland. In addition to the nucleus, these cells contain the endoplasmic reticulum, Golgi apparatus, numerous mitochondria, lipid droplets, and occasional lysosomes. *Arrows,* Many junctional complexes between the ductal cells. (**A** and **B,** Alcian blue and fast red procedure; **C,** Uranyl acetate and lead citrate stain; **A** to **C,** ×1600, ×2400, ×6900.)

autonomic axons, together with general sensory components, are supplied to the maxillary sinus from the maxillary nerve complex. Numerous nonmyelinated and fewer myelinated axons are readily observable in the subepithelial layer of the sinus (Fig. 14-12). They are related here to the blood capillaries, fibroblasts, fibrocytes, collagen bundles, and other connective tissue elements.

## FUNCTIONAL IMPORTANCE

Very little is known about the participation of the paranasal sinuses in the functioning of either the nasal cavity or the respiratory system as a whole. This is partially because of the relative inaccessibility of the sinuses to the systemic functional studies, as well as because of the great variation in size of sinuses and their relationship to and communication with the nasal cavity. It is not surprising,

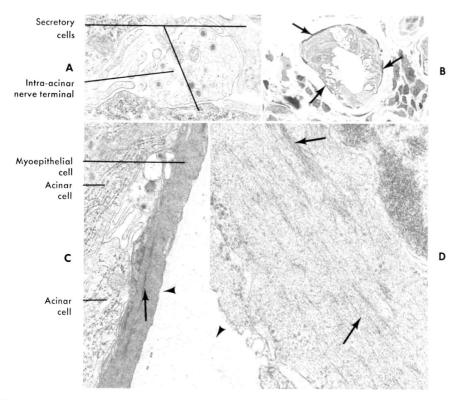

Secretory
cells

**A**

Intra-acinar
nerve terminal

**B**

Myoepithelial
cell

Acinar
cell

**C**

**D**

Acinar
cell

Fig. 14-11. **A,** Electron micrograph of intra-acinar nerve terminal in juxtaposition to two secretary cells taken from human maxillary gland. Note, in addition to mitochondria, two populations of small vesicles, dense and translucent, inside the nerve terminal. **B,** Thin section (0.5 microns) of several mucous and ductal cells from human maxillary gland. Periphery of this acinus is surrounded by dark-appearing myoepithelial cells *(arrows).* **C** and **D** illustrate relationship between acinar cells and myoepithelial cell and numerous bundles of filaments *(arrows)* that occupy most of the cytoplasm of the myoepithelial cells, respectively. In both instances basement lamina adjacent to myoepithelial cell is indicated by *arrowhead.* (**A, C,** and **D,** Uranyl acetate and lead citrate stain; **B,** toluidine blue stain; **A** to **D,** ×37,500, ×1600, ×27,000, ×96,000.)

then, that the theories of the functional importance of the sinuses range from no importance on the one hand to a multitude of involvements on the other hand.

The sinus is regarded by some as an accessory space to the nasal cavity, occurring only as a result of an inadequate process of ossification (Negus). In contrast others report the functional contributions of the maxillary sinus in many aspects of olfactory and respiratory physiology. In individuals in whom the maxillary ostium is large enough and conveniently situated in the uncibullar groove, the air pressure in the sinus fluctuates from ± 0.7 to ± 4 mm. of water between the nasal expiration and inspiration (Lamm). This dependence of the pressure in the sinus on the wave of respiration is, however, less probable in

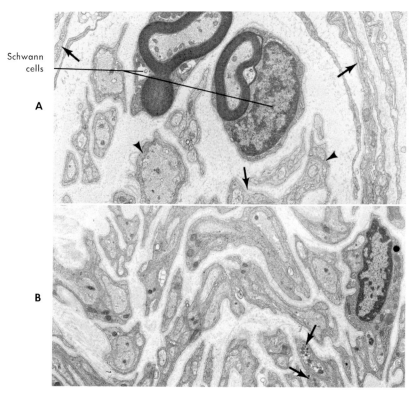

Schwann cells

A

B

**Fig. 14-12. A,** Electron micrograph of two myelinated and several nonmyelinated axons in mucoperiosteal layer of human maxillary sinus. Schwann cells *(labeled and at arrowheads)* are intimately related to axons which contain individual mitochondria and microtubules or microfilaments cut in different planes. *Arrows,* Connective tissue elements surrounding either individual axon or entire nerve. **B,** Nonmyelinated axons isolated from human mucoperiosteal layer of maxillary sinus. Most of them contain the same organelles as in **A.** However, some *(arrows)* are occupied by dense or translucent vesicles. ( **A** and **B,** Uranyl acetate and lead citrate stain; **A,** ×11,200; **B,** ×19,200. )

instances of either the small maxillary ostium or the ostium hidden in the depth of the uncibullar groove. On the basis of the same two conditions related to the structure and topography of the ostium some suggested functions attributed to the sinus by Koertvelyessy, Allen, Döderlein, Latkowski, and Doiteau ( humidification and warming of inspired air and contribution to the olfaction, for instance ) are subject to controversy. However, it is possible that if air is arrested in the sinus for a certain time, it quickly reaches body temperature and thus protects the internal structures, particularly the brain, against exposure to cold air ( Koertvelyessy, Allen, Latkowski, Maurer ). The other contribution by paranasal cavities to the resonance of voice, lightening of the skull weight ( Merideth, Nemours ), enhancement of faciocranial resistance to mechanical shock, and the production of bactericidal lysozyme to the nasal cavity are reviewed in detail by Latkowski and by Blanton and Biggs.

## CLINICAL CONSIDERATIONS

The section on developmental anomalies discusses several modifications of genetic and other origins in the developmental pathways of the maxillary sinus (agenesia, aplasia, hypoplasia, and supernumerary sinus). Some other criteria that correlate the extent of pneumatization by sinuses to the general disfunctions of the endocrine system are by now developed. In the case of pituitary giantism, for example, all sinuses assume a much larger volume than in healthy individuals of the same geographic environment (Püschel et al.). It is also known that in some congenital infections, such as by spirochetes in congenital syphilis, the pneumatic processes are greatly suppressed, resulting in small sinuses (Richter).

In most respects the pathogenic relationship of the maxillary sinus to the orodental complexes is the result of topographic arrangement and of the functional and systemic association between the two territories. The transfer of a pathologic condition from the sinus to the orodental apparatus, or vice versa, is achieved either by mechanical connections or by way of the blood or lymphatic pathways. Since the upper first molar tooth is most often closest to the floor of the maxillary sinus, surgical manipulation on this tooth is most likely to break through the partitioning bony lamina and thus to establish an oroantral fistula (2.19% of all such fistulas are caused by first molars, 2.01% by second molars). If untreated, the lumen of such fistulas might epithelialize and permanently connect the maxillary space with the oral cavity. A similar condition might arise as a result of either a molar or a premolar radicular cyst, granuloma, or abscess. Hypercementosis of root apices and subsequent extraction of the affected tooth may also lead to a perforation. It is necessary, therefore, to consider on a radiograph the relationship between any such premolar or molar tooth with the floor of the maxillary sinus prior to surgical intervention.

The chronic infections of the mucoperiosteal layer of the sinus, on the other hand, might involve superior alveolar nerves, if these nerves are closely related to the sinus, and cause the neuralgia that mimics possible dental origin (Osmont). In this instance the diagnosis must be based on a careful inspection of all the upper teeth as well as of the maxillary sinus to differentiate cause and eventual result of this condition. The neuralgia of the maxillary nerve (tic douloureux) could also have an etiologic origin in either the superior dental apparatus or the mucoperiosteal layer of the sinus, or both. For the diagnosis and treatment of this condition, it is most important to determine precisely the causal focus. Because of overlap of innervated territories and close topographic relationships between the teeth and the sinus, however, the causal focus is often difficult to assess.

The pathogenic association of the sinus with the orodental system, or vice versa, is based, in addition to a close topographic relationship, on an extensive vascular connection between these two regions by the superior alveolar vessels. As a consequence of this vascular arrangement, nonspecific bacterial sinusitis may be followed by some oral manifestations. Also the infections caused by the streptococci, staphylococci, pneumococci, or the virus of common cold are likely to spread from either of the two regions to involve the other one. Finally, malignant lesions (adenocarcinoma, squamous cell carcinoma, osteosarcoma, fibrosarcoma, lymphosarcoma, etc.) of the maxillary sinus may produce their primary manifestation in the maxillary teeth. This may consist of pain, loosening, supraeruption, or bleeding in their gingival tissue.

## REFERENCES

Allen, B. C.: Applied anatomy of paranasal sinuses, J. Am. Osteopath. Assoc. **60**:978, 1961.

Ardouin, P.: Étude embryologique du développement du sinus maxillaire, Rev. Laryngol. Otol. Rhinol. **79**:834, 1958.

Blair, V. P., Brown, J. B., and Byars, L. T.: Observations on sinus abnormalities in congenital total and hemiabsence of the nose, Ann. Otol. Rhinol. Laryngol. **46**:592, 1937.

Blanton, P. L., and Biggs, N. L.: Eighteen hundred years of controversy: The paranasal sinuses, Am. J. Anat. **124**:135, 1969.

Blumenstein, G.: Die Entwicklung der Kieferhöhlen bei Rachenmandelhyperplasie, Nasenrachenfibrom, Choanalatresia und Dysostosis mandibulofacialis im Vergleich zur normalen Entwicklung, Hals-Nasen-Ohrenklinik der Westfälischen Wilhelms Universität (Thesis), Münster, Germany, 1963.

Cheraskin, E.: Diagnostic stomatology. A clinical pathologic approach, New York, 1961, The Blakiston Division, McGraw-Hill Book Co.

Colby, R. A., Kerr, D. A., and Robinson, H. B. G.: Color atlas of oral pathology, Philadelphia, 1961, J. B. Lippincott Co.

Cullen, R. L., and Vidić, B.: The dimensions and shape of the human maxillary sinus in the perinatal period, Acta Anat. **83**: 411, 1972.

Delaney, A. J., and Morse, H. R.: Inferior meatal accessory ostia; report of a case, Ann. Otol. Rhinol. Laryngol. **60**:635, 1951.

Döderlein, W.: Experimentelle Untersuchungen zur Physiologie der Nasen und Mundatmung und über die physiologische Bedeutung der Nasennebenhöhlen, Z. Hals-Nasen-u. Ohrenheilk. **30**:459, 1932.

Doiteau, R.: Contribution à l'étude de la physiologie des sinus de la face. Renouvellement de l'air intrasinusien échanges gazeux permuqueux, Rev. Laryngol. Otol. Rhinol. **77**:900, 1956.

Eckel, W., and Beisser, D.: Untersuchungen zur Frage eines Einflusses der Gaumenspaltbildung auf die Kieferhöhlengrösse, Z. Laryngol. Rhinol. Otol. **40**:23, 1961.

Fatin, M.: A rare case of congenital malformation. Total absence of half the nose, probably supporting the theory of bilateral nasal origin, J. Egypt. Med. Assoc. **38**(8): 470, 1955.

Gouzy, J., Voilgue, G., and Jakubowicz, B.: A propos de deux cas d'agénésie du sinus maxillaire, J. Fr. Otorhinolaryngol. **17**:759, 1968.

Hajniš, K., Kustra, T., Farkaš, L. G., and Feiglová, B.: Sinus maxillaris, Z. Morph. Anthropol. **59**:185, 1967.

Koertvelyessy, T.: Relationships between the frontal sinus and climatic conditions: A skeletal approach to cold adaptation, Am. J. Phys. Anthropol. **37**:161, 1972.

Lamm, H., and Schaffrath, H.: Druckmessungen im gesunden Sinus maxillaris bei verschiedenen Atmungstypen, Z. Laryngol. Rhinol. Otol. **46**:172, 1967.

Latkowski, B.: Poglądy na znaczenie zatok bocznych nosa, Pol. Tyg. Lek. **19**:1206, 1964.

Maurer, R.: Zur Physiologie der Schädelpneumatisation, Arch. Ohren-Nasen-u. Kehlkopfheilk. **163**:471, 1953.

Merideth, H. W.: The paranasal sinuses, Rocky Mountain Med. J. **49**:343, 1952.

Mocellin, L.: Um caso de pan-agenesia dos seios paranasais, Rev. Bras. Cirurg. **48**(4): 283, 1964.

Negus, V.: The function of the paranasal sinuses, A.M.A. Arch. Otolaryngol. **66**:430, 1957.

Nemours, P. R.: A comparison of the accessory nasal sinuses of man with those of the lower vertebrates, Trans. Am. Laryngol. Otol. Rhinol. Soc. **37**:195, 1931.

Osmont, J., Jars, G., and Ged, S.: Anatomie chirurgicale du sinus maxillaire, Rev. Odontostomatol. Midi Fr. **25**:50, 1967.

Perović, D.: Medicinska Enciklopedija, vol. 6,

Zagreb, 1962, Naklada Leksikografskog Zavoda F.N.R.J.

Püschel, L., and Schlosshauer, B.: Ueber den Einfluss des somatotropen und androgenen Hormons auf die Pneumatisation, Arch. Ohren-Nasen-u. Kehlkopfheilk. **167**:595, 1955.

Richter, H.: Ueber exogene Einflüsse auf die Entwicklung der Nasennebenhöhlen, Arch. Ohren-Nasen-u. Kehlkopfheilk. **143**:251, 1937.

Rosenberger, H. C.: Does sinus infection affect sinus growth? Laryngoscope **55**:62, 1945.

Satir, P.: How cilia move, Sci. Am. **231**:45, 1974.

Schaeffer, J. P.: The nose, paranasal sinuses, nasolacrimal passageways, and olfactory organ in man, Philadelphia, 1920, P. Blakiston's Son & Co.

Schaeffer, J. P.: The anatomy of the paranasal sinuses in children, Arch. Otolaryngol. **15**:657, 1932.

Schaeffer, J. P.: The clinical anatomy and development of the paranasal sinuses, Penn. Med. J. **65**:395, 1935.

Schürch, O.: Ueber die Beziehungen der Grössenvariationen der Highmorshöhle zum individuellen Schädelbau und deren praktische Bedeutung für die Therapie der Kieferhöhleneiterungen, Arch. Laryngol. Rhinol. **18**:229, 1906.

Scopp, I. W.: Oral medicine. A clinical approach with basic science correlation, St. Louis, 1969, The C. V. Mosby Co.

Terracol, J., and Ardouin, P.: Anatomie des fosses nasales et des cavités annexes, Paris, 1965, Librairie Maloine S.A.

Van Alyea, O. E.: The ostium maxillare, Arch Otolaryngol. **24**:553, 1936.

Vidić, B.: The morphogenesis of the lateral nasal wall in the early prenatal life of man, Am. J. Anat. **130**:121, 1971.

Vidić, B., and Tandler, B.: Ultrastructure of the secretory cells of the submucosal glands in the human maxillary sinus, J. Morphol. (In press.)

# 15 Histochemistry of oral tissues

Histochemistry is generally considered to be an empirical extension of routine histologic staining methods. However, this is not necessarily so since most histochemical techniques have had their origin with a chemist in collaboration with a cell biologist or a biochemist. Histochemical techniques generally have a precise chemical rationale for their ability to stain different biochemical substances. These techniques preclude, as much if not more, stringent precautions to preserve the chemical integrity of the tissues, as does a biochemical assay. In fact the histochemical techniques provide a more exact in situ information on the chemical composition of a cell or groups of cells than do most biochemical methods. As a consequence, histochemistry has been very advantageously utilized with increasing frequency in the diagnosis of disease or in studying changes in metabolic pathways of tissues under normal and altered physiologic environments.

Most histochemical techniques have been generally used for qualitative analysis of chemical substances in cells and tissues. However, many sophisticated techniques have been devised recently for quantitative analysis of histochemical reactions. (These include use of the original microphotocell counter, double-beam recording microdensitometry, and more recently the scanning and integrating microdensitometry using the Barr and Strond GN2 and Vickers M85 microdensitometer models. This later method has been successfully used by

Chayen in measuring lysosomal membrane permeability and by Stuart and Stuart and by Simpson in measuring the activity of dehydrogenase enzymes in single cells from bone marrow biopsies of normal and leukemic patients.)

Many new techniques, not precisely histochemical, are frequently utilized by histochemists in making qualitative as well as quantitative analysis of tissue substances, particularly mineral elements. These include roentgen-ray and interference microscopy for measuring the dry mass of a biologic substance or a reaction product, roentgen-ray diffraction, roentgen-ray spectrophotometry, and electron-probe microanalysis for qualitative and quantitative distribution of metals. Neiders and his co-workers have made conjunctive use of the electron probe with a scanning electron microscope attachment for obtaining a visual surface-texture image of tooth cementum analyzed for its mineral content. Techniques of polarized light and roentgen-ray analysis have been used for study of enamel. Phosphorescence of calcified tissues has been demonstrated in bone, dentin, and enamel at liquid nitrogen temperatures. Laser spectroscopy has been recently used for qualitative and quantitative microanalysis of inorganic components of calcified tissues. Fluorescent-antibody technique and the fluorescence of tetracycline have also been applied to the study of oral tissues (Fig. 15-1).

In the last 10 years, light microscopic histochemical techniques have been

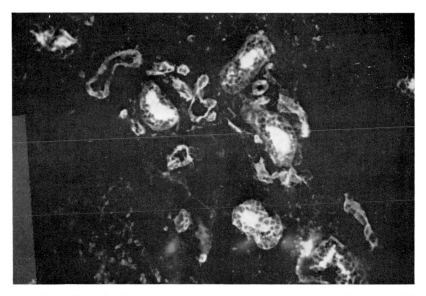

**Fig. 15-1.** Submaxillary gland secreting mucus in which the A antigen is demonstrated by immunofluorescence using rabbit anti-A serum and goat antirabbit serum: fluorescein. Human fetus, 8 cm. crown-rump length. This secretion and the mucus-borne antigen persist throughout life. (Courtesy Dr. A. E. Szulman, Pittsburgh, Pa.)

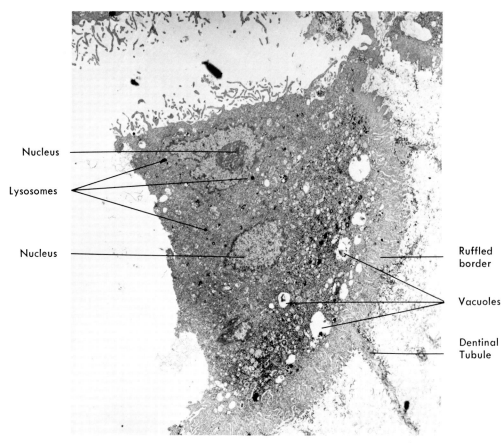

Nucleus

Lysosomes

Nucleus

Ruffled
border

Vacuoles

Dentinal
Tubule

**Fig. 15-2.** Electron micrograph of an odontoclast from mongrel-puppy primary tooth under-going resorption. Notice acid phosphatase reaction product in the form of a black precipitate along dentinal tubule, ruffled border, and vacuoles and in lysosomes. (Gluteraldehyde fixation, Gomori's metal substitution method; ×6250.) (From Freilich, L. S.: A morphological and histological study of the cells associated with physiological root resorption in human and canine primary teeth, Ph.D. thesis, Georgetown University, Washington, D.C., 1972.)

increasingly adapted for use in electron microscopic histochemistry. The visualization of carbohydrates, specific proteins, and phosphatases are some examples of such adaptive use (Fig. 15-2).

The role of radioautographic techniques in histochemistry cannot be over-emphasized in its ability to elucidate the uptake of chemical substances into the metabolic pathways of different tissues and in different regions of the cytoplasm (Figs. 15-3 and 15-4). Tissue sections taken from animals injected with a radioisotope are covered with a photographic film or emulsion and left in the dark. Radiowaves emitted by the isotope hit the silver halides of the film, and these tracks are later developed by processing of the slide or the metal grid like a photographic film. The radioisotope appears as dark granules in the light micro-

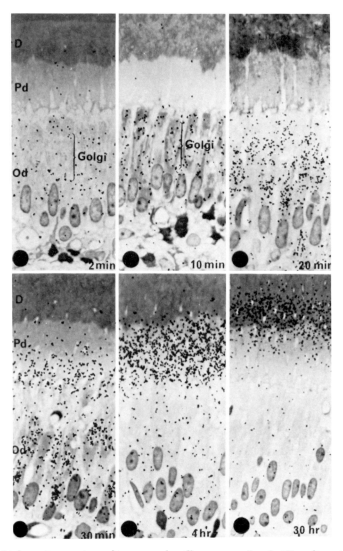

Fig. 15-3. Light microscopic radioautographs illustrate path of ³H-proline (injected into young rat) over odontoblasts, *OD;* predentin, *PD;* and dentin, *D,* at growing end of incisor tooth. Notice that silver grains representing path of ³H-proline appear first in the granular endoplasmic reticulum at 2 minutes and subsequently at 10 and 20 minutes in the Golgi region of the odontoblasts. Thirty minutes after injection silver grains start appearing in odontoblastic processes and predentin, whereas at 4 hours entire radioactivity is located in predentin. Thirty hours after injection, dentin is completely labeled with ³H-proline, now incorporated into the collagen fibrils of the dental matrix. (×1000.) (From Weinstock, M., and Leblond, C. P.: J. Cell Biol. **60**:92, 1974.)

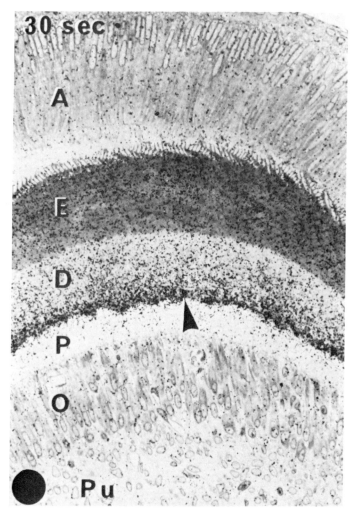

**Fig. 15-4.** Radioautograph of incisor tooth (undecalcified cross section) at its growing end in a young rat killed 30 seconds after intravenous injection of $^{45}$Ca. *A*, Ameloblasts; *E*, enamel; *D*, dentin; *P*, predentin; *O*, odontoblasts; *Pu*, pulp. Notice that $^{45}$Ca is immediately incorporated into the dentin over the predentin-dentin junction at *arrow*. Some $^{45}$Ca activity in form of few grains is seen in odontoblasts and predentin. (×250.) (From Munhoz, C. O. G., and Leblond, C. P., Cal. Tissue Res. **15:**221, 1974.)

scope and as linear tracks of the radiowaves in the electron microscopic autoradiographs.

## STRUCTURE AND CHEMICAL COMPOSITION OF ORAL TISSUES

Oral structures are primarily composed of connective tissue and epithelial linings, and associated glands. An understanding of these structures and their chemical composition is important in the consideration of biologic problems related to oral health. Significant chemical constituents of these tissues are glyco-proteins (mucoproteins), mucopolysaccharides, mucins, and enzymes.

## Connective tissue

Connective tissue is derived from the mesenchyme and consists of various types of cells and fibers that are embedded in an amorphous, semigel, colloidal, ground substance.

The connective tissue ground substance is generally rich in glycoproteins and acid mucopolysaccharides, e.g., hyaluronic acid and chondroitin sulfates. Glyco-proteins are chemically constituted of polysaccharide hexosamine, protein, and frequently hexuronic acid, e.g., sialic acid. Glycoproteins can be histochemically demonstrated by reactions involving the glycol groups or residual groups of pro-teins. Hyaluronic acid exists in polymeric form and, because of its capacity to hold water, is responsible for transport or diffusion of metabolic substances across tissues. Bacterial infections may occur as a consequence of the hydrolytic action of the bacterial enzyme hyaluronidase on the polymeric integrity of hyaluronic acid.

Chondroitin sulfates differ from hyaluronic acid in having acetylgalactosamine sulfate instead of acetylglucosamine in their molecules. Both of these acid mucopolysaccharides are widely distributed in connective tissue, with chondroitin sulfates being predominant in the cartilage. Chondroitin sulfates constitute only 1% of total bone tissue, whereas only 0.5% is present in dentin.

Other organic constituents of bone consist of approximately 93% collagen, 5% resistant protein, and 1.7% citrate. Histochemical visualization of acid mucopolysaccharides is related to the binding of cationic dye molecules to the anionic residues.

The levels of glycoproteins and mucopolysaccharides in connective tissue undergo alterations in various pathologic states; i.e., during inflammation or in early stages of wound healing there is a histochemically detectable increase in both the glycoproteins and acid mucopolysaccharides. However, as wound heal-ing progresses, there is a decline in the levels of both these substances.

Fibroblasts are the most common cell type in connective tissues. They are responsible for the elaboration of the glycoproteins and acid mucopolysaccharides that form the amorphous ground substance. They also elaborate the fibrous com-ponents of ground substance in the form of collagen, reticular fibers, and elastin.

Electron microscopic radioautography has been used to elucidate the manner of the synthesis and secretion of collagen. Current evidence suggests that col-lagen elaboration is initiated by the release of 30 to 160 Å microfibrils on the cell surface. These microfibrils serve as templates for initiation and extension of polymerization and the accretion of more monomeric tropocollagen into fibrils. Collagen is an albuminous protein, rich in the amino acids proline and hydroxy-proline. The latter amino acid is obtained by hydroxylation of proline in the presence of vitamin C. Hydroxylation of proline provides stability to the tropocollagen molecule. In vitamin C deficiency this stability is lost, resulting in the formation of an abnormal, immature collagen with consequent collagen disease.

The newly elaborated collagen fibrils, formed during development or in wound healing, are equivalent to reticular fibers in their electron microscopic structure. Both of these fibers stain positively for glycoproteins with silver stains and the periodic acid–Schiff (PAS) method. These reactions indicate the presence of a considerable packing of glycoprotein between aligned microfibrils of tropocollagen macromolecules.

Elastic fibers are elaborated by fibroblasts and also possibly by smooth muscle cells in the walls of blood vessels. They are composed of a protein component characterized by the presence of the amino acids desmocine and isodesmocine and acid mucopolysaccharides. Unlike collagen and reticular fibers, elastic fibers are not considered to be important constituents of the fully repaired tissues. Elastic fibers are stained specifically by the dye orcein in histologic preparations. A fluorescent staining method, using tetraphenylporphine sulfonate in combination with silver or gold, has been recently developed by Albert and Fleischer for electron microscopic visualization of elastic fibers.

Besides fibroblasts, other cellular elements of connective tissue are macrophages, which scavenge on tissue debris; mast cells, which are rich in the sulfated mucopolysaccharide heparin, an anticoagulant, and histamine, a vasodilator; and plasma cells, which elaborate immunoglobulins.

### Epithelial tissues and derivatives

Salivary glands elaborate the so-called mucins or mucoids. The definition of these substances is exclusively chemical from the biochemical standpoint, but from a histochemical point of view this definition is in part based on color reactions. Histochemical detection of mucins is generally based upon their acid mucopolysaccharide content, which affects certain staining reactions. The acidic nature is attributable to the presence of glucuronic acid, sulfate, or sialic acids. Histochemical observations show that a number of acid mucins lack sulfate esters. Histochemical characteristics of the oral epithelium, the epithelial components of the tooth germ, and the salivary glands will be considered in another section of this chapter.

Several histochemical studies have been made on the structural proteins of the salivary gland leukocytes or the so-called salivary corpuscles. Histochemical techniques are also being utilized in oral exfoliative cytology for the detection of oral cancer. Identification of lung carcinoma by analysis of normal and abnormal cells present in sputum is used clinically.

### Enzymes

Histochemistry has enabled the histologists to demonstrate the actual sites of cellular enzymic activity. The topographic distribution of enzymes may be ascertained by the quantitative microchemical techniques developed by the

Linderstrøm-Lang group or by techniques that result in the formation of visible reaction products in tissue sections. It is the latter approach that is widely used in histochemical demonstrations of enzymes.

Most frequently studied enzymes in oral tissues are those related to the transfer of phosphate esters (specific and nonspecific phosphatases) in the organic matrix of bone, dentin, and enamel (alkaline phosphatase) and to resorption of bone and of dentin (acid phosphatase). Oxidases and dehydrogenases, reflecting the metabolic activity of different tissues in oral structures, have also been studied extensively. Esterases, generally associated with the hydrolysis of carboxylic acid esters of alcohol, have been studied in salivary glands and in the taste buds. More recently, studies on lysosomal sulfatase and on adenyl cyclase involved in the formation of cyclic adenosine monophosphate (cAMP) have been reported.

## HISTOCHEMICAL TECHNIQUES
### Fixation procedures

For histochemical study, a tissue block must be preserved in such a way that it causes minimal changes in the reactivity of the cytoplasmic and extracellular macromolecules, e.g., enzymes, structural proteins, protein-carbohydrate complexes, lipids, and nucleic acids. This is accomplished by using optimum osmotic conditions, cold temperatures, controlled pH of the fixing solutions, and minimum possible exposure to the fixative.

Formaldehyde is considered to be one of the ideal fixatives, especially for enzymes and other proteins. This is because of its ability to react with major reactive groups of proteins to form polymeric or macromolecular networks, without affecting their native reactivity to histochemical procedures. Formaldehyde has a preservative effect on lipids by altering their relationship with the proteins. Use of electrolytes such as calcium or cadmium in formaldehyde or chromation of tissue blocks subsequent to fixation prevents dissolution of phospholipids. Formaldehyde is generally used as a 10% solution buffered to a pH range of 7 at cold temperatures in the range of 0° to 4° C.

Acrolein and gluteraldehyde are other frequently used aldehydes, with the latter being routinely used for electron microscopy. Conjunctive use of colloids like sucrose, ficoll, polyvinylpyrrolidone, and dextrans in the fixing solutions is often made to prevent osmotic rupture of cell organelles. This helps to improve the in situ localization of the histochemical reactions.

Other fixatives used for the study of glycogen, glycoproteins, mucopolysaccharides, and nucleic acids are frequently mixtures of many chemical ingredients. *Rossman's fluid*, used for visualization of glycogen, glycoproteins, and mucopolysaccharides, contains formaldehyde, alcohol, picric acid, and acetic acid. *Carnoy's mixture*, used for histochemical staining of nucleic acids, is composed of ethyl alcohol, acetic acid, and chloroform. Alcohol denatures proteins without causing irreversible chemical changes in the active groups but, being a poor fixative, is used in combination with acetic acid and chloroform. Feulgen's reaction, used for visualizing deoxyribosenucleic acids (DNA), requires acid hydrolysis of the DNA polymers so as to expose the deoxyribose sugar residues of DNA molecules. The aldehyde groups thus exposed (on the deoxyribose sugar residues) are then chemically reacted with leucofuchsin (Schiff's reagent) to form a reddish purple reaction product.

Some enzyme systems like cytochrome oxidases are highly labile and therefore cannot be preserved by chemical fixation. Visualization of such enzymes is performed on fresh frozen (cryostat) sections. However, to prevent diffusion and to preserve the in vivo status of the tissue macromolecules, one must fix the tissue blocks by a freeze-drying procedure. Tissues are frozen rapidly at very low temperatures, usually in liquid nitrogen, and then placed in a refrigerated vacuum chamber where ice, formed in the tissues, is removed by sublimation, i.e., by direct transformation into vapor without going through a liquid phase. After dehydration in vacuum, tissue blocks are embedded in paraffin and sectioned routinely with a microtome. Freeze-dried tissues exhibit optimal enzyme activity, show excellent histologic characteristics, and do not show any shrinkage artifacts that are seen with routine fixation. Besides oxidative enzymes, freeze-drying is used for visualization of other enzyme systems, e.g., phosphatases and dehydrogenases, and also for the precise localization of otherwise diffusible inorganic ions.

Techniques of freeze-fracture and freeze-etching have now been devised for use in electron microscopy to avoid use of chemicals in tissue preparation. This technique has enabled biologists to obtain excellent three-dimensional images of the surfaces of various cell membranes not previously observed.

Histochemical study of teeth and bone requires careful fixation and controlled decalcification procedures. Simultaneous fixation and decalcification with formaldehyde or glutaraldehyde and Versene (ethylenediaminetetraacetate, EDTA) has been successfully employed in the study of teeth and bone for light and electron microscopic histochemistry. Techniques have been developed for sectioning freeze-dried, undecalcified tissues. Decalcified ground sections have also been employed in histochemical studies of teeth and bone. Gray and Opdyke have described a saw for the preparation of 10- to 50-micron sections of undecalcified tissue. Such sectioning has been employed for histochemical studies of dental decay.

### Specific histochemical methods

Histochemical techniques primarily used in the study of oral tissues may be categorized as (1) glycogen, glycoprotein, and mucopolysaccharide methods; (2) protein and lipid methods; and (3) enzyme methods. They are all characterized by a direct staining reaction or by the formation of an insoluble dye or precipitate at the reactive sites.

*Glycogen, glycoproteins, and mucopolysaccharides.* The best known and most frequently used technique for detection of carbohydrate groupings is the periodic acid–Schiff (PAS) technique. The chemical basis of this method lies in the fact that periodic acid oxidizes the glycol groups to aldehydes and these in turn are revealed as a reddish purple dye product on treatment with leuco-fuchsin (Schiff reagent). Treatment of tissue sections with amylase prior to oxidation removes glycogen from the tissues, and this is reflected in a reduced Schiff reaction product. A comparison of the amylase digested and undigested sections is used in estimating the amounts of glycogen or other carbohydrate-protein molecules. Electron microscopic visualization of carbohydrates has been achieved, among other techniques, by use of phosphotungstic acid and lead citrate after oxidation with periodic acid.

Acid mucopolysaccharides are well demonstrated by thiazine dyes like toluidine blue, azure A, and alcian blue. Toluidine blue produces a metachro-matic reaction ranging from a purple to a red reaction product. This change of color (metachromasia) from the original (orthochromatic) blue color of the monomeric form of toluidine blue reflects the extent of polymerization of the dye molecules as they tag onto the anionic residues on the acid mucopolysaccharide molecule. Thus heparin present in the mast cell granules and chondroitin sulfates present in the intercellular ground substance of the cartilage or developing bone, give an intense red metachromasia demonstrating the highly acidic or sulfated nature of these acid mucopolysaccharides. A technique employing silver tetra-phenylporphine sulfonate has been used for electron microscopic demonstration of acid mucopolysaccharides.

*Proteins and lipids.* Histochemistry of proteins is based on classical reactions of protein chemistry involving various amino acid groups, i.e., amino, imino, carboxyl, disulfide, and sulfhydryl groups. Reagents such as dinitrofluorbenzene, ninhydrin, or ferric ferricyanide are utilized to give insoluble colored reaction products.

Histochemical study of lipids frequently imply use of frozen or freeze-dried sections. Total lipids are studied by using fat colorant dyes such as Sudan dyes. Chromation of formol-calcium–fixed tissues and their subsequent staining with Sudan black has been employed for the identification of phospholipids. Extraction procedures with various lipid solvents are considered essential to accompany most histochemical staining procedures for lipids.

*Enzymes.* The enzyme techniques utilize many different principles. Some of the criteria used in deciding the application of a technique are related to avoidance of inhibition by the substrate, insolubility of the primary reaction product, and its immediate coupling to the capture reagent, to prevent diffusion and false localization of enzyme activity.

The Gomori method for phosphatases uses phosphoric esters of glycerol, glucose, or adenosine. The enzymatically liberated phosphate ion is converted into an insoluble salt, which can be visualized by polarized light or phase contrast, or the salt can be transformed into a cobalt or lead compound, which is black. Riboflavin-5'-phosphate has been used as substrate, which at the site of phosphatase activity results in the formation of a fluorescent precipitate. Electron microscopic demonstration of phosphatase is also based on Gomori's original method of metal substitution with some modification. A technique employing ruthenium red has been used for demonstration of acid phosphatase in electron microscopic studies.

Another procedure employed for demonstration of phosphatases is the simultaneously coupling azo dye technique. This employs a naphthol phosphate or other type of ester. The enzmatically released naphthol is coupled in situ with a diazonium salt to form an insoluble colored reaction product. With regard to the original Gomori's glycerophosphate technique, it has been shown that the calcium phosphate formed may diffuse and give false localization. Because of this and other considerations in calcified tissues, the azo dye techniques are better suited for the study of phosphatases in teeth and bones. Sophisticated new substrates for use with azo dye techniques have been developed in recent years. They facilitate precise microscopic localization of alkaline and acid phosphatases as well as esterases. Aminopeptidases can also be detected by an azo dye method.

## HISTOCHEMISTRY OF ORAL HARD TISSUES
### Carbohydrates and protein

The PAS method is employed more than any other in studying the ground substance of teeth and bones. Under specific conditions, this method is believed to demonstrate the carbohydrate moiety as well as the glycoprotein complexes. The ground substance of normal mature bone and dentin exhibit little or no reactivity with the PAS technique (Fig. 15-5). However, developing or resorbing bone and dentin stain intensely with PAS. Newly formed bone and dentin are also rich in PAS-reactive carbohydrates. Besides the presence of glycogen and glycoproteins, the mineralizing zone of developing bone and dentin matrix is also rich in chondroitin sulfate.

Interglobular less-calcified dentin exhibits a distinct PAS reaction (Fig. 15-5) as does abnormally and poorly calcified dentin matrix in dentinogenesis imperfecta and in odontomas (Plate 4, *B*).

Enamel matrix is essentially nonreactive with the PAS method. However, enamel lamellae are intensely stained in ground sections (Fig. 15-6). In some areas the rod interprismatic substance exhibits some reactivity.

Specific protein methods identify certain amino acids or their groupings, i.e., amino, carboxyl, or sulfhydryl. Only a few of these techniques have been applied in the study of teeth and bone. Of interest are the dinitrofluorobenzene (DNFB) and ninhydrin-Schiff methods. The DNFB reagent combines with α-amino groups of proteins in tissue sections to form a pale yellow complex. An intense reddish color is subsequently revealed by a reduction and diazotization technique, which results in the formation of an azo dye (Plate 4, *A*). The pattern of staining is essentially the same as seen with the PAS method in both normal

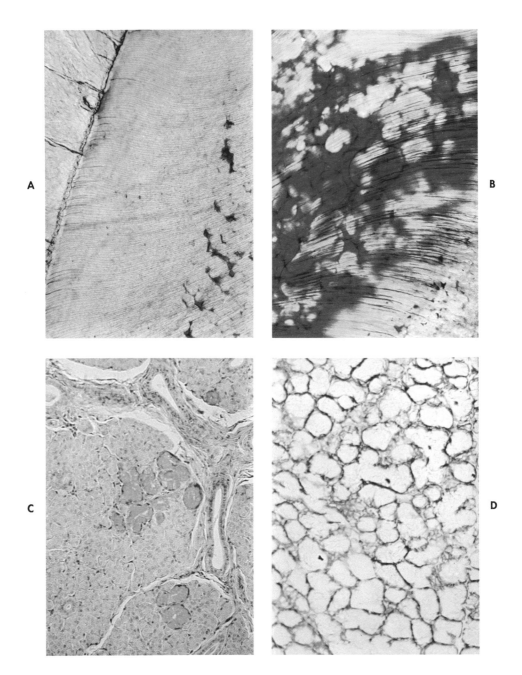

**Plate 4.** Photographs of several histochemical reactions. **A,** Ground section of human dentin. Dinitrofluorobenzene (DNFB) technique reveals reactive protein groups of interglobular areas *(arrows).* (×143.) **B,** Ground section of human odontoma showing PAS reaction of poorly calcified dentin. (×85.) **C,** Alcian blue staining of isolated group of mucous cells in a dog parotid gland. Mucicarmine counterstain. (×143.) **D,** Alkaline phosphatase activity of basement membranes of rat sublingual gland. (×143.)

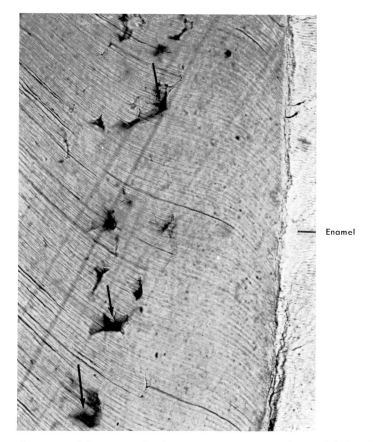

Enamel

**Fig. 15-5.** Ground section of human tooth showing PAS reactivity of interglobular dentin *(arrows).* (×143.)

and abnormal dentin. A modification of DNFB method wherein the final reaction product is a mercaptide of lead or silver has been used for electron microscopic histochemistry of amino groups. The ninhydrin-Schiff method is dependent on the formation of imino groups that decompose to a keto acid to form aldehyde groups, and these are reacted with leucofuchsin (Schiff reagent) to form a final red-colored reaction product. Some of these techniques have been applied to the study of dental caries in bone and in dentin resorption.

Histochemical reactions imply a need for some specific protein groups to initiate the mineralization of predentin and osteoid. Everett and Miller have noted the absence of carboxyl and amino complexes in predentin and osteoid in contradistinction to the presence of these complexes in dentin and bone. Sulfhydryl groups are present optimally at the mineralizing front in predentin and osteoid while being present minimally in the mineralized regions of these tissues.

Immature, newly formed enamel in rats shows histochemical staining for sulf-

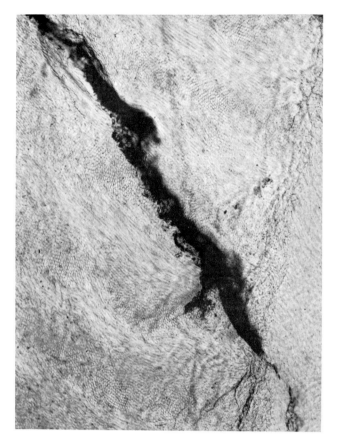

**Fig. 15-6.** Ground section of human enamel. Lamella stains with PAS method. (×143.)

hydryls and tyrosine residues characteristic of keratin. However, these protein residues are not demonstrable in the mature enamel.

### Lipids

Biochemical studies indicate a rather low lipid content in the organic matrix of dentin. Lipids have been demonstrated by the sudanophilic reaction in the odontoblastic processes and enamel rod sheaths. Sudanophilia is based upon the solubility of Sudan dyes with lipids of varied description. Sudanophilia is widespread in the developing tooth, being present in the zone of mineralization and predentin, and in the basal zone of the ameloblasts. These reactive zones of the predentin and ameloblasts imply a role to phospholipids in the process of mineralization of dentin and enamel matrices.

### Enzyme histochemistry of hard tissue

Histochemical techniques are extremely useful in demonstrating specific enzymes in specific cellular and intercellular locations in bone and teeth.

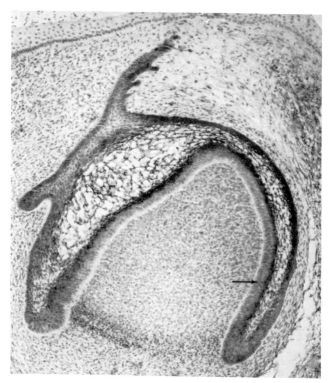

**Fig. 15-7.** Alkaline phosphatase reaction of a tooth of a monkey embryo. Ameloblastic layer (*arrow*) is nonreactive. (×87.)

*Alkaline phosphatase.* Alkaline phosphatase is capable of hydrolyzing phosphoric acid esters. In hard tissues, alkaline phosphatase has been implicated in the process of mineralization. However, some recent studies have projected some doubts on this assumption and instead suggest that the enzyme is involved in the synthesis of organic matrix only.

Alkaline phosphatase is observed to be associated with osteogenesis and dentinogenesis (Figs. 15-7 and 15-8). The osteoblasts and odontoblasts give an intense staining reaction for the enzyme (Figs. 15-8 and 15-9). No enzyme activity is found in bone or dentin matrices per se, except in close association with the matrix-synthesizing cells. At sites of intramembraneous bone development, alkaline phosphatase activity is observed in the endosteum, periosteum, and osteocytes (Table 6). Wergedal and Baylink report no enzyme activity at the actual calcification sites. However, conflicting views are reported in endochondral bone formation where the enzyme is localized in matrices and cells of the hypertrophic and provisional zones of calcification. The view that alkaline phosphatase is involved in actual calcification is also strengthened by observations in vitamin D treatment of human rickets wherein the increase in the calcification zone parallels an increase in serum alkaline phosphatase.

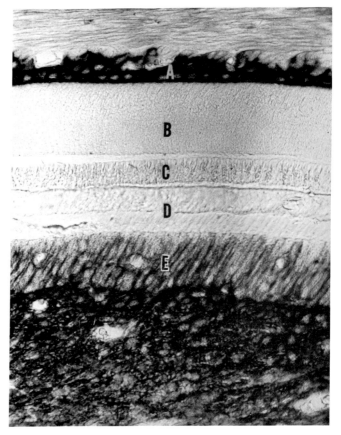

**Fig. 15-8.** Freeze-dried undecalcified incisor of hamster. *A*, Stratum intermedium; *B*, ameloblasts; *C*, enamel matrix; *D*, dentin matrix; *E*, odontoblasts. Note alkaline phosphatase reactivity of Korff's fibers and subjacent pulp. (×87.)

In the developing molar and incisor teeth, alkaline phosphatase is present in the stratum intermedium, odontoblasts (Fig. 15-8) and subjacent Korff's fibers, and the ground substance. No activity is observed in the ameloblasts (Fig. 15-8). However, in the incisors of rodents, enzyme activity is present in the ameloblasts and the reduced enamel organ at the growing end of the tooth (Table 6), with the remaining ameloblasts of the incisor being unreactive, as in the molars. The existence of alkaline phosphatase in the dentin proper has been reported.

*Acid phosphatase.* Acid phosphatase is less widely distributed than its alkaline counterpart (Table 6). Histochemical localization of intracellular acid phosphatase is generally more discrete than that of alkaline phosphatase because it is localized mainly in specific membrane-bound organelles, the lysosomes.

Osteoclasts in bone and odontoclasts in resorbing dentin exhibit an intense acid phosphatase activity (Figs. 15-9 and 15-10). The enzyme is localized in the part of the cytoplasm that lies apposed to the resorbing surface of bone and

**Table 6.** Enzyme activity of cells associated with bones and teeth

| | Alkaline phosphatase° | Acid phosphatase° | Amino-peptidase† | Cytochrome oxidase† | Succinic de-hydrogenase† |
|---|---|---|---|---|---|
| **Bone** | | | | | |
| Osteoblasts | ++ | 0 | + | + | + |
| Osteocytes | ++ | 0 | + | + | + |
| Osteoclasts | 0 | ++ | ? | ++ | ++ |
| **Cartilage** | | | | | |
| Active chondrocyte | ++ | 0 | ++ | ++ | ++ |
| Resting chondrocyte | 0 | 0 | + | + | + |
| Hypertrophic chondrocyte | ++ | 0 | + | + | + |
| **Tooth** | | | | | |
| Stellate reticulum | ++ | 0 | + | + | + |
| Stratum intermedium | ++ | 0 | + | + | + |
| Ameloblasts (molar) | 0 | 0 | 0 | 0 or + | 0 |
| Odontoblasts | + or ++ | 0 | + | + | + |

0 = No staining. + = Less active. ++ = More active.
°Freeze-dried paraffin-embedded tissues.
†Fresh-frozen tissues.

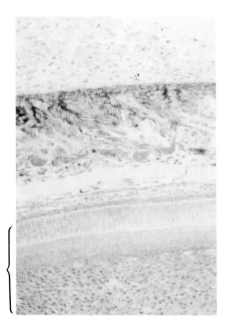

**Fig. 15-9.** Alkaline phosphatase *(dark areas)* in osteoblasts and acid phosphatase *(dark areas)* reaction in the osteoclasts in resorbing bone adjacent to incisor tooth *(brace)* in a 3-day-old hamster. (Mx naphthol phosphate and red-violet LB salt incubation for alkaline phosphatase; GR naphthol phosphate and blue BBN salt incubation for acid phosphatase; ×143.) (From Burstone, M. S.: In Sognnaes, R. F., editor: Calcification in biological systems, 1960, American Association for the Advancement of Science Publications, p. 64.)

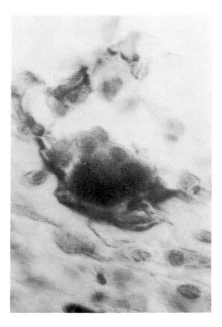

**Fig. 15-10.** Hamster osteoclast showing cytoplasmic acid phosphatase reaction *(dark)*, with some enzyme activity also present in the resorbing bone matrix. (AS-BI naphthol phosphate and red-violet LB salt incubation. Nuclear counterstain is hematoxylin; ×750.) (From Burstone, M. S.: In Sognnaes, R. F., editor: Calcification in biological systems, 1960, American Association for the Advancement of Science Publications, p. 64.)

dentin (Figs. 15-10 and 15-11). Electron microscopic studies reveal that the enzyme is localized in the lysosomes, though activity is also seen extracellularly between the microvillus-like projections of the ruffled border (Fig. 15-2). Uptake of resorbed mineral, hydrolyzed collagen fibrils, and injected radioactive substances at the site of resorption has been observed.

Several recent studies imply that acid phosphatase may (in addition to its function in bone and dentin resorption) confer calcifiability to the organic matrix by its hydrolytic action on the protein-polysaccharide granules present in the zone of mineralization.

*Esterase.* According to histochemical definition, esterases hydrolyze simpler fatty acid esters in comparison to lipases, which hydrolyze complex fatty acid esters.

Most histochemical techniques for esterases do not reveal any activity in bone or dentin. However, with use of specific naphthol esters like naphthol AS-D acetate, an intense staining reaction is observed in the calcifying matrices of bone and dentin. This reactive zone, situated in the tooth between predentin and dentin, is also sudanophilic, indicating the presence of phospholipids.

Considerable esterase activity has also been found in the cells and microorganisms associated with the formation of calculus deposits on teeth.

*Aminopeptidase.* Aminopeptidases are proteolytic enzymes that hydrolyze

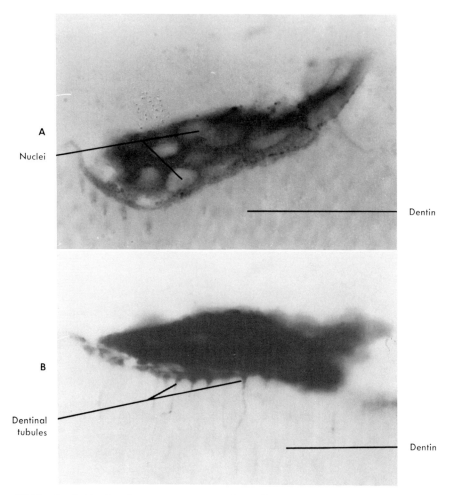

A

Nuclei

Dentin

B

Dentinal
tubules

Dentin

**Fig. 15-11.** **A,** Acid phosphatase activity in odontoclasts of mongrel-puppy primary tooth undergoing resorption. Notice reaction product is localized in descrete granules in cytoplasm. No reaction is seen in nuclei. **B,** Acid phosphatase activity in the odontoclast and dentinal tubules of a mongrel-puppy primary tooth undergoing resorption. (**A** and **B,** Alpha-naphthyl acid phosphatase and fast Garnet GBC salt incubation; ×1060.) (From Freilich, L. S.: A morphological and histological study of the cells associated with physiological root resorption in human and canine primary teeth, Ph.D. thesis, Georgetown University, Washington, D.C., 1972.)

certain terminal peptide bonds. Azo dye techniques using L-leucyl-β-naphthyl-amide or DL-alanyl-β-naphthylamide have been developed for histochemical demonstration of this enzyme. Human osteoclasts give a strong reaction. Although no staining reaction occurs in the osteoclasts of rodents, the enzyme is demonstrated in the stratum intermedium and odontoblasts during dentinogenesis. Some staining reaction is also noticed in the periosteum, perichondrium, and chondrocytes (Table 6). It is significant that aminopeptidase has also been localized in the macrophages and certain sites associated with the breakdown of connective tissues.

*Cytochrome oxidase.* Cytochrome oxidase is an iron-porphyrin protein that enables cells to utilize molecular oxygen. Its histochemical localization therefore reflects the oxygen requirements of the cells and tissues and the levels of their metabolic and physiologic activity.

The original histochemical reaction, the "nadi" reaction, employing α-naphthol and N,N-dimethyl-p-phenylenediamine, is now considered inadequate because of the instability of the substrate solution, lipid solubility, crystallization, and fading of the reaction product—indophenol blue. New techniques using p-amino-diphenylamine in conjunction with p-methoxy-p-aminodiphenylamine or 8-aminotetrahydroquinoline have overcome these technical problems so that the reaction is discretely localized in the mitochondria.

Both osteoclasts and osteoblasts show oxidase activity, with the reaction being more predominant in the former. Stratum intermedium of both molars and incisors also exhibit oxidase activity (Table 6).

*Succinic dehydrogenase.* Succinic dehydrogenase is closely associated with cytochrome oxidase in the mitochondria. It is one of a series of citric acid cycle enzymes that catalyzes the removal of hydrogen, which in turn is removed by a hydrogen acceptor or carrier. This serves as the basis of the histochemical reaction used in demonstrating this enzyme. The enzyme present in the tissues acts on the substrate (usually sodium succinate), causing the removal of hydrogen, which is picked up by a synthetic acceptor (a tetrazolium compound) present in the incubating medium. The reduced acceptor substance, called formazan, appears as a colored reaction product.

The distribution of succinic dehydrogenase in oral hard tissues is essentially similar to that of cytochrome oxidase. The dehydrogenase activity is relatively high in osteoclasts as compared to the osteoblasts. The stratum intermedium and the odontoblasts in developing teeth also reveal a positive reaction (Table 6).

*Citric acid cycle in osteoblasts and osteoclasts.* Besides observations on succinic dehydrogenase, studies on isocitric dehydrogenase, α-ketoglutaric dehydrogenase, and DPN-TPNH-diaphorases have also been reported. It is indicated that osteoclasts maintain a high rate of citrate and lactate production at the expense of glutamate and thereby actively promote decalcification of bone matrix and calcified cartilage.

*Summary.* A survey of the distribution of various enzymes associated with bone and teeth is given in Table 6. It is interesting to note that although acid phosphatase activity is associated with the osteoclasts only, distribution of other enzymes is widespread in hard oral tissues.

## HISTOCHEMISTRY OF ORAL SOFT TISSUES
### Polysaccharides, proteins, and mucins

*Polysaccharides.* The dye carmine is often used to demonstrate glycogen, but it is not as specific as the PAS method. Epithelial glycogen is known to increase during inflammation and repair. Attached human gingiva shows variation in the extent of its keratinization, and this variability is reflected in the glycogen content of the tissue. On the other hand, the nonkeratinized alveolar mucosa virtually always shows constant levels of glycogen. Animal experiments involving benign and malignant epithelial proliferations demonstrate an increase in glycogen.

When oral soft tissues are stained with the metachromatic dye, toluidine blue, mast cells become visible in varying numbers in the loose connective tissue, particularly along the blood vessels. The metachromatic reaction given by the cytoplasmic granules of these cells is caused by the presence of heparin—a sulfated acid mucopolysaccharide. The cytoplasmic granules also contain histamine—a vasodilator that can be demonstrated by fluorescent microscopy. Mast cells are present in particularly large numbers in the tongue and in the gingiva. The lack of these cells in acute necrotizing gingivitis is significant.

***Proteins and protein groups.*** Keratinization is one of the important characteristics of the epidermis. Although under normal circumstances it occurs only in some areas of the oral epithelium, in pathologic conditions, it occurs anywhere in the mouth. The mechanism by which the cells of the malpighian layer are altered to form keratin has been only partly elucidated. The disulfide bridges present in keratin are believed to result from the oxidation of sulfhydryl groups

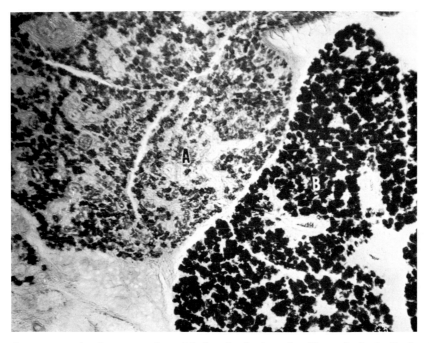

**Fig. 15-12.** Freeze-dried mouse submandibular gland, *A,* and sublingual gland, *B,* showing PAS reactivity of mucins. (×140.)

of cysteine. Sulfhydryl groups are demonstrated histochemically by the ferric ferricyanide method in which this compound is reduced to a Prussian blue color by these protein groups. Thus the extent of the blue reaction product reflects the degree of keratinization. Attempts to demonstrate sulfhydryl groups in electron microscopy have not been completely successful. However, electron microscopic demonstration of disulfide groups, using alkaline methenamine silver, has been made.

*Mucins.* Salivary mucins form semiviscous protective coatings over oral mucous membranes. They are composed of high molecular weight carbohydrate-protein complexes. Two types of mucins are recognized by the predominant carbohydrate component in their molecules—fucomucins rich in L-fucose and sialomucin rich in sialic acid. The latter is believed to confer acidity on certain types of mucins. Both of these mucins are present together in saliva, with one predominating over the other.

Histochemical techniques have been very useful in our understanding of the salivary mucins present in various salivary glands and their chemical composition. The dyes mucicarmine and mucihematin are frequently used for non-specific staining of mucins. PAS technique is used to identify neutral mucins (Fig. 15-12). Alcian blue, toluidine blue, colloidal iron, and aldehyde fuchsin methods are used to localize the acid mucins (Plate 4, *C*). These techniques reveal species differences in the mucins of different salivary glands.

## Enzyme histochemistry

*Alkaline phosphatase.* Alkaline phosphatase activity in human gingiva is specifically demonstrable in the capillary endothelium of the lamina propria (Fig. 15-13). The reaction product, observed in the gingival epithelium and in the collagen fibers, seems to be a diffusion artifact.

Oral epithelium of the rat exhibits an increased alkaline phosphatase activity during the estrous cycle, correlated to phosphatase changes in the vaginal epithelium. Alkaline phosphatase is implicated in the mechanism of keratinization, though its precise role in this process is still uncertain.

The basement membranes associated with salivary gland acini exhibit high alkaline phosphatase activity (Plate 4, *D*). Similar activity in taste buds of several species of animals has also been reported.

*Acid phosphatase.* Acid phosphatase activity in human gingiva seems related to the degree of keratinization, being very high in the zone of keratinization and low in nonkeratinized regions. This pattern corresponds with that observed in the skin epidermis. Cells of the functional epithelium in the gingival sulcus have been reported by Lange and Schroeder to be rich in lysosomal enzymes in the normal healthy tissue.

*Esterase.* Little information is available on the esterase activity of human gingiva. Superficial layers including keratinizing zone show the presence of some esterase activity.

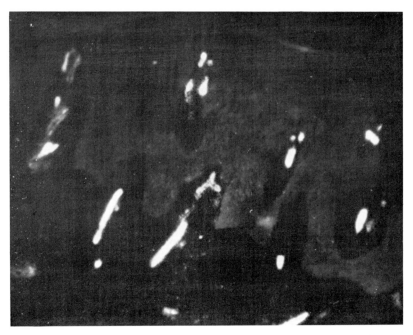

**Fig. 15-13.** Alkaline phosphatase activity of capillaries of the lamina propria of human gingiva revealed by ultraviolet fluorescence. (×80.)

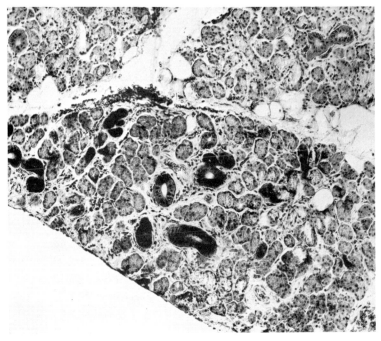

**Fig. 15-14.** Esterase activity of ducts of freeze-dried human parotid gland (nuclear counterstain). (×110.)

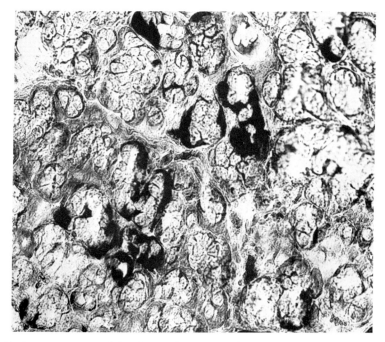

**Fig. 15-15.** Esterase activity of demilune cells of freeze-dried human sublingual gland. (×210.)

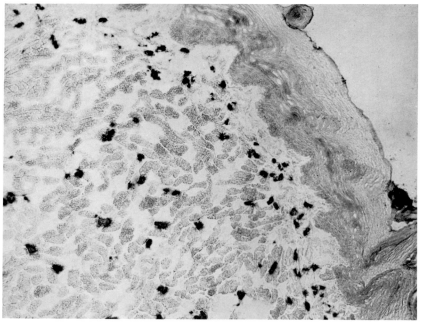

**Fig. 15-16.** Mast cells of rat tongue incubated with substrate solution containing naphthol AS-D chloroacetate. (×250.)

High esterase activity is demonstrable in the salivary gland ducts and also in the serous demilunes of the sublingual gland (Figs. 15-14 and 15-15). Similar activity is observed in the taste buds of several animal species and this has been implicated in gustatory discrimination. Mast cells in oral tissues also contain esterase activity (Fig. 15-16).

*Aminopeptidase.* The activity of this enzyme in human gingiva is low and is localized primarily in the basal cell layers of the epithelium and in the underlying connective tissue. An increase in aminopeptidase activity during inflammation and in hyperplasia caused by diphenylhydantoin has been reported.

Aminopeptidase is also observed in the salivary gland ducts.

*β-Glucuronidase.* β-Glucuronidases hydrolyze the β-glycoside linkage of glucuronides and are involved in conjugation of steroid hormones and in hydrolysis of conjugated glucuronides and play a role in cellular proliferation. The enzyme has been localized in the basal cell layers of the oral epithelium in man and rat.

*Cytochrome oxidase and succinic dehydrogenase.* Histochemical techniques

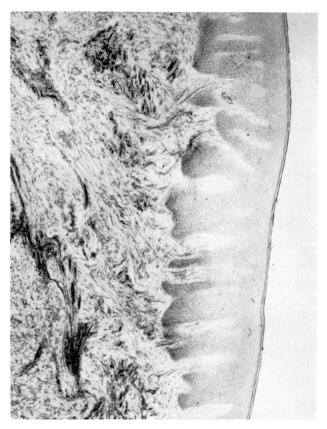

**Fig. 15-17.** Human attached gingiva showing cytochrome oxidase activity of basal cell layer and in connective tissue of lamina propria.

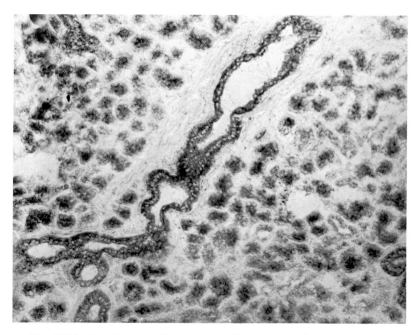

**Fig. 15-18.** Cytochrome oxidase activity of human parotid gland. (×143.)

demonstrate low levels of cytochrome oxidase activity in human gingiva. Specifically, this activity is localized in the basal layers of the free and attached gingiva, crevicular epithelium, and epithelial attachment (Fig. 15-17). In chronic gingivitis a striking increase in oxidase activity is observed in the epithelium from the free gingival groove through to the epithelial attachment. In chronic gingivitis, the underlying connective tissue also shows a variable increase in oxidase activity.

Cytochrome oxidase activity is also demonstrated in the salivary glands, especially in the duct system (Fig. 15-18).

The distribution pattern of succinic dehydrogenase is similar to that of cytochrome oxidase. This dehydrogenase is observed primarily in the basal cell layers of the gingival epithelium and in the ducts of the salivary glands.

## CLINICAL CONSIDERATIONS

Histochemical techniques are not only an important tool in dental research but they are frequently used in histopathologic diagnosis. Although the tissue biopsy materials are usually stained with hematoxylin and eosin, there are numerous occasions when this type of a staining technique does not permit a definitive diagnosis. In a differential diagnosis of an epithelial tumor in or around the oral cavity a histochemical stain for mucin may assist the oral pathologist in distinguishing a tumor of salivary gland origin from an odontogenic tumor or tumor arising from nonglandular epithelium. Since these tumors often require different types of treatment, this distinction is of great practical importance.

A variety of fungi that infect man contain mucopolysaccharides. The hyphae and spores of these fungi are present in the infected tissues, and their correct diagnosis can often be made only after special histochemical stains for mucin has been accomplished. In the human oral cavity diagnosis of histoplasmosis, actinomycosis, blastomycosis, and coccidioidomycosis can often be made only after special histochemical stains.

Histochemical stains that reveal lipids are of value in correctly diagnosing tumors that arise from the fat cells (lipoma and liposarcoma). They are also an important aid in establishing the identity of vacuoles that may appear in tumor cells of various benign and malignant lesions. Since cytoplasmic vacuoles may represent lipid, mucin, glycogen, or intracellular edema, their true identity is sometimes important for correct diagnosis and therapy.

## REFERENCES

Albert, E. N., and Fleischer, E.: A new electron dense stain for elastic tissue, J. Histochem. Cytochem. **18**:697, 1970.

Argyris, T. S.: Glycogen in the epidermis of mice painted with methylchol-anthrene, J. Natl. Cancer Inst. **12**:1159, 1952.

Arnold, J. S., and Jee, W. S. S.: Bone growth and osteoclastic activity as indicated by radioautographic distribution of plutonium, Am. J. Anat. **101**:367, 1957.

Baer, P. N., and Burstone, M. S.: Esterase activity associated with formation of deposits on teeth, Oral Surg. **12**:1147, 1959.

Balough, K.: Decalcification with Versene for histochemical study of oxidative enzyme systems, J. Histochem. Cytochem. **10**:232, 1962.

Balough, K.: Histochemical study of oxidative enzyme systems in teeth and peridental tissues, J. Dent. Res. **42**:1457, 1963.

Baradi, A. F., and Bourne, G. H.: Gustatory and olfactory epithelia. In Bourne, G. H., and Danielli, J. F., editors: International review of cytology, New York, 1953, Academic Press Inc., vol. 2, p. 289.

Baradi, A. F., and Bourne, G. H.: Histochemical localization of cholinesterase in gustatory epithelia, J. Histochem. Cytochem. **7**:2, 1959.

Baradi, A. F., and Bourne, G. H.: New observations on alkaline glycophosphatase reaction in the papilla foliata, J. Biophys. Biochem. Cytol. **5**:173, 1959.

Barka, T., and Anderson, P. J.: Histochemistry, theory, practice, and bibliography, New York, 1965, Harper & Row, Publishers.

Birkedal-Hansen, H.: Effect of fixation on detection of carbohydrates in demineralized paraffin sections of rat jaw, Scand. J. Dent. Res. **82**:99, 1974.

Bourne, G. H., editor: The biochemistry and physiology of bone, New York, 1956, Academic Press Inc.

Bradfield, J. R. G.: Glycogen of the vertebrate epidermis, Nature **167**:40, 1951.

Burstone, M. S.: A cytologic study of salivary glands of the mouse tongue, J. Dent. Res. **32**:126, 1953.

Burstone, M. S.: The ground substance of abnormal dentin, secondary dentin, and pulp calcification, J. Dent. Res. **32**:269, 1953.

Burstone, M. S.: Esterase of the salivary glands, J. Histochem. Cytochem. **4**:130, 1956.

Burstone, M. S.: Histochemical observations on enzymatic processes in bones and teeth, Ann. New York Acad. Sci. **85**:431, 1960.

Burstone, M. S.: Postcoupling, noncoupling and fluorescence techniques for the demonstration of alkaline phosphatase, J. Natl. Cancer Inst. **24**:1199, 1960.

Burstone, M. S.: Histochemical study of cytochrome oxidase in normal and inflamed gingiva, Oral Surg. **13**:1501, 1960.

Burstone, M. S.: Hydrolytic enzymes in dentinogenesis and osteogenesis. In Sognnaes, R. F., editor: Calcification in biological systems, Washington, D.C., 1960, American

Association for the Advancement of Science, p. 217.

Burstone, M. S.: Enzyme histochemistry and its application in the study of neoplasms, New York, 1962, Academic Press Inc.

Burstone, M. S.: Enzyme histochemistry and cytochemistry. In Bourne, G. H., editor: Cytology and cell physiology, New York, 1964, Academic Press Inc.

Burstone, M. S., and Folk, J. E.: Histochemical demonstration of aminopeptidase, J. Histochem. Cytochem. 4:217, 1956.

Cabrini, R. L., and Carranza, F. A.: Histochemical distribution of acid phosphatase in human gingiva, J. Periodontol. 29:34, 1958.

Cabrini, R. L., and Carranza, F. A.: Histochemical localization of β-glucuronidase in stratified squamous epithelium, Naturwissenschaften 22:553, 1958.

Cabrini, R. L., and Carranza, F. A.: Histochemical distribution of beta-glucuronidase in gingival tissue, Arch. Oral Biol. 2:28, 1960.

Carranza, F., and Cabrini, R. L.: Mast cells in human gingiva, Oral Surg. 8:1093, 1955.

Chan, J. F. Y., and Saleyddin, A. S. M.: Acid phosphatase in the mantle of the shell-regenerating snail *Helisoma duryi duryi*, Calc. Tissue Res. 14:213, 1974.

Chapman, J. A.: Fibroblasts and collagen, Br. Med. Bull. 18:233, 1962.

Chayen, J., and Bitensky, L.: Lysosomal enzymes and inflammation with particular references to rheumatoid diseases, Ann. Rheum. Dis. 30:522, 1971.

Chayen, J., Bitensky, L., and Butcher, R. G.: Practical histochemistry, New York, 1973, John Wiley & Sons, Inc.

Comar, C. L., and Bronner, F., editors: Mineral metabolism, vol. 1, New York, 1960, Academic Press Inc.

Dorfman, A.: The biochemistry of connective tissues, J. Chronic Dis. 10:403, 1959.

Eastoe, J. E.: The organic matrix of bone. In Bourne, G. H., editor: The biochemistry and physiology of bone, New York, 1956, Academic Press Inc.

Eichel, B.: Oxidative enzymes of gingiva, Ann. New York Acad. Sci. 85:479, 1960.

Eveland, W. C.: Fluorescent antibody technique in medical diagnosis, Curr. Med. Dig. 31:351, 1964.

Everett, M. M., and Miller, W. A.: Histochemical studies on calcified tissues, I.:

Amino acid histochemistry of fetal calf and human enamel matrix, Calc. Tissue Res. 14:229, 1972.

Everett, M. M., and Miller, W. A.: Histochemical studies on calcified tissues. II: Amino acid histochemistry of developing dentin and bone, Calc. Tissue Res. 16:73, 1974.

Felton, J. H., Person, P., and Stahl, S. S.: Biochemical and histochemical studies of aerobic oxidative metabolism of oral tissues. II: Enzymatic dissection of gingival and tongue epithelia from connective tissues, J. Dent. Res. 44:392, 1965.

Fisher, E. R.: Tissue mast cells, J.A.M.A. 173:171, 1960.

Freilich, L. S.: Ultrastructure and acid phosphatase cytochemistry of odontoclasts: Effects of parathyroid extract, J. Dent. Res. 50:1047, 1971.

Freilich, L. S.: A morphological and histological study of the cells associated with physiological root resorption in human and canine primary teeth, Ph.D. thesis, Department of Anatomy, Georgetown University, Washington, D.C., 1972.

Gersh, I., and Catchpole, J.: The organization of ground substance and basement membrane and its significance in tissue injury, disease, and growth, Am. J. Anat. 85:457, 1949.

Gersh, I., and Stephenson, J.: Freezing and drying of tissues for morphological and histochemical studies. In Harris, R. J. C., editor: Biological applications of freezing and drying, New York, 1954, Academic Press Inc., p. 329.

Gerson, S.: Activity of glucose-6-phosphate dehydrogenase and acid phosphatase in nonkeratinized and keratinized oral epithelia and epidermis in rabbit, J. Periodontol. Res. 8:151, 1973.

Goldman, H. M., Ruben, M. P., and Sherman, D.: The application of laser spectroscopy for the qualitative and quantitative analysis of the inorganic components of calcified tissues, Oral Surg. 17:102, 1964.

Gomori, G.: Microscopic histochemistry: principles and practice, Chicago, 1952, University of Chicago Press.

Gray, J. A., and Opdyke, D. L.: A device for thin sectioning of hard tissues, J. Dent. Res. 41:172, 1962.

Gregg, J. M.: Analysis of tooth eruption and alveolar bone growth utilizing tetracycline fluorescence, J. Dent. Res. 43(suppl.):887, 1964.

Greep, R. O., Fischer, C. J., and Morse, A.: Alkaline phosphatase in odontogenesis and osteogenesis and its histochemical demonstration after demineralization, J. Am. Dent. Assoc. 36:427, 1948.

Gustafson, G.: The histopathology of caries of human dental enamel, Acta Odontol. Scand. 15:13, 1957.

Hancox, N. M., and Boothroyd, B.: Structure-function relationship in the osteoclast. In Sognnaes, R. F., editor: Mechanism of hard tissue destruction, Washington, D.C., 1963, American Association for the Advancement of Science.

Hess, W. C., Lee, C. Y., and Peckham, S. C.: The lipid content of enamel and dentin, J. Dent. Res. 35:273, 1956.

Hoerman, K. C., and Mancewicz, S. A.: Phosphorescence of calcified tissues, J. Dent. Res. 43(suppl.):775, 1964.

Holliday, T. D.: Diagnostic exfoliative cytology, its value as an everyday hospital investigation, Lancet 1:488, 1963.

Jackson, D. S.: Some biochemical aspects of fibrogenesis and wound healing, New Eng. J. Med. 259:814, 1958.

Lange, D. E., and Schroeder, H. E.: Structural localization of lysosomal enzymes in gingival sulcus cells, J. Dent. Res. 51:272, 1972.

Larmas, L. A., Makinen, K. K., and Paunio, K. U.: A histochemical study of arylaminopeptidases in hydantoin induced hyperplastic, healthy and inflamed human gingiva, J. Periodont. Res. 8:21, 1973.

Laskin, D. M., and Engel, M. B.: Relation between the metabolism and structure of bone, Ann. New York Acad. Sci. 85:421, 1960.

Leblond, C. P., and Warren, K. B., editors: The use of radioautography in investigating protein synthesis, New York, 1965, Academic Press Inc.

Luft, J. H.: Ruthenium red and violet. 1. Chemistry, purification, methods of use for electron microscopy and mechanism of action, Anat. Rec. 171:347, 1971.

Matsuzawa, T., and Anderson, H. C.: Phosphatases of epiphyseal cartilage studied by electron microscopic cytochemical methods, J. Histochem. Cytochem. 19:801, 1971.

Matukas, V. J., and Krikos, G. A.: Evidence

for changes in protein-polysaccharide association with the onset of calcification in cartilage, J. Cell. Biol. 39:43, 1968.

McCrea, J. F.: Studies on influenza virus receptor-substance and receptor-substance analogues. I. Preparation and properties of a homogeneous mucoid from the salivary gland of sheep, Biochem. J. 55:132, 1953.

Millard, H. D.: Oral exfoliative cytology as an aid to diagnosis, J. Am. Dent. Assoc. 69:547, 1964.

Mörnstad, H., and Sundström, B.: Cytochemical demonstration of adenyl cyclase in rat incisor enamel organ, Scand. J. Dent. Res. 82:146, 1974.

Munhoz, Cassio O. G., and Leblond, C. P.: Deposition of calcium phosphate into dentin and enamel as shown by radioautography of sections of incisor teeth following injection of $^{45}$Ca into rats, Cal. Tissue Res. 14:221, 1974.

Neiders, M. E., Eick, J. D., Miller, W. A., and Leitner, J. W.: Electron probe microanalysis of cementum and underlying dentin in young permanent tooth, J. Dent. Res. 51:122, 1972.

Opdyke, D. L.: The histochemistry of dental decay, Arch. Oral Biol. 7:207, 1962.

Palen, V. W.: Electron microscopy, Biomed. Instrum. 1:7, 1964.

Pearse, A. G. E.: Histochemistry, theoretical and applied, vol. 1, Boston, 1968, Little Brown & Co.

Pearse, A. G. E.: Histochemistry, Theoretical and applied, vol. 2, Baltimore, 1972, The Williams & Wilkins Co.

Perry, M. M.: Identification of glycogen in thin sections of amphibian embryos, J. Cell. Sci. 2:257, 1967.

Person, P., and Burnett, G. W.: Dynamic equilibria of oral tissues. II. Cytochrome oxidase and succinoxidase activity of oral tissues, J. Periodontol. 26:99, 1955.

Philips, F. R.: A short manual of respiratory cytology—a guide to the identification of carcinoma cells in the sputum, Springfield, Ill., 1964, Charles C Thomas, Publisher.

Porter, K. R., and Pappas, G. D.: Collagen formation by fibroblasts of the chick embryo dermis, J. Biophys. Biochem. Cytol. 5:153, 1959.

Rabinowitz, J. L., Ruthberg, M., Cohen, D. W., and Marsh, J. B.: Human gingival lipids, J. Periodont. Res. 8:381, 1973.

Rasmussen, H., and Bordier, P.: The physiological and cellular basis of metabolic bone disease, Baltimore, 1974, The Williams & Wilkins Co.

Riley, J. F.: The mast cells, London, 1959, E. & S. Livingstone, Ltd.

Rovalstad, G. H., and Calandra, J. C.: Enzyme studies of salivary corpuscles, Dent. Progr. **2**:21, 1961.

Sandritter, W., and Schreiber, M.: Histochemie von Sputumzellen. I. Qualitative histochemische Untersuchungen, Frankfurt. Z. Pathol. **68**:693, 1958.

Schajowicz, F., and Cabrini, R. L.: Histochemical studies on glycogen in normal ossification and calcification, J. Bone Joint Surg. **40**:1081, 1958.

Shackleford, J. M., and Klapper, C. E.: Structure and carbohydrate histochemistry of mammalian salivary glands, Am. J. Anat. **111**:825, 1962.

Shimizu, M., Glimcher, M. J., Travis, D., and Goldhaber, P.: Mouse bone collagenase: Isolation, partial purification, and mechanism of action, Proc. Soc. Exp. Biol. Med. **130**:1175, 1969.

Smith, C. W., Metzger, J. F., and Hoggan, M. D.: Immunofluorescence as applied to pathology, Am. J. Clin. Path. **38**:26, 1962.

Sognnaes, R. F.: Mechanism of hard tissue destruction, Washington, D.C., 1963, The American Association for the Advancement of Science.

Soyenkoff, R., Friedman, B. K., and Newton, M.: The lipids of dental tissues: A preliminary study, J. Dent. Res. **30**:599, 1951.

Spicer, S. S.: A correlative study of the histochemical properties of rodent acid mucopolysaccharides, J. Histochem. Cytochem. **8**:18, 1960.

Spicer, S. S.: Histochemical differentiation of mammalian mucopolysaccharides, Ann. New York Acad. Sci. **106**:379, 1963.

Spicer, S. S., and Warren, L.: The histochemistry of sialic acid containing mucoproteins, J. Histochem. Cytochem. **8**:135, 1960.

Steinman, R. R., Hewes, C. G., and Woods, R. W.: Histochemical analysis of lesions in incipient dental caries, J. Dent. Res. **38**: 592, 1959.

Stoward, P. J.: Fixation in histochemistry, London, 1973, Chapman & Hall.

Stuart, J., and Simpson, J. S.: Dehydrogenase enzyme cytochemistry of unfixed leucocytes, J. Clin. Path. **23**:517, 1970.

Symons, N. B. B.: Alkaline phosphatase activity in the developing tooth of the rat, J. Anat. **89**:238, 1955.

Symons, N. B. B.: Lipid distribution in the developing teeth of the rat, Br. Dent. J. **105**:27, 1958.

Szulman, A. E.: The histological distribution of the blood group substance in man as disclosed by immunofluorescence. II. The H antigen and its relation to A and B antigens, J. Exp. Med. **115**:97, 1962.

Szulman, A. E.: Histological distribution of the blood group substance in a man as disclosed by immunofluorescence. II. The A, B, and H antigens in embryos and fetuses from 17 mm in length, J. Exp. Med. **119**:503, 1964.

Turesky, S., Glickman, I., and Litwin, T.: A histochemical evaluation of normal and inflamed human gingiva, J. Dent. Res. **30**: 792, 1951.

Turesky, S., Crowly, J., and Glickman, I.: A histochemical study of protein-bound sulfhydryl and disulfide groups in normal and inflamed human gingiva, J. Dent. Res. **36**:255, 1957.

Vallotton, C.: Étude bio-histologique de la phosphatase dans la gencive humaine normale et dans les gingivites, Schweiz. Monatsschr. Zahnheilkd. **52**:512, 1942.

Van Scott, E. J., and Flesh, P.: Sulfhydryl groups and disulfide linkages in normal and pathological keratinization, Arch. Derm. Syph. **70**:141, 1954.

Veterans Administration Cooperative Study: Oral exfoliative cytology, Washington, D.C., 1962, U.S. Government Printing Office.

Walker, D. G.: Citric acid cycle in osteoblasts and osteoclasts, Bull. Johns Hopkins Hosp. **108**:80, 1961.

Weinmann, J. P., Meyer, J., and Mardfin, D.: Occurrence and role of glycogen in the epithelium of the alveolar mucosa and of the attached gingiva, Am. J. Anat. **104**: 381, 1959.

Weinstock, A., Weinstock, M., and Leblond, C. P.: Autoradiographic detection of $^3$H-glucose incorporation into glycoprotein by odontoblasts and its deposition at the site of the calcification front in dentin, Calc. Tissue Res. **8**:181, 1972.

Weinstock, M., and Leblond, C. P.: Synthesis, migration, and release of precursor collagen by odontoblasts as visualized by radioautography after [$^3$H] proline administration, J. Cell. Biol. **60**:92, 1974.

Wergedal, J. E., and Baylink, D. J.: Distribution of acid and alkaline phosphatase activity in undemineralized sections of the rat tibial diaphysis, J. Histochem. Cytochem. **17**:799, 1969.

Wied, G. L., editor: Introduction to quantitative cytochemistry, New York, 1965, Academic Press Inc.

Wisotzky, J.: Effects of neo-tetrazolium chloride on the phosphorescence of teeth, J. Dent. Res. **43**:659, 1964.

Yoshiki, S., and Kurahashi, Y.: A light and electron microscopic study of alkaline phosphatase activity in the early stage of dentinogenesis in the young rat, Arch. Oral Biol. **16**:1143, 1971.

Zander, H. A. L.: Distribution of phosphatase in gingival tissue, J. Dent. Res. **20**:347, 1941.

# APPENDIX Preparation of specimens for histologic study

PREPARATION OF SECTIONS OF PARAFFIN-
EMBEDDED SPECIMENS

PREPARATION OF SECTIONS OF PARLODION-
EMBEDDED SPECIMENS

PREPARATION OF GROUND SECTIONS OF TEETH
OR BONE

PREPARATION OF FROZEN SECTIONS

TYPES OF MICROSCOPY

The morphologic study of oral tissues involve the preparation of tissue sections for microscopic examination. Knowledge of various types of microscopes and related histologic techniques will assist the student in interpretation of the structure and function of oral tissues.

The fundamental methods of tissue preparation for various types of microscopy, although basically similar to those for light microscopy, show differences in specific procedures. For example, differences in the tissue preparation for electron microscopy are necessitated by the lower penetrating power of electrons compared with the light and the greater resolving power of the electron microscope. Tissues for light microscopic study must be sufficiently thin to transmit light, and its components must have sufficient contrast for the parts to be distinguishable from each other. Routine histologic techniques involve the fixation of tissues in protoplasmic coagulating solution, dehydration in organic solvents, embedding in paraffin or plastics, and cutting of thin sections on a microtome. The sections are mounted on an appropriate supporting structure, stained, and examined under a microscope. The basic procedures are modified depending on the nature of the specimen and the type of microscope to be utilized for examination of structures of particular interest.

Four methods of preparation of oral tissues for microscopic examination are commonly used:

1. *Specimens may be embedded in paraffin and sectioned.* The most commonly used method of perparing soft tissues for study with an ordinary light microscope is that of embedding the specimen in paraffin and then cutting sections 4 to 10 microns thick. The sections are mounted on microscope slides, passed through a selected series of stains, and covered with a cover glass.

2. *Specimens may be embedded in parlodion and sectioned.* Specimens containing bone or teeth require different preparation. Such specimens must be decalcified (the mineral substance removed) and usually embedded in parlodion rather than in paraffin prior to being sectioned on a microtome.

452

3. *Specimens of calcified tissue may be ground into thin sections.* Sections of undecalcified tooth or bone may be obtained by preparing a *ground section.* This is done by slicing the undecalcified specimen, which is ground down to a section of about 50 microns on a revolving stone or disc.
4. *Specimens of soft tissue may be frozen and sectioned.* When it is important that pathologic tissue specimens be examined immediately, or if the reagents used for paraffin or parlodion embedding would destroy the tissue characteristics that are to be studied, the fresh, unfixed or fixed soft tissue may be frozen and sectioned without being embedded. Such tissue sections are usually referred to as *frozen sections.*

These four methods of specimen preparation will now be described in more detail.

## PREPARATION OF SECTIONS OF PARAFFIN-EMBEDDED SPECIMENS

The method of preparing a specimen for sectioning by embedding it in paraffin is suitable for oral specimens that contain no calcified tissue, such as specimens of gingiva, cheek, and tongue.

*Obtaining the specimen.* Specimens taken from humans or an experimental animal must be removed carefully, without crushing, either while the animal is alive or immediately after it has been killed. Specimens taken from human beings for biopsy must be removed carefully to avoid crushing.

*Fixation of the specimen.* Immediately after removal of the specimen it must be placed in a *fixing solution.* Specimens that have not been placed in such a solution are seldom any good. There are many good fixing solutions available. Sometimes the kinds of stains subsequently to be used determine the kind of solution to be chosen. One of the most commonly used fixatives for dental tissues is 10% neutral formalin.

The purposes of fixation are to coagulate the protein, thus reducing alteration by subsequent treatment, and to make the tissues more readily permeable to the subsequent applications of reagents. The fixation period varies from several hours to several days, depending on the size of density of the specimens and on the type of fixing solution used.

After fixation in formalin, the specimen is washed overnight in running water.

*Dehydration of the specimen.* Since it is necessary that the specimen be completely infiltrated with the paraffin in which it is to be embedded, it must first be infiltrated with some substance that is miscible with paraffin. Paraffin and water do not mix. Therefore, after being washed in running water to remove the formalin, the specimen is gradually dehydrated by being passed through a series of increasing percentages of alcohol (40, 60, 80, and 95% and absolute alcohol), remaining in each dish for several hours. (The time required for each step of the process depends on the size and density of the specimen.) To ensure that the water is replaced by alcohol, two or three changes of absolute alcohol are used. Then, since paraffin and alcohol are not miscible, the specimen is passed from alcohol through two changes of xylene, which is miscible with both alcohol and paraffin.

*Infiltration of the specimen with paraffin.* When xylene has completely replaced the alcohol in the tissue, the specimen is ready to be infiltrated with paraffin. It is removed from the xylene and placed in a dish of melted embedding paraffin, and the dish is put into a constant-temperature oven regulated to about 60° C. (The exact temperature depends on the melting point of the paraffin used.) During the course of several hours the specimen is changed to two or three successive dishes of paraffin so that all of the xylene in the tissue is replaced by paraffin. The time in the oven depends on the size and density of the specimen: a specimen the size of a 2 or 3 mm. cube may need to remain in the oven only a couple of hours, whereas a larger, firmer specimen may require 12 to 24 hours to ensure complete paraffin infiltration.

*Embedding the specimen.* When the specimen is completely infiltrated with paraffin, it is embedded in the center of a block of paraffin. A small paper box, perhaps a ¾-inch cube for a small specimen, is filled with melted paraffin, and with warm forceps the specimen is removed from the dish of melted paraffin and placed in the center of the box of paraffin. Attention must be given here to the orientation of the specimen so that it will be cut in the plane desired for examination. A good plan is to place the surface to be cut first toward the bottom of the box. The paper box containing the paraffin and the specimen is then immersed in cool water to harden the paraffin. The hardened paraffin block is removed from the paper box and is mounted to a paraffin-coated wooden cube (about a ¾-inch cube). The mounted paraffin block is trimmed with a razor blade so that there is about ⅛ inch of paraffin surrounding the specimen on all four sides so that the edges are parallel. The specimen is now ready to be sectioned on a microtome.

*Cutting the sections of the specimen.* The wooden cube to which the paraffin block is attached is clamped on a percision rotary microtome, the microtome is adjusted to cut sections of the desired thickness (usually 4 to 10 microns), and the perfectly sharpened microtome knife is clamped into place for sectioning.

*Mounting the cut sections on slides.* Suitable lengths of the paraffin ribbon are then mounted on prepared microscope slides. The preparation of the slides is done by the coating of clean slides with a thin film of Meyer's albumin adhesive (egg albumin and glycerin). A short length of paraffin ribbon is floated in a pan of warm water (about 45° C.). A prepared slide is slipped under the ribbon and then is lifted from the water with the ribbon, which of course contains the tissue sections, arranged on its upper surface. The slide is placed on a constant temperature drying table, which is regulated to about 42° C., so that the sections will adhere to the slide. The slide is then allowed to dry on this table.

*Staining the sections.* There are innumerable tissue stains, methods of using stains, and methods of preparing tissues to receive stains. Some of the many factors that influence the choice of stains are the kind or kinds of tissue to be studied and the particular characteristics of immediate interest.

**Table 7.** Staining of sections

| | | |
|---|---|---|
| 1. Xylene | 2 min. | To remove paraffin from sections |
| 2. Xylene | 2 min. | To remove paraffin from sections |
| 3. Absolute alcohol | 2 min. | To remove xylene |
| 4. 95% alcohol | 1 min. | Approach to water |
| 5. 80% alcohol | 1 min. | Approach to water |
| 6. 60% alcohol | 1 min. | Approach to water |
| 7. Distilled water | 1 min. | Water precedes stains dissolved in water |
| 8. Hematoxylin (Harris's) | 3-10 min. | To stain nuclei |
| 9. Distilled water | Rinse | To rinse off excess stain |
| 10. Ammonium alum (saturated solution) | 2-10 min. | To differentiate; nuclei will retain stain |
| 11. Sodium bicarbonate (saturated solution) | 1-2 min. | Makes stain blue |
| 12. Distilled water | 1 min. | Removes $NaHCO_3$ |
| 13. 80% alcohol | 1 min. | Partially dehydrates |
| 14. 95% alcohol | 1 min. | Alcohol precedes stains dissolved in alcohol |
| 15. Eosin (alcohol soluble) | 1-2 min. | To stain cytoplasm and intercellular substance |
| 16. 95% alcohol | Rinse, or longer | Alcohol destains eosin and should be used as long as needed |
| 17. 95% alcohol | Rinse, or longer | To remove excess eosin |
| 18. Absolute alcohol | 1 min. | To dehydrate |
| 19. Absolute alcohol | 2 min. | To dehydrate |
| 20. Xylene | 2 min. | To remove alcohol and clear |
| 21. Xylene | 2 min. | To clear |

One combination of stains often used for routine microscopic study is hematoxylin and eosin, commonly known as H & E. A usual procedure for staining sections with hematoxylin and eosin is a follows.

The dried slides are placed vertically in glass staining trays, and the trays are passed through a series of staining dishes that contain the various reagents (Table 7).

The slides are removed one at a time from the xylene, the sections are covered with a mounting medium, and a cover glass is affixed. When the mounting medium has hardened, the slides are ready for examination.

## PREPARATION OF SECTIONS OF PARLODION-EMBEDDED SPECIMENS

Specimens that contain bone and teeth cannot be cut with a microtome knife unless the calcified tissues are first made soft by decalcification. Furthermore, if a specimen contains any appreciable amount of bone or teeth, the decalcified specimen is better embedded in parlodion (celloidin, pyroxylin) than in paraffin. It is extremely difficult, if not impossible, to get good sections of a large mandible containing teeth in situ if the specimen is embedded in paraffin.

Let us suppose that we are to section a specimen of dog mandible bearing two premolar teeth. One method of procedure is a follows.

*Obtaining the specimen.* The portion of the mandible containing the two premolar teeth is separated as carefully as possible from the rest of the mandible by means of a sharp scapel and a bone saw. Unwanted soft tissue is removed. If the area of the specimen next to the line of sawing will be seriously damaged by the saw, the specimen should be cut a little larger than needed and then trimmed to the desired size after partial decalcification. It is better to have the mandible cut into several pieces before placing it in the fixative because a smaller specimen allows quicker penetration of the fixing solution to its center. If the tooth pulp is of interest, a bur should be used to open the root apex of the teeth to permit entrance of the fixing solution into the pulp chamber. This operation must be done with care so that too much heat does not burn the pulp tissue.

*Fixation of the specimen.* The specimen so cut and prepared is quickly rinsed in running water and for fixation is placed immediately in about 400 ml. of 10% neutral formalin. It should remain in the formalin not less than a week preferably longer. It may be stored in formalin for a long period.

*Decalcification of the specimen.* When fixation is complete, the specimen is then decalcified. Decalcification may be accomplished in several ways. One way is to suspend the specimen in about 400 ml. of 5% nitric acid. The acid is changed daily for 8 to 10 days, and then the specimen is tested for complete decalcification.

One way to test for complete decalcification is to pierce the hard tissue with a needle. When the needle enters the bone and tooth easily, the tissue is probably ready for further treatment.

Another way to test for complete decalcification is to determine by a precipitation test whether there is calcium present in the nitric acid in which the specimen is immersed. This is done by placing in a test tube 5 or 6 ml. of the acid in which the specimen has been standing and then adding 1 ml. of concentrated ammonium hydroxide and several drops of a saturated aqueous solution of ammonium oxalate. A precipitate will form if any appreciable amount of calcium is present. If a precipitate forms, the acid covering the specimen should be changed and a couple of days later the test for complete decalcification should be repeated. If no precipitate is detected after the test tube has stood for an hour and after several additions of ammonium oxalate, it may be assumed that the specimen is almost completely decalcified. The specimen should be allowed to remain in the same acid for 48 hours longer and the test repeated.

The end point of decalcification is sometimes difficult to determine, but it is important. Specimens left in the acid too short a time are not completely decalcified and cannot be cut successfully and specimens left in the acid too long a time do not stain well. Because of the adverse effect of prolonged exposure to acid on the staining quality of tissues, specimens should be reduced to their minimum size before decalcification is begun in order to keep the time necessary for acid treatment as short as possible.

***Washing the specimen.*** When decalcification is complete, the specimen must be washed in running water for at least 24 hours to remove all of the acid.

***Dehydration of the specimen.*** After washing, dehydration is accomplished by the placement of the specimen successively in increasing percentages of alcohol (40, 60, 80, and 95% and absolute alcohol). The specimen should remain in each of the alcohols up to and including 95% for 24 to 48 hours, and it should then be placed in several changes of absolute alcohol over a period of 48 to 72 hours. It is necessary to remove, as much as possible, all of the water from the tissues in order to have good infiltration of parlodion.

From absolute alcohol the specimen is transferred to ether-alcohol (1 part anhydrous ether, 1 part absolute alcohol), because parodion is dissolved in ether-alcohol. There should be several changes of ether-alcohol over a period of 48 to 72 hours.

***Infiltration of the specimen with parlodion.*** Parlodion is purified nitrocellulose dissolved in ether-alcohol. From the ether-alcohol in which it has been standing, the specimen is transferred to 2% parlodion, covered tightly to prevent evaporation, and allowed to stand for a period of from 2 weeks to a month.

From 2% parlodion the specimen is transferred to increasing percentages of parlodion (4, 6, 10, and 12%). The estimation of the time required for the infiltration of a specimen is a matter of experience, with the determining factors being the size of the specimen and the amount of bone and tooth material present. For the specimen of mandible being described here, the time required for complete parlodion infiltration might vary from several weeks to several months.

***Embedding the specimen in parlodion.*** When infiltration with parlodion is complete, the specimen is embedded in the center of a block of parlodion. A glass dish with straight sidewalls and a lid is a good container to use for embedding. Some 12% parlodion is poured into the dish, and the specimen is placed in the parlodion. Then more parlodion is added so that there is about ½ inch of parlodion above the specimen, the additional amount being necessary to allow for shrinkage during hardening.

Orientation of the specimen at this point to ensure the proper plane of cutting is important. If this piece of dog mandible is to be sectioned in such a way that the premolar teeth are cut in a mesiodistal plane and the first sections are cut from the buccal surface, then the buccal surface of the mandible should be placed toward the bottom of the dish when the specimen is embedded.

The dish is now covered with a lid that fits loosely enough to permit very slow evaporation of the ether-alcohol in which the parlodion is dissolved. As the ether-alcohol evaporates, the parlodion will become solidified and will eventually acquire a consistency *somewhat* like that of hard rubber.

This process of hardening the parlodion may require 2 or 3 weeks. When the block is very firm, it is removed from the dish and placed in chloroform until it sinks. It is then transferred to several changes of 70% alcohol to remove the chloroform.

Blocks of parlodion-embedded material must never be allowed to dry out. The blocks should be stored in 70% alcohol to allow the parlodion to harden further. Blocks that are to be stored for many months or years should eventually be transferred to a mixture of 70% alcohol and glycerin for storage.

*Cutting the sections of the specimen.* The hardened block of the parlodion-embedded specimen is fastened with liquid parlodion to a fiber block or to a metal object holder so that it can be clamped onto the precision sliding microtome. (This is a different instrument from the rotary microtome used for cutting paraffin.) Sections are cut with a very sharp microtome knife. For the specimen of dog mandible being described here, the sections may have to be cut at a thickness of as much as 15 microns. Unlike paraffin sections, these parlodion sections must be handled one at a time. As each section is cut, it is straightened out with a camel's hair brush on the top surface of the horizontally placed microtome knife and is then removed from the knife and placed flat in a dish of 70% alcohol. It must not be allowed to become dry. If it is important that the sections be kept in serial order, a square of paper should be inserted after every fourth or fifth section as they are stored in the dish of alcohol.

*Staining the sections.* Ordinarily the parlodion is not removed from the sections, and the sections are not mounted on slides until after staining, dehydrating, and clearing are completed. The sections are passed through the series of reagents separately or in groups of three or four, using a perforated section lifter to make the transfer.

From the 70% alcohol in which they are stored when cut, the sections may be stained with hematoxylin and eosin as follows.

Referring to Table 8, omit steps 1 to 3 and start with step 4; i.e., transfer the parlodion sections from 70% to 95% alcohol. Follow each step down through step 17, which is 95% alcohol. At this point, for the absolute alcohol specified in steps 18 and 19, substitute carbolxylene (75 ml. xylene plus 25 ml. melted carbolic acid crystals). This substitution is made bacause the parlodion is slightly soluble in absolute alcohol. From carbolxylene the sections are transferred to xylene (steps 20 and 21).

The sections should not be allowed to become folded or rolled up during the staining process. When they are put into the carbolxylene, they must be flattened out carefully, because the xylene that follows will slightly harden the parlodion sections so that they cannot easily be flattened.

To mount the stained section on a slide, slip the clean slide (no adhesive is used) into the dish of xylene beneath the section, and lift the section onto the slide from the liquid, straightening it carefully, and quickly and firmly press it with a small piece of filter paper. The slide bearing the section is then quickly dipped back into the xylene and drained, and mounting medium is flowed over the section and a cover glass is dropped into place.

A modification of this embedding method, using acid celloidin instead of parlodion, will preserve much of the organic matrix of tooth enamel during the process of decalcification.

For variations in the hematoxylin and eosin stain and for information on the many other kinds of stains useful for both paraffin-embedded and parlodion-embedded specimens, the student of histology must refer to books on microtechnique.

## PREPARATION OF GROUND SECTIONS OF TEETH OR BONE

Decalcification of bone and teeth often obscures the structures. Teeth in particular are damaged because tooth enamel, being about 96% mineral substance, is usually completely destroyed by ordinary methods of decalcification. Undecalcified teeth and undecalcified bone may be studied by making thin ground sections of the specimens.

The equipment used for making ground sections includes a laboratory lathe, a coarse and a fine abrasive lathe wheel, a stream of water directed onto the rotating wheel and a pan beneath to catch the water, a wooden block (about a 1-inch cube), some ½-inch adhesive tape, a camel's hair brush, ether, mounting medium, microscope slides, and cover glasses.

Let us suppose that a thin ground section is to be prepared of a human mandibular molar tooth cut longitudinally in a mesiodistal plane. The coarse abrasive lathe wheel is attached to the lathe, water is directed onto the wheel, the tooth is held securely in the fingers, and its buccal surface is applied firmly to the flat surface of the rapidly rotating wheel. The tooth is ground down nearly to the level of the desired section.

The coarse wheel is now exchanged for a fine abrasive lathe wheel, and the cut surface of the tooth is ground again until the level of the desired section is reached.

At this point a piece of adhesive tape is wrapped around the wooden block in such a way that the sticky side of the tape is directed *outward*. The ground surface of the tooth is wiped dry and then is pressed onto the adhesive tape on one side of the wooden block. It will stick fast. With the block held securely in the fingers, the lingual surface of the tooth is applied to the coarse adhesive lathe wheel and the tooth is ground down to a thickness of about 0.5 mm. Then the coarse wheel is again exchanged for the fine-abrasive lathe wheel, and the grinding is continued until the section is as thin as desired.

The finished ground section is soaked off of the adhesive tape with ether and then dried for several minutes. Drying for too long will result in cracking. It is then mounted on a microscope slide. To do this, a drop of mounting medium is placed on the slide, the section is lifted with a camel's hair brush and placed on the drop, another drop of mounting medium is put on top of the section, and a cover glass is affixed for microscopic study.

The teeth used for ground sections should not be allowed to dry out after extraction, because drying makes the hard tissues brittle and the enamel may chip off in the process of grinding. Extracted teeth should be preserved in 10% formalin until used.

Precision equipment for making ground sections with much greater accuracy is available. The method described here is one in which equipment at hand in almost any laboratory is used. The technical literature contains a number of articles on the preparation of sections of undecalcified tissues.

## PREPARATION OF FROZEN SECTIONS

Fixed soft tissues or fresh unfixed soft tissues may be cut into sections 10 to 15 microns thick by freezing the block of tissue with either liquid or solid carbon dioxide and cutting it on a freezing microtome. Frozen sections can be quickly prepared and are useful if the immediate examination of a specimen is required. Frozen sections are also useful when the tissue characteristics to be studied would be destroyed by the reagents used in paraffin embedding.

Details of the preparation of frozen sections can be obtained from books on microtechnique.

## TYPES OF MICROSCOPY

A thin tissue section has the property to modify the color or intensity of light passing through it. The modified light containing information from the section is amplified through the lens system of a microscope and transmitted to the eye. Since the unstained tissues do not absorb or modify the light to a useful degree, tissue staining is utilized to induce differential absorption of light so that tissue components may be seen.

Many types of microscopes are used for the study of tissues. The most common is the bright-field microscope, which is a complex optical instrument and uses visible light. Modifications of this instrument have provided the phase-contrast, interference, dark-field, and polarizing microscopes. The optical systems that utilize invisible radiations include the ultraviolet microscope, roentgen-ray, and electron microscope. Each of these instruments have been valuable tools in the study of oral tissues.

## REFERENCES

Bodecker, C. F.: The Cape-Kitchin modification of the celloidin decalcifying method for dental enamel, J. Dent. Res. **16**:143, 1937.

Brewer, H. E., and Shellhamer, R. H.: Stained ground sections of teeth and bone, Stain Techn. **31**:111, 1956.

Davenport, H. A.: Histological and histochemical technics, Philadelphia, 1960, W. B. Saunders Co.

Fremlin, J. H., Mathieson, J., and Hardwick, J. L.: The grinding of thin sections of dental enamel, J. Dent. Res. **39**:1103, 1960.

Gatenby, J. B., and Beams, H. W., editors: The microtomist's vade-mecum (Bolles Lee), ed. 11, Philadelphia, 1950, The Blakiston Co.

Guyer, M. F.: Animal micrology, Chicago, 1953, University of Chicago Press.

Koehler, J. K.: Advanced techniques in biological electron microscopy, New York, 1973, Springer-Verlag.

Krajian, A. A., and Gradwohl, R. B. H.: Histopathological technic, ed. 2, St. Louis, 1952, The C. V. Mosby Co.

Mallory, F. B.: Pathological technique, Philadelphia, 1938, W. B. Saunders Co.

Morse, A.: Formic acid–sodium citrate decalcification and butyl alcohol dehydration of teeth and bones for sectioning in paraffin, J. Dent. Res. **24**:143, 1945.

Nikiforuk, G., and Sreebny, L.: Demineralization of hard tissues by organic chelating agents at neutral pH, J. Dent. Res. **32**:859, 1953.

Pearce, A. G. E.: Histochemistry, ed. 3, vol. 1, Baltimore, 1973, The Williams & Wilkins Co.

Sognnaes, R. F.: Preparation of thin serial ground sections of whole teeth and jaws and other highly calcified and brittle structures, Anat. Rec. **99**:134, 1947.

Sognnaes, R. F.: The organic elements of the enamel, J. Dent. Res. **27**:609, 1948; **28**:549, 558, 1949; **29**:260, 1950.

Weber, D. F.: A simplified technique for the preparation of ground sections, J. Dent. Res. **43**:462, 1964.

Yaeger, J. A.: Methacrylate embedding and sectioning of calcified bone, Stain Techn. **33**:229, 1958.

# Index